AF779808

To Sheldon –

with thanks for everything!

Len

International Review of RESEARCH IN MENTAL RETARDATION

Language and Communication in Mental Retardation

VOLUME 27

International Review of

RESEARCH IN MENTAL RETARDATION

EDITED BY

LARAINE MASTERS GLIDDEN

DEPARTMENT OF PSYCHOLOGY
ST. MARY'S COLLEGE OF MARYLAND
ST. MARY'S CITY, MARYLAND

Language and Communication in Mental Retardation

A Volume in

International Review of
RESEARCH IN MENTAL RETARDATION

VOLUME 27

EDITED BY

Leonard Abbeduto

WAISMAN CENTER AND
DEPARTMENT OF EDUCATIONAL PSYCHOLOGY
UNIVERSITY OF WISCONSIN-MADISON
MADISON, WISCONSIN

ACADEMIC PRESS

An imprint of Elsevier, Inc.

Amsterdam Boston Heidelberg London New York Oxford
Paris San Diego San Francisco Singapore Sydney Tokyo

This book is printed on acid-free paper. ♾

Academic Press
An Elsevier Imprint.
525 B Street, Suite 1900, San Diego, California 92101-4495, USA
http://www.academicpress.com

Academic Press
84 Theobald's Road, London WC1X 8RR, UK
http://www.academicpress.com

International Standard Book Number: 0-12-366227-3

PRINTED IN THE UNITED STATES OF AMERICA
03 04 05 06 07 08 9 8 7 6 5 4 3 2 1

Contents

Language and Communication in Fragile X Syndrome

Melissa M. Murphy and Leonard Abbeduto

On Becoming Socially Competent Communicators: The Challenge for Children with Fetal Alcohol Exposure

Truman E. Coggins, Lesley B. Olswang, Heather Carmichael Olson, and Geralyn R. Timler

Memory, Language Comprehension, and Mental Retardation

Edward C. Merrill, Regan Lookadoo, and Stacy Rilea

Reading Skills and Cognitive Abilities of Individuals with Mental Retardation

Frances A. Conners

Language Interventions for Children with Mental Retardation

Nancy C. Brady and Steven F. Warren

Augmentative and Alternative Communication for Persons with Mental Retardation

MaryAnn Romski, Rose A. Sevcik, and Amy Hyatt Fonseca

Atypical Language Development in Individuals with Mental Retardation: Theoretical Implications

Jean A. Rondal

Contributors

Numbers in parentheses indicate the pages on which the authors' contributions begin.

Leonard Abbeduto (83), *Waisman Center and Department of Educational Psychology, 1500 Highland Avenue, University of Wisconsin-Madison, Madison, Wisconsin 53705*

Angela M. Becerra (35), *Department of Psychological and Brain Sciences, University of Louisville, Louisville, Kentucky 40292*

Nancy C. Brady (231), *Schiefelbusch Institute for Life Span Studies, University of Kansas, Lawrence, Kansas 66045*

Heather Carmichael Olson (121), *Psychiatry and Behavioral Sciences, University of Washington, Seattle, Washington 98195*

Robin S. Chapman (1), *Waisman Center, 1500 Highland Avenue, University of Wisconsin-Madison, Madison, Wisconsin 53705*

Truman E. Coggins (121), *Center on Human Development and Disability, University of Washington, Seattle, Washington 98195*

Frances A. Conners (191), *Department of Psychology, University of Alabama, 348 Gordon Palmer, Box 870348, Tuscaloosa, Alabama 35487-0348*

Amy Hyatt Fonseca (255), *Georgia State University, Atlanta, Georgia 30303*

Bonita P. Klein-Tasman (35), *Department of Psychology, University of Wisconsin-Milwaukee, Milwaukee, Wisconsin 53201*

Regan Lookadoo (151), *Department of Psychology, University of Alabama, 348 Gordon Palmer, Box 870348, Tuscaloosa, Alabama 35487-0348*

Edward C. Merrill (151), *Department of Psychology, University of Alabama, 348 Gordon Palmer, Box 870348, Tuscaloosa, Alabama 35487-0348*

Carolyn B. Mervis (35), *Department of Psychological and Brain Sciences, University of Louisville, Louisville, Kentucky 40292*

Melissa M. Murphy (83), *Waisman Center and Department of Educational Psychology, University of Wisconsin-Madison, Madison, Wisconsin 53705*

Lesley B. Olswang (121), *Speech and Hearing Sciences, University of Washington, Seattle, Washington 98195*

Stacy Rilea (151), *Department of Psychology, University of Alabama, 348 Gordon Palmer, Box 870348, Tuscaloosa, Alabama 35487-0348*

Byron F. Robinson (35), *Department of Psychological and Brain Sciences, Georgia State University, Atlanta, Georgia 30303*

MaryAnn Romski (255), *Department of Communication, Georgia State University, Atlanta, Georgia 30303*

Jean A. Rondal (281), *Laboratory for Psycholinguistics, B-32, 4000 Sart Tilman, University of Liege, Liege, Belgium*

Melissa L. Rowe (35), *Department of Psychological and Brain Sciences, University of Louisville, Louisville, Kentucky 40292*

Rose A. Sevcik (255), *Department of Communication, Georgia State University, Atlanta, Georgia 30303*

Geralyn R. Timler (121), *Department of Communicative Disorders, SUNY at Buffalo, New York 14214*

Steven F. Warren (231), *Schiefelbusch Institute for Life Span Studies, University of Kansas, Lawrence, Kansas 66045*

Foreword

This volume on *Language and Communication in Mental Retardation* is the first in the 37-year history of the *International Review of Research in Mental Retardation* that has been proposed, designed, and assembled by a guest editor. The *Review* began a new tradition in 2001 with the first publication of a theme-oriented volume. All eleven chapters of Volume 23 had autism as their focus. That volume has been received with substantial enthusiasm and that reception encouraged me to continue the practice with the plan being to publish one theme volume, usually guest-edited, approximately every two years. The next one, on *Motivation in Mental Retardation*, is being guest-edited by Harvey Switsky of Northern Illinois University; Phil Davidson of University of Rochester has already started the planning for a volume with a focus on *Neurotoxicity*.

When I began thinking about the value of a special issue on *Language and Communication*, I knew immediately who would be the best choice for guest editor. Len Abbeduto had substantial editorial experience and was also a productive investigator working in the area of language and mental retardation. Fortunately, when I approached him about taking on this project he recognized at once that the rapid advances in this field made it a propitious time to bring together those individuals who were responsible for the progress that we've seen in the last 20 years. What has resulted is a remarkable volume, with chapters from investigators who have shaped this field during the last several decades. Contributors have focused on language and communication abilities and disabilities in individuals with mental retardation of varying etiology in addition to issues with regard to both theory and intervention. I predict that this volume will be read, consulted, and cited, both now and for years to come, and I want publicly to acknowledge and thank Len Abbeduto for his work in bringing it to fruition. It was delightful to collaborate with him and I am grateful for his expertise, acumen, persistence, and good humor, all of which contributed to this outstanding product.

LARAINE MASTERS GLIDDEN
SERIES EDITOR

Preface

This volume contains nine articles, all addressing the theme of language and communication challenges in persons with mental retardation. Such challenges have long figured prominently in the measurement of intelligence and adaptive behavior and thus in the definition of mental retardation. Not surprisingly, therefore, there is a long tradition of empirical research designed to document the extent, nature, and amenability to intervention of problems in learning and using language amongst persons with mental retardation. At the same time, however, the pace of research on language learning and use in mental retardation has quickened and taken new directions in recent years. The chapters in this volume represent an opportunity to take stock of what these new directions have yielded and what remains to be learned.

This "revitalization" of research on language and communication in mental retardation can be traced to three sources. The first source is a more general shift in behavioral research on mental retardation, from an approach focused on variations in severity of mental retardation to one focused on differences amongst subtypes of mental retardation, especially those defined by differences in etiology. This shift has been made possible in part by technological advances in molecular genetics that have led to the identification of more than 1000 genetic syndromes associated with mental retardation. The shift toward etiology-based research, however, has also been fueled by the discovery of interesting differences in the behavioral phenotypes of these syndromes. In this volume, there are chapters documenting the three most intensely investigated genetic syndromes: Williams syndrome (Mervis et al.), Down syndrome (Chapman), and fragile X syndrome (Murphy & Abbeduto). These syndromes have long been thought to contrast in interesting ways from a behavioral perspective, with language thought to be a strength in Williams syndrome and, to a lesser extent, fragile X syndrome, but a glaring weakness in Down syndrome. The authors in these chapters present research suggesting that although there are differences among these syndromes, a more complicated and nuanced view of their development of language and communication is in order. In their chapter, Coggins et al. focus on the linguistic dimensions of fetal alcohol syndrome (and the more milder fetal alcohol effects), which result from environmental rather than genetic effects. Although fetal alcohol syndrome is among the most frequent causes of mental retardation, research on the language and communication challenges associated with the syndrome has been rare until just recently.

The second source of the increased interest in language and communication in mental retardation is an ongoing controversy in the typical development literature concerning the relationship between language and thought. This controversy is one of several sparked by the nativist approach espoused originally by Noam Chomsky. The nativists claim, among other things, that language development is driven by learning mechanisms that operate with little input from more general faculties of the mind. This claim of modularity, or independence of language and thought, has led to an intense interest in syndromes that appear to provide evidence of (relatively) spared language in the face of substantial limitations in cognitive functioning. Indeed, as can be seen in the chapter by Mervis et al., Williams syndrome has, over the past two decades, become the battleground for many of the arguments about modularity. Also relevant to the issue of modularity are case studies of individuals with mental retardation who are thought to be "exceptional" (e.g., possess age-appropriate skills) in one or more domains of language. These case studies are presented in exquisite detail in the chapter by Rondal, who also grounds the modularity position in recent work on neuroscience. Many theoretical alternatives to the nativist position have been forthcoming, most of which view language learning and use as being intimately connected to the larger architecture of the human information processing system. Indeed, these more cognitively oriented theories have provided the framework for much of the research on language and communication (and language disorders, more generally) over the past decade. Some of this research is summarized in the chapter by Merrill et al., who focus on the role of memory in language comprehension. Interestingly, because the goal has been to investigate the relationship between variations in memory and variations in linguistic performance, etiological subtypes have not always figured prominently in research in this area. The role of memory, especially auditory memory, is also a topic considered in the chapter on the development of reading in persons with mental retardation (Conners).

The third source of the increased interest in language and communication in mental retardation is the change throughout our society in attitudes about the contexts in which persons with mental retardation have a right to live and in expectations concerning what people with mental retardation can achieve with appropriate environmental supports. This has led researchers to focus on approaches to intervention that provide greater support for the development of language and communication within "natural" settings rather than within the "contrived" setting of an isolated therapy room and on skills such as reading, which were previously thought to be beyond the ken of people with mental retardation and of little functional value for them. In their chapter, Brady and Warren focus on recent research on language intervention, most conducted within a milieu, or naturalistic contexts, approach. Romski and Sevick also focus on intervention, but on augmentative approaches for people with mental retardation who largely lack the capacity for speech. Both chapters provide evidence that communication in persons with mental retardation is amenable to intervention in the form of an appropriately structured and supportive environment. Both sets of authors, however, also describe the personal and environmental constraints on intervention effectiveness. In her chapter, Conners reviews research focused on the factors promoting and constraining acquisition of reading skills in persons with mental retardation. Here too, personal and environmental factors are found to be important.

The chapters in this volume provide a comprehensive picture of the most active areas of research on language and communication in persons with mental retardation. The authors are leading scholars in their areas and all were invited to participate in this special issue. Each chapter was also reviewed by one or two other scholars, and the authors revised their chapters in accordance with the feedback provided by the reviewers. I am indebted to the following scholars who served as reviewers: Valerie Ahl, Donna Boudreau, Mina Johnson-Glenberg, Howard Goldstein, Jon F. Miller, Pat Mirenda, Joe Reichle, Lisa Turner, and Krista Wilkinson. Thanks also to Laraine Masters Glidden, who is the editor of this series, for inviting me to edit this special issue. It has been a rewarding experience. I would like to dedicate this volume to the faculty, staff, and students of the Waisman Center, for their collegiality and commitment to improving the lives of people with developmental disabilities, and to Terrence R. Dolan and Marsha Mailick Seltzer, for their leadership, vision, support, and friendship.

LEONARD ABBEDUTO
GUEST EDITOR

Language and Communication in Individuals with Down Syndrome

ROBIN S. CHAPMAN

WAISMAN CENTER,
UNIVERSITY OF WISCONSIN-MADISON
MADISON, WISCONSIN

I. INTRODUCTION

In this chapter the emphasis is on our own program of research on language and communication skills in children with Down syndrome, rather than the broader literature. We will review a number of our longitudinal and cross-sectional research findings on language development in children and adolescents with Down syndrome. We begin by describing Child Talk, the model of normal language development that gave rise to our questions of how language can come apart. We then summarize our research on the behavioral phenotype in Down syndrome within the broader context of others' research findings and the predictions of our model of language learning. We summarize our longitudinal study of individual differences in language development in the context of prior beliefs about limited language learning in Down syndrome, particularly the beliefs that language learning plateaus in adolescence or is limited to simple syntax. And we review our studies of incidental lexical learning—fast mapping of new vocabulary—in the contexts of the phenotypic account and the Child Talk model. Implications for intervention and methodological issues are considered briefly at the end of the chapter.

II. THE CHILD TALK MODEL AND LANGUAGE LEARNING

We began our research on language development in children with Down syndrome working from a contextual, developmental process model of

INTERNATIONAL REVIEW OF RESEARCH IN
MENTAL RETARDATION, Vol. 27

0074-7750/2003 $35.00

language production and comprehension (Chapman et al., 1992). Within this model, speaker intent, affect, actions, the event context and topic, in addition to the ongoing record of talk, determine the child's comprehension and production of utterances. Thus, what is understood reflects one's expectations in the communicative context. What is said reflects contextual biasing of available lexicon and syntax. And what is active contextually reflects both short-term memory systems and long-term knowledge.

A. The Role of Novelty

Within the model, novel information—such as is encountered in novel objects, actions, or words—is assumed to be more learnable in context than familiar information. Children's tracking of what is novel, or unexpected, as action unfolds is assumed to be ongoing and automatic, localized in part in the hippocampus, which maintains spatial information and generates predictions of what will happen next, inhibiting the brain stem's *locus coeruleus* activity until unexpected, moderately novel information occurs. On release from inhibition, the locus coeruleus, a center in the brain stem, fires (e.g., upon encounters with moderately novel events), dosing the whole cortex with norepinephrine, a neurotransmitter that appears to plasticise synapses for the next 2–10 s. This brief increase in norepinephrine creates a brief window of time—a "learning moment"—in which learning of what comes next is more probable, and in which associated context is connected with novel elements (Hebbian learning) (see Chapman, 2000).

B. The Role of Phonological Memory

The available evidence shows that infants can learn the statistical properties of syllables that regularly succeed one another—or not—by 8 months (Saffran, Aslin, & Newport, 1996), thus developing expectations about acoustic sequences likely to be words and formulaic elements and making these elements available for mapping to meaning. Even earlier expectations about the mapping of acoustic stream to familiar speaker, parental mouth movements to speech sounds, and intonation contour to speaker affect have been demonstrated (see Jusczyk, 1997). Acoustic perception and production become linked for the child as prototypic categories of speech sounds perceived in the language, develop and come to guide the child's attempted vocalizations (Kent, 1992) in the first year of life.

This "tuning" of speech production by perception is thought to persist life-long, but necessarily through the years up to adulthood as face, jaw, and laryngeal structures change and grow at differing rates, requiring modification of production programming to produce the same perceptual effect.

This mapping of speech production onto perception, we believe (Seung & Chapman, 2000), constitutes an automatic loop that serves as the refresher of auditory short-term memory as well as the source of early motor programming "practice" upon hearing speech, and constitutes the principle means by which phonological memory affects speech production. Such a mapping is different from the intentional rehearsal postulated as the articulatory loop in Baddeley's (1992) model, but it is needed in the model to explain developmental increases in span prior to intentional rehearsal (Baddeley, Gathercole, & Papapgno, 1998; Jarrold, Baddeley, & Phillips, 2002) as well as to account for the contributions of comprehension to production. A selectively smaller neural network serving such a loop, or a more slowly functioning one, would then contribute both to delays in learning expressive language and to impairments of comprehension when short-term memory demands were high.

Learning of "what comes next" in the auditory stream, as word-size recognition develops, can then expand to multiword sequences, lexical and utterance scripts, and within them, their variable grammatical morpheme inflections. Thus, either a novel phonological form or a novel (unnamed) referent—or both—can initiate the "learning moment" in which attention is focused and a mapping is likely to be learned. On this view, language learning is not modular—that is, dissociated from social and cognitive development—but mapped onto learning in the latter spheres, and hence multiply determined. The syntactic structures characteristic of skilled adult use are assembled over long time periods on early, lexical bases and conditioned by communicative context.

C. The Role of Other Mappings

In addition to the mapping of sounds heard onto sounds produced and back again, other streams of information are also being mapped to encounters with language, in the Child Talk view (see Figure 1). These include the speaker (her affect, goals, focus of attention, actions); referent objects (their identities, sensorimotor affordances, locations in relation to other objects and the viewer); and actions on objects (one's own and others'). The developmental emergence of these sensorimotor mappings, illustrated schematically in Figure 1, includes both the evolving schemas representing prototypic or categorical knowledge within domains (e.g., the construction of person identity and permanence, object identity and permanence, sensorimotor schemes) and the mapping of one domain upon another—and back again, as represented by the two-way arrows.

A selective deficit in the processing of any one information stream, then, can slow the multiple mapping of meaning in learning. For individuals

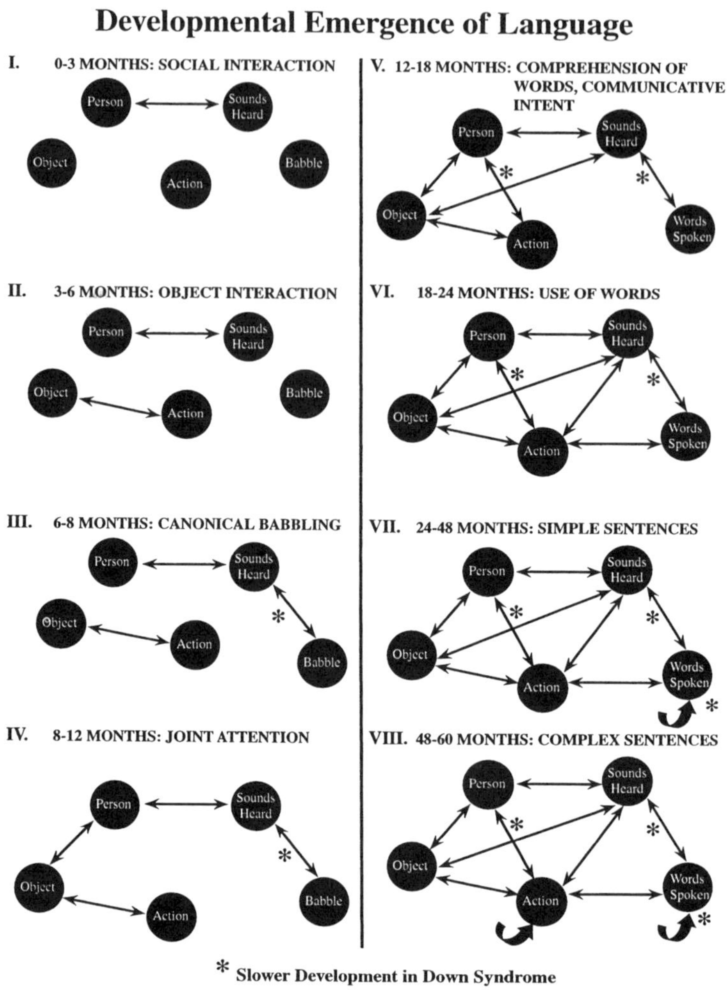

FIG. 1. Language development in typical children.

with Down syndrome, the information reviewed here suggests that, in addition to a generalized slowness of mappings, the links between speech production and speech perception are selectively slow to develop, as is the link between nonverbal requesting and the other person (see Figure 1). Such deficits would then contribute to deficits in comprehension or production when the child must rely on information in the affected stream. For example, failure to track speaker attention to referents, reported for individuals with autism, can impair the mapping of object and auditory word and the mapping of object and produced word. Or selective deficits in event representation within the hippocampus (a possibility raised for individuals with Down syndrome by Pennington, Edgin, Moon, Stedron, & Nadel, in press) might impair the meaning representation of an action verb and its associated elements of agent and object. A selective deficit in the perception–production loop subserving auditory short-term memory would impair all aspects of learning "what comes next" in the auditory stream, beginning at the level of developing syllable and word-level expectations, and continuing in the slower development of grammatical morphology, representation of phonologically complex words, utterance frames, and syntactic structures. The result would be a "computational deficit," compared to spared semantic content, but its locus would shift from phonological to lexical to syntactic with child language level.

D. Questions Raised About Language Development in Children with Down Syndrome

Children's language disorders afford a test of this process view in revealing how language skills can diverge in acquisition. Our research with individuals with Down syndrome began, then, with the desire to characterize how language learning could "come apart." We asked whether production and comprehension skills diverged in this population, as they do for some individuals with specific language impairment (SLI) in expressive language. In addition, we asked whether expressive grammatical morphology was particularly affected, as it is in SLI. And we asked whether expressive language development continued beyond the onset of adolescence or simple syntax, when Fowler, Gelman, and Gleitman (1994) proposed that it plateaued. Beyond that, we wished to examine group differences in word learning, sentence construction, and story-level skills in both comprehension and production. And we asked whether hearing, visuospatial cognition, visuospatial short-term memory, or auditory short-term memory, in particular, were predictors of variation in comprehension, production, and language learning.

III. THE BEHAVIORAL PHENOTYPE OF DOWN SYNDROME

Descriptions of the behavioral phenotype of specific syndromes have been particularly helpful in the last decade in contrasting the ways in which language, cognition, and communication skills can diverge from one another. These descriptions are useful in understanding the strengths and weaknesses of children's skills, in planning adequate assessment and intervention programs, and in testing our theories of the causal underpinnings of language learning. Accounts of groups with Down syndrome, fragile X syndrome, Williams syndrome, and fetal alcohol syndrome can be found in this volume, and the behavioral phenotype associated with Down syndrome has been a particular focus of our own research (Chapman & Hesketh, 2000).

Down syndrome typically arises from triplication of chromosome 21 (Hassold & Sherman, 2000; see Hattori et al., 2000, for the DNA sequence of chromosome 21) in whole or part (Shapiro, 1999), with an attendant cascade of gene dosage effects in development that result in the 80 or more physical and behavioral characteristics of the syndrome (Epstein et al., 1991; Korenberg, 1993; Korenberg et al., 1994; Pritchard & Kola, 1999; Reeves, Baxter, & Richtsmeier, 2001). Mouse models have helped investigators to characterize the functional genetic systems associated with physical (Kola & Herzog, 1998) and behavioral (Reeves et al., 1995) characteristics of some aspects of chromosome 21 trisomy (the mouse chromosome 16 is largely homologous). Down syndrome's genetic sources will involve the functional interaction of a number of the 225 genes triplicated on chromosome 21, rather than the alteration of a single gene, as in fragile X syndrome, or a small set of genes, as in Williams syndrome.

The behavioral phenotype of people with Down syndrome as it emerges developmentally is summarized in Table I, based on the work of a number of investigators (Abbeduto et al., 2001; Bergland, Eriksson, & Johansson, 2001; Chapman, 1995, 1997a,b, 1999; Chapman, Schwartz, & Kay-Raining Bird, 1991; Chapman, Seung, Schwartz, & Kay-Raining Bird, 1998, 2000; Cunningham, Glenn, Wilkinson, & Sloper, 1985; Dykens, Hodapp, & Evans, 1994; Eadie, Fey, Douglas, & Parsons, 2002; Epstein et al., 1991; Fowler et al., 1994; Laws, 1998; Miller, 1995, 1999; Pueschel & Sustrova, 1997; Rondal, 1998; Rosin, Swift, Bless, & Vetter, 1988; Vicari, Caselli, & Tonucci, 2000). Briefly put, cross-sectional and longitudinal evidence suggests that individuals with Down syndrome typically show an expressive language deficit, compared to comprehension and nonverbal visual cognition, with expressive syntax and grammatical morphology most severely affected. Additionally, syntax comprehension skills lag behind nonverbal visuospatial cognition in adolescence, and lexical comprehension exceeds it. Deficits in auditory short-term memory, compared to visual short-term memory or nonverbal mental age, have been reported (Chapman et al., 1991; Jarrold & Baddeley, 1997; Jarrold et al., 2002; Laws, 1998; Marcell & Armstrong, 1982; Marcell & Weeks, 1988; Seung & Chapman, 2000; Varnhagen, Das, & Varnhagen, 1987), although some individuals have normal auditory memory spans and good language skills (Rondal, 1998). Visual short-term memory falls behind visual cognition in adolescence, when the Stanford-Binet subtests of Pattern Analysis and Bead Memory are

TABLE I

DEVELOPMENTAL EMERGENCE OF THE BEHAVIORAL PHENOTYPE OF DOWN SYNDROME (adapted from Chapman & Hesketh, 2000)

Age	Domain	Behavioral phenotype
Infancy (0–4 years)	Cognition	Learning delays at ages 0–2 accelerating at ages 2–4
	Speech	No difference in vocalization types; slower in transition from babbling to speech; poorer intelligibility
	Language	Delays relative to cognition in frequency of nonverbal requesting, rate of expressive vocabulary development, rate of increase in mean length of utterances; but not comprehension
Childhood (4–12 years)	Cognition	Selective deficits in verbal short-term memory
	Speech	Longer period of phonological errors and more variability; poorer intelligibility
	Language	Expressive language delays continue relative to comprehension
	Adaptive behavior	Fewer behavior problems compared to controls with cognitive disability; more behavior problems than siblings without Down syndrome. Anxiety, depression, and withdrawal correlate positively with increasing age
Adolescence (13–18 years)	Cognition	Deficits in verbal working-memory and delayed recall
	Speech	More variability in fundamental frequency, rate control, and placement of sentential stress
	Language	Expressive language deficit in syntax greater than expressive language deficit in the lexicon
		Comprehension of words typically more advanced than nonverbal cognition
		Syntax comprehension beginning to lag nonverbal cognition
	Adaptive behavior	Fewer behavior problems compared to controls with cognitive disability
		Anxiety, depression, and withdrawal correlate positively with increasing age
Adulthood	Cognition	Behavioral symptoms of dementia beginning to emerge at 50 years for up to 50%
	Speech	Higher incidence of stuttering and hypernasality
	Language	Comprehension of syntax continues to lag cognition
	Adaptive behavior	Fewer maladaptive behaviors than controls with cognitive disability
		Higher rates of depression with increased age
		Dementia in Down syndrome is not associated with increased rates of aggression

taken as indicators, respectively, of these skills (Chapman et al., 1991). The Bead Memory task requires reconstruction of a series of objects after a delay; Pattern Analysis, reproduction with the pattern present. When both tests are included in the characterization of nonverbal mental age, syntax comprehension appears commensurate with the average value. When visual short-term memory (Bead Memory) is excluded, syntax comprehension in adolescence shows deficits relative to Pattern Analysis. (A similar finding is reported by Rosin et al. (1988), comparing syntax comprehension to performance on the Columbia Test of Mental Maturities, which requires perceptual and conceptual matching but not short-term visual memory.) Speech intelligibility (Kumin, 2001) and hearing (Marcell & Cohen, 1992) are also frequent areas of parental concern and affect communicative success. Some 60% of the population have mild hearing impairment (Marcell & Cohen, 1992).

A. Contrasts with Other Groups

In evaluating the cognitive and communication profile of individuals with Down syndrome, it is helpful to contrast the pattern of results with those from other groups. Comparison with the profiles from typically developing children, for example, controls for possible differences between standardization samples on different tests. Comparison with individuals with autism allows the role of social cognition in language learning to be more closely examined. For example, compared to individuals with autism, the performance of individuals with Down syndrome reveals their greater skill in joint attention (following the other person's gaze or focus of attention) and emotional responsiveness (Sigman & Ruskin, 1999). Comparison with individuals with Williams syndrome, who show superior auditory-verbal short-term memory skills, allows predictions of the role of phonological short-term memory to be evaluated. For example, compared to those with Williams syndrome (Bellugi, Wang, & Jernigan, 1994), individuals with Down syndrome show poorer expressive language form and reduced auditory short-term memory but comparable comprehension skills. The comparisons with individuals with fragile X syndrome discussed by Murphy and Abbeduto elsewhere in this book offer another test of the role of auditory short-term memory in the two profiles.

Within-individual comparison of skills in Down syndrome reveals that individuals often have better comprehension and problem solving behavior than their spoken communicative behavior would suggest. Conversational partners and teachers may be misled by their shorter utterances and grammatical omissions and errors to underestimate the other skills of an individual with Down syndrome, and consequently offer fewer learning opportunities at developmentally appropriate levels; indeed, the challenge is to offer opportunities appropriate to differing skill levels within the same individual.

IV. INDIVIDUAL DIFFERENCES IN SYNTAX DEVELOPMENT OF INDIVIDUALS WITH DOWN SYNDROME

Although we have described a general behavioral phenotype for Down syndrome, the description fails to capture the wide range of individual variability within the population. For example, IQ ranges between 30 and 90, with an average of approximately 50. Institutional or home environments had differing consequences for language learning, when institutionalization was common. Further, individual differences in mild hearing loss, auditory short-term memory deficit, and visual short-term memory skills may contribute to the level of language skill achieved. To an unknown degree, individual and age-related deficits associated with cumulative oxidative damage (the SOD1 gene), the toxic early effects of beta-amyloid precursor (APP) over-production, or cumulative effects of other gene expression might alter the developmental course (see, e.g., Lott & Head, 2001). Conversely, age-related strengths associated with cumulative experience might improve performance on vocabulary tests based on frequency of exposure, such as the Peabody Picture Vocabulary Test (PPVT), rather than conceptual complexity, such as the Boehm Test of Basic Concepts.

A. Longitudinal Study of Language Acquisition

Longitudinal designs that examine individual growth trajectories, and the predictors of those trajectories, allow the full range of individual differences in performance to be explored (Chapman, Hesketh, & Kistler, 2002). These analyses are particularly important to evaluate claims that language learning plateaus in adolescence, either as a function of chronological age or a ceiling at the level of simple syntax (Fowler et al., 1994). In our longitudinal study, 31 individuals with Down syndrome, ages 5–20 in approximately equal distribution across the range at study outset, participated in four language assessments across a six-year span, with approximately two years between assessments (Chapman et al., 2002). Hierarchical linear modeling (Raudenbush & Bryk, 2002) was the method chosen for analysis of developmental change. Using mean length of utterance of spontaneous utterances (MLU-S) in 12-min narratives as a measure of syntax production, we fit growth trajectories for individuals as a function of time in study (linear trajectories were used because we had only four data points). This yielded parameters for initial status and slope for each individual. Predictors considered included gender, chronological age at study start, hearing status, visuospatial cognition (the Pattern Analysis subtest of the Stanford-Binet), visual short-term memory (the Bead Memory subtest of the Stanford-Binet), and auditory short-term memory (from the ITPA, administered at times 2–4). For the cognitive and short-term memory measures we had values at each test time; to obtain predictors we also fit these measures as a function of time in the study, and used initial status and slope as the predictors of the MLU-S parameters. Although hearing was also evaluated at each time, it did not show any rate of improvement or loss, so global scores reflecting the number of frequencies passed at 25 db HL in the better ear, or whether the 25 db HL screening was passed in at least one ear on all visits, were used as predictors. We systematically evaluated models containing one or more of these predictors to determine the best-fitting model of MLU-S initial status and slope; and compared that model to one that also included syntax comprehension (initial status and slope) as predictors.

B. Expressive Language Learning Continues in Adolescence

Our longitudinal analysis of change in the MLU of spontaneous utterances (i.e., not answers to questions) revealed that individuals with Down syndrome continued to make progress in expressive language across the 6 years of observation, with mean MLU-S (*SD*) across the four time periods of 3.48 (1.76), 3.84 (1.83), 4.04 (1.84), and 4.93 (2.14). In contrast, slopes for syntax comprehension (measured by age-equivalent scores on the TACL-R) slowed and actually became negative for the older teenagers, indicating an actual drop in the corresponding raw score. When individual data were fit linearly as a function of time in the study, initial study performance in MLU-S was best predicted by age at study start, visual short-term memory at study start, and auditory short-term memory at study start. Age at study start predicted growth trajectory, or slope. When comprehension parameters were added to the predictor set, the best model, accounting for 94% of the variability in study-start parameters and 22% of the variance in slope parameters, contained only comprehension at study start, predicting initial status, and comprehension slope, predicting production slope. Thus expressive language acquisition continues in adolescence and is predicted by the initial status and growth rates in syntax comprehension, though these are slower or declining. Comprehension, in turn, is predicted by age at study start, and visual and auditory short-term memory.

C. Complex Sentence Acquisition Continues with Increasing MLU

Detailed analyses of the syntactic structure of utterances produced by individuals with Down syndrome at Time 1 by MLU level revealed almost as many syntactically complex utterances for a given length as typically developing children demonstrated, with the same wide range of structures (Thordardottir, Chapman, & Wagner, 2002). Thus we can refute the claim that expressive language development plateaus with simple syntax. Analyses of verb use in narratives revealed, however, more frequent omission of verbs, particularly mental verbs, than a typically developing comparison group matched for MLU (Hesketh & Chapman, 1998). Additionally, we found that individuals with DS were more likely to omit grammatical words and morphemes than the typically developing comparison group matched for MLU (Chapman et al., 1998), revealing that the expressive language deficit was not simply a delay, but included particular difficulty in using grammatical morphology, a finding also characteristic of typically developing children with SLI (Bedore & Leonard, 1998; Paul & Alforde, 1994; Steckol & Leonard, 1979). Sources of the verb and grammatical morpheme deficits may differ. The verb differences, in particular, seem less attributable to the problems of auditory-verbal short-term memory or hearing loss that appear to contribute to grammatical morpheme learning for individuals with Down syndrome (Miolo, Chapman, & Sindberg, submitted). Abbeduto et al. (2001) have reported difficulties for DS participants in the Theory of Mind task, attributing differing knowledge states to other people, that would suggest a potential explanation for the slower acquisition of mental state verbs.

D. Sources of Variation in MLU

Our finding of expressive language growth from each time period to the next, rather than plateauing, we attribute to our use of a narrative language sample. We asked participants to retell their favorite stories, television shows, or movies; to create stories completing story stems (Stein & Glenn, 1982); to recount personal event narratives associated with photographs from home; and to describe a complex event picture (the Cookie Theft Picture). At time 4 we also asked them to tell a story supported by a wordless picture book, *Frog, Where Are You?* (Mayer, 1969). Our method was in contrast to Fowler et al.'s (1994), who worked from samples gathered in conversation with younger adolescents. Conversation does not offer the same obligatory contexts for complex content and the complex syntax needed to convey it that narrative does.

We found that CA, visual, and auditory short-term memory tasks were the best predictors of expressive language performance in the longitudinal sample when comprehension was not included as a predictor (Chapman, Hesketh, & Kistler, 2002). This finding was surprising with respect to the nonverbal cognitive measures: the short-term visual memory task (Stanford-Binet's Bead Memory), rather than the visual pattern analysis task, offered the best fit. The role for auditory short-term memory is consistent with the observation that, for exceptional individuals with DS who also have good auditory short-term memory, excellent expressive language skills have been reported (Rondal, 1998). It is also consistent with the observations of contrasting syndromes—e.g., Williams syndrome—in which high auditory short-term memory scores are accompanied by unusually good computational aspects of expressive language (Bellugi, Wang, & Jernigan, 1994; Bellugi, Lichtenberger, Jones, Lai, & St George, 2000). As reported earlier, the inclusion of syntax comprehension as a predictor of expressive language MLU-S provided a more successful model of expressive language, with syntax comprehension status at the beginning of the study predicting variation in expressive language status at the study start; and the growth trajectory (slope) of comprehension skills predicting individual differences in growth trajectory (slope) of expressive syntax (Chapman, Hesketh, & Kistler, 2002). This link between syntax comprehension and production suggests an important implication for clinical intervention: the need to address comprehension, as well as production, goals to achieve results in later expressive language.

V. EFFECTS OF VISUAL SUPPORT ON NARRATIVES

A. Mean Length of Utterance

Our subsequent work with a new cohort of individuals with Down syndrome (Miles, Sindberg, Bridge, & Chapman, in preparation) using narratives gathered from wordless picture books led, initially, to a puzzling failure to replicate expressive language deficits of the same magnitude as our own and earlier studies. One factor at work was the entry criterion for the DS group of an MLU of at least 2.0, as the tasks required considerable narrative skill. A second was the restriction of participants from 12 to 20 years, a range when the gap between syntax comprehension and expressive language narrows. However, we also asked whether the practice of supporting narrative with a wordless picture text differentially improved utterance length for individuals with Down syndrome more than typically developing children. At this point we turned to the other source of narrative in our current protocol, an interview (Evans & Craig, 1992) soliciting talk about family, school, favorite activities and favorite videos or movies with prompting but not questioning or picture depiction: here, the expressive language deficit re-emerged. We confirmed this effect directly in a time 3 study of the prior cohort, in which the participants with DS were matched to a typically developing group on the basis of MLU in narrative from memory, and then compared on MLU for a complex event-picture description with the picture in front of them: the DS group's MLU was significantly higher than the typically developing MLU-matched group, and comparable to typically developing nonverbal mental age- and syntax comprehension-matched groups, for the pictures but not the memory-based narrative (Seung & Chapman, 2002).

Thus, we have learned an important fact about language production by speakers with DS: picture support for narration benefits the complexity of their syntactic constructions (Miles et al., in prep.). This finding must also temper, however, our report of expressive language improvement in adolescence, which would have been more modest at time 4 if we had not included the wordless picture book in the sampling protocol.

B. Story Content

Narratives can be compared not only on length and complexity of utterances, but on content. The comparison is interesting from the point of view of the Child Talk model because a differing mix of information sources contributes to content rather than form. In particular, visual cognition and visual short-term memory, knowledge of person, affect, and event—episodic information generally, play important roles in content, and many of these are strengths for individuals with Down syndrome. Two narratives gathered from the longitudinal sample were analyzed for story content: the time 4 wordless picture book, *Frog, Where Are You?* (Mayer, 1969), narrated from the pictures; and a time 3 recounting of a 6-min wordless film used for cross-linguistic study, *The Pear Story*. *The Pear Story* study revealed that the DS group's memory for event structure was more similar to typically developing children matched for comprehension than typically developing children matched for MLU from remembered stories. At the same time, the syntactic form of recall was more limited in the DS group than in the typically developing comparison group matched for comprehension (Boudreau & Chapman, 2000). Put differently, despite a deficit in expressive language syntax, individuals with DS mentioned more of the content of the filmed episode than the typically developing children at the same MLU level. The *Frog, Where Are You?* study revealed that plot line, search theme, and the misadventures of the protagonist and his dog were more often included in narration by the DS group than the typically developing MLU-matched group (Miles & Chapman, 2002); here, too, is a dissociation between the amount of content conveyed and the average utterance length used to express it.

These findings, taken together, identify two loci for the DS group's language difficulties. Auditory short-term memory plays a role in sentence comprehension (Miolo et al., submitted) as well as in production (Chapman, Seung, & Kistler, 2002). In the latter part of this chapter we will show that auditory short-term memory also plays a role in learning phonological production forms of novel words. Visual short-term memory appears to be a second factor contributing to expressive language complexity. Its slowed rate of development in adolescence may limit the degree to which prior visual information can be recalled in complex language (e.g., *The Pear Story* vs The Frog Story narratives), and the adolescents with Down syndrome appear to benefit more than an MLU-matched group from the presence of pictures depicting the story. Why these two short-term memory systems show deficits in adolescents with Down syndrome is a question for future investigation from both behavioral and biological perspectives.

C. Implications for the Child Talk Model

The findings of the longitudinal study of syntax are consistent with the Child Talk's process-based model in which general learning mechanisms rather than the presence of linguistically based modules determine language performance. The mechanisms appear to reside in the short-term memory systems supporting visual and auditory aspects of learning, with visual support freeing resources for more complex syntax. Deficits in auditory short-term memory are linked to deficits in expressive syntax. The Child Talk model applied to lexical learning would predict the same split in comprehension and production of words that is revealed for syntax. We have also carried out studies of vocabulary learning, including an evaluation of auditory short-term memory contributions to comprehension and production of novel words. To preview the conclusion of the "fast mapping" studies described in the following section, production of novel words after one to a few encounters is poorer in groups with Down syndrome than in the typically developing comprehension-matched group; and production, but not comprehension, of vocabulary is predicted by auditory short-term memory.

VI. FAST MAPPING OF NOVEL WORDS

The Child Talk model introduced at the beginning of the chapter also has implications for the learning of new vocabulary, when multiple mappings must be established between the speaker's utterance, focus of attention, intended referent, actions, and the event context. The term "fast mapping," (Carey & Bartlett, 1978) or "quick incidental learning" (Rice, 1990; Rice, Buhr, & Nemeth, 1990), refers to the incidental learning that takes place in the first few encounters with a novel word in context. In the case of novel words for nouns or verbs, receptive representation and production of the novel phonological sequence must be linked to each other and to the object or action the speaker intends (e.g., Tomasello & Barton, 1994; Tomasello & Kruger, 1992). Further, as comprehension develops, emerging syntactic cues come to play a role in the child's understanding of the category of meaning—verb, name, noun, adjective—intended by the speaker of the novel word.

On this view, object word learning can be decomposed into a series of paired sensory and sensorimotor mappings that emerge developmentally (see Figure 1), through successive stages of: (1) initial mapping of sounds to the mother's face; (2) mapping of actions on objects; (3) sounds heard to sounds produced; (4) the object-focus of the speaker; (5) the referent intended by the speaker's words; (6) the use of words to name objects and actions; (7) the combination of words in early sentences; and (8) the combination of actions in complex sentences. A number of these mappings are already accomplished for learners in the stages we studied, but word–object or –action mappings may be established in the course of one or more trials in the fast-mapping task. What is important in the fast-mapping paradigm from the Child Talk point of view is that if the word and its link to an object are novel in some way, learning is thought to be more likely because attention mechanisms are more likely to be engaged and because synaptic plasticity is enhanced. Extensive training sessions that involve already familiar objects (and rapidly familiar phonological forms) lack the novelty that underlies these enhanced "moments of learning," although reinforcement contingencies may keep the child focused on the elements to be mapped; and mapping of phonological forms for production may indeed require more repeated exposure than mapping for comprehension.

Other theorists have viewed fast-mapping tasks from the perspective of constraint theories that invoke particular principles of comprehension, or comprehension strategies, to account for the mapping of word to object meaning. For example, the Principle of Contrast (Clark, 1993) implies that a novel word must map some meaning not already named in the child's repertoire, so that a novel word used in the context of an object whose label is already known is associated with some contextual difference in speaker dialect, language, or is understood to designate some part, quality, or other taxonomic level of the object, rather than the object itself. The tendency to associate word and object (or rather, the conceptual category to which the object belongs for the child) has been designated the Principle of Whole Object correspondence, or the N3C Principle (Mervis & Bertrand, 1995): novel name–nameless category. Other research and debate has recast these rules of inference as probabilistic biases in children's responding (Merriman & Bowman, 1989). The Child Talk model's view is similar to their recasting—in early word learning, expectations based on context can determine the referent attended to and the action carried out; but expectations are based on specific experience in specific contexts.

Our view of early conceptual categories for objects is that they typically reflect object–action mappings. Perceptual attributes of novel objects may mislead the child about the appropriate action mapping, and lead to overgeneralizations of functional categories based on perceptual attributes—round candles called "balls," for example. Though objects may be unfamiliar, many of their properties—substance, weight, graspability, texture, animated features—will be familiar, and associated with action mappings—even if only looking—that constitute an initial conceptual categorization and set of expectations about future behaviors.

A. Fast Mapping in Children with Down Syndrome

The children and adolescents in the longitudinal study took part in a study of fast mapping of new vocabulary at each of four test times. The learning that takes place in one to a few encounters with new word–object pairings can be tested by seeing whether the child has inferred a connection between a novel word and the novel referent, by testing his or her ability to pick out the referent subsequently among other novel referents (*comprehension*, as it is typically measured), and ability to name the referent (*production*) or select the name among several alternatives (*word recognition*). Other control conditions that researchers have used include testing of phonologically related novel words to see whether comprehension performance depends on the word's phonological representation, and how complete it is (e.g., Kay-Raining Bird & Chapman, 1998). Testing can also be carried out with other versions of the novel object, to see whether the novel word is generalized to new instances, and which object features govern its generalization. Additional controls may incorporate object and novel word alternatives that have been equated for familiarity (number of prior encounters in the task), or variations in the cues provided by linguistic context to word category (e.g., unique names vs class nouns, nouns vs verbs).

The fast-mapping paradigm has been extended to "theory of mind" domains by tasks in which the novel referent is revealed later, or earlier, than the label; or is mistakenly labeled by the examiner (e.g., Tomasello & Barton, 1994; Tomasello & Kruger, 1992). These versions of the fast-mapping task require the child to keep track of speaker intent in identifying the referent. The paradigm has also been extended from nouns to action verbs and other open and closed morpheme classes. Additional control tasks for verbs may test for the way in which the linguistic context signals which action is the referent (e.g., past or future), and what critical features the associated action is expected to have. Our tasks, described subsequently, varied in their make-up and experimental goals across the four test times, but we attempted to probe a variety of these questions cumulatively. In the studies to be described, the samples of participants with DS are overlapping and the number of comparison groups varies.

VII. THE ROLE OF WORKING MEMORY IN FAST MAPPING OF VOCABULARY

We used Baddeley and Hitch's (1974, Baddeley, 1998; Baddeley & Hitch, 2000) model of working memory in conceptualizing the specific role of short-term memory in our studies. In this model, "slave" systems of short-term store with limited capacity subserve visual and phonological input: that is, visual and auditory information are briefly maintained and coupled in memory. Thus, it represents the two most important aspects of the Child Talk model for the mapping of new vocabulary. The visual scratch-pad is estimated to have a capacity of three items. The phonological loop is estimated to hold about 2 s of spoken language, and is refreshed by the articulatory loop, which overtly or subvocally rehearses the content of phonological store. Attentional shift between short-term stores (and the individual's action goals) is accomplished by a central executive process that allocates resources and selects actions such as intentional rehearsal of the contents of phonological short-term store (the articulatory loop). This model was attractive because it captured the early evidence of fractionated working memory skills identified in the behavioral phenotype of Down syndrome (Chapman & Hesketh, 2000). Although assessment of executive function often requires performance on tasks too difficult for many individuals with Down syndrome (e.g., backward digit repetition), a selective deficit in auditory short-term memory (repetition of digit strings, nonsense words, or sentences), and, to a lesser degree, visual short-term memory has been frequently reported and confirmed in our own and others' work (Kay-Raining Bird & Chapman, 1994; Seung & Chapman, 2000).

Recent research (Gathercole & Martin, 1996) has modified this view of short-term memory, demonstrating the role of long-term learning in the span of both visual and auditory scratch-pad store, as the Child Talk model also proposes. Further, the intentional rehearsal processes of the model appear too late developmentally (5–7 years in typically developing children) to account for the early childhood increases in memory span (Jarrold & Baddeley, 1997, 2001; Jarrold et al., 2002). Our own view, summarized earlier, is that the perceptual–production mappings established in babbling and early word learning provide for an automatic rehearsal link, subject to a more limited network subserving the link in Down syndrome, relative to other cortical development. This is a speculative interpretation, confirmed only in that imaging studies of intellectually typical adults reveal activity in the early speech-motor area when listening to word lists (Price et al., 1996) but it integrates the two key findings: expressive language lags production, and comprehension predicts production.

From the Child Talk view, working memory will also be required to represent the event context—speaker, affect, referent, goal, action, topic—as well as the talk about a referent; such representation, especially in its spatial aspect, is thought to be the province of the hippocampus, whose "feed forward" activation of expectations constitute the model of the world based on past experience, whose disconfirmation by moderate novelty leads to focused attention and increased synaptic plasticity. Thus, the hippocampal deficits, relative to other brain volumes, recently identified in Down syndrome (Pennington et al.) may be related to reduced visuo-spatial representations as well as phonological ones. Deficits in central executive processes, usually associated with prefrontal cortex functioning, remain another possibility in this conceptual fractionating of short-term learning skills.

The role of working memory (in our current understanding of it) becomes one of linking past learning to the current context. Deficits—or strengths—in any one of the paired mappings outlined in Figure 1 could conceivably contribute to impairment—or improvement—on selected tests of word learning. We began our studies, however, with a particular focus on auditory working memory and its role in comprehension and production of novel phonological forms. Auditory short-term memory in individuals with SLI has been related to deficits in fast mapping, particularly to deficits in producing the novel word (Dollaghan, 1987; Rice et al., 1990). Thus we hypothesized that the expressive language deficit in Down syndrome might include problems in fast mapping the production, but not the comprehension, forms of words, and that individual differences in word production might be predicted by auditory memory span.

VIII. FAST MAPPING IN EVENT CONTEXTS

The first study of fast mapping compared the performance of 48 children and adolescents with DS (age range 5–20 years) to 48 typically developing children (age range 2–6 years) matched for nonverbal mental age (Chapman, Kay-Raining Bird, & Schwartz, 1990). No significant differences in fast mapping skill were found. The task was modeled after Dollaghan's (1985), in including a single item. Children and adolescents with Down syndrome, whose expressive language was delayed compared to the typically developing group matched for nonverbal mental age, succeeded in fast mapping a single, phonologically simple word such as "koob" (rhymes with "rube") for a novel object in the context of a simple hiding game. All participants succeeded in inferring the relation between the novel word and the novel object, which co-occurred on the last hiding trial when other objects, including another novel object, had already been hidden. Their willingness to hide the object was the test of this inference. Comprehension was tested by having participants pick out the referent from among two familiar objects and two novel objects, all previously used in the hiding task, and an additional new novel object; thus, they at least had to remember which of the novel objects had co-occurred in the presence of the novel word. The single exposure led 83% of the typically developing comparison group matched for nonverbal mental age and 73% of the DS group to succeed on this comprehension task.

Memory for the location in which they had hidden the novel object was equally as good (83 and 75%); four separate hiding locations, a black box, a cloth, a cup, and a tissue box were used. Ability to produce the novel word (defined as producing at least two out of the three phonemes in correct order, to take the intelligibility problems of individuals with Down syndrome and the phonological processes of young children's articulatory skills into account) was poorer for both groups, but again not significantly different (48 vs 40%). Comparing the youngest and oldest quarters of the DS group, there was a significant improvement with age in memory for location and in comprehension. Among the typically developing children in the comparison group matched for nonverbal mental age, memory for location and production improved with age.

Retesting an hour later yielded similar results, although a substantial decrement in production labeling occurred in both groups. No auditory short-term memory measure was available at time 1 to test its role in predicting individual differences. This study failed to identify fast-mapping of a phonological word form as an area of specific deficit in individuals with Down syndrome, but it included only one very simple item. For all individuals, as for those in Dollaghan's studies (1986, 1987), production was a harder task than comprehension or memory for location. Strikingly, a large proportion of the children remembered over a short interval the labeled object and its location after a single encounter in context.

Why, then, has it been so hard in intervention studies to teach novel object labels in traditional paradigms that present a number of objects and a number of novel words, with multiple trials being necessary? Competition among phonological forms, or incomplete phonological representations, are likely to be major sources of difficulty; competition among the object representations another. A third potential contributing source, in the view of the Child Talk model, would be the interference induced by embedding all objects and words in the same action context, thus reducing the event context cues that might provide some protection from competition. Finally, it matters how we test learning: must the child demonstrate comprehension? How? Production? How? Producing the word is a harder task than recognizing its referent, and fast-mapping of the production form is far less likely than some connection of the novel word to its referent.

IX. FAST MAPPING NOVEL WORDS OF VARYING PHONOLOGICAL COMPLEXITY AND UTTERANCE POSITION

We hypothesized that fast mapping of the novel phonological form would be harder when it was embedded within a series than when it was in initial or final position in a list; and that words with more syllables (two or three) would be harder than words of only one syllable. Given the deficits in auditory short-term memory associated with Down syndrome, we also hypothesized that the DS group would have more difficulty fast-mapping the difficult items than typically developing groups matched for nonverbal mental age or comprehension. We investigated these questions with the 35 continuing study participants with Down syndrome (now aged 9–24 years) in a series of six fast mapping tasks, each similar to the hiding task of the first fast-mapping study (Chapman, Miller, Sindberg, & Seung, 1996a). The array of four hiding places changed for each task, as did the array of six objects, four being familiar and two novel. Thus we provided differing event context cues for each novel word encountered. Children were asked to hide three objects on a first trial, including an unnamed novel object; and the other three, including the fast mapped novel object, on a second trial, with the hiding locations indicated by pointing. For three of the tasks, the order of mention of a monosyllabic novel word was varied in the list; for three other tasks, the novel word was in final position but varied in syllabic complexity (one to three syllables). Task order was randomized. Production, comprehension, and memory for location was tested immediately after each hiding task and, for each task, an hour later.

We compared the group with Down syndrome to typically developing comparison groups matched for nonverbal mental age ($n = 35$), syntax comprehension ($n = 35$), or syntax production ($n = 35$). Neither utterance position nor syllable length had a significant effect for any group on any measure. The objects were visible while the examiner gave instructions, and it is likely that participants located the referent objects visually as the examiner named them, as adults in eye-gaze studies have been shown to do (Tanenhaus, Spivey-Knowlton, Eberhard, & Sedivy, 1995). This may have mitigated the auditory short-term memory demands of the stimuli.

In memory for location, the group comparisons of performance on all six tasks revealed no differences among groups, which averaged approximately 70% correct responses. The group with DS, however, performed significantly better than the MLU-matched group in delayed memory for hiding location (52 vs 34%).

In comprehension, the group with DS performed significantly more poorly than the typically developing comparison group matched for nonverbal mental age (56 vs 76%). The MLU-matched group (44%) performed more poorly than the comprehension (65%) and typically developing group matched on nonverbal mental age (76%). On delayed testing, no group contrasts were significant; performance declined to 54% overall.

In production, as indicated by 2/3 of the phonemes in correct order, the DS group averaged 26% correct and the comprehension group 25%. The mental age matched group performed significantly better (39%) than the MLU matched group (14%). After an hour's delay, performance declined sharply, averaging 7% in the DS group to 1% in the MLU group, despite the presence of the differentiating sets of hiding places.

We concluded that fast-mapping skills of individuals with Down syndrome in the 9- to 24-year age range show evidence of deficits in comprehension compared to a typically developing group matched on nonverbal mental age. Production performance is comparable to the typically developing group matched for syntax comprehension, not to the typically developing group matched for MLU. This is not the production deficit we expected that multiple items might reveal, although our subsequent longitudinal analyses of syntax showed continued growth in syntax production in adolescence, and actual loss of performance on syntax comprehension tests in the same period, a pattern of divergence similar to that observed here for lexical fast mapping.

A. Relation to Auditory Short-term Memory

Is there any other evidence that auditory short-term memory plays a role in fast-mapping performance? We carried out stepwise regression analyses in which the predictors evaluated were chronological age, nonverbal cognition, auditory memory, syntax comprehension, and syntax production (Chapman, Miller, Sindberg, & Seung, 1996b). Nonverbal cognition was indexed, as before, by the mean of the age-equivalent scores on the Bead Memory and Pattern Analysis subtests of the Stanford-Binet, 4th ed. Auditory memory was evaluated by the age-equivalent score on the digit span task of the Illinois Test of Psycholinguistic Ability. Syntax comprehension was evaluated by total age-equivalent score on the Test of Auditory Comprehension of Language—Revised. Syntax production was evaluated by mean length of utterance in morphemes (MLU) in a 12-min sample of narration.

For the DS group, these measures were moderately (0.5–0.6) correlated with the exception of syntax comprehension and cognition (0.8) and syntax production and comprehension (0.86). Memory for hiding location was predicted by nonverbal cognition and auditory memory, accounting for 43% of the variance. Comprehension of novel words was predicted by syntax comprehension, accounting for 45% of the variance. Production of novel words was predicted by auditory short-term memory, accounting for 41% of the variance.

For the combined typically developing control groups, predictor measures were more highly intercorrelated. Memory for hiding location was predicted by syntax production, accounting for 22% of the variance. Comprehension of novel words was predicted by age and syntax comprehension, accounting for 51% of the variance. Production of novel words was predicted by age and auditory memory, accounting for 45% of the variance.

Thus, in both the DS group and the typically developing groups, auditory short-term memory predicts production, rather than comprehension, of novel words. Comprehension of fast-mapped novel words, in contrast, is predicted by a syntax comprehension measure. These results suggest that it is the perception–production loop indexed by the auditory short-term memory task that plays an important role in fast mapping, and that these differences contribute to the learning of the production form more importantly than to the amount of phonological representation needed to succeed on the fast-mapping comprehension tests.

B. What's Happening in Our Comprehension Tests of Novel Words?

Failure of the auditory short-term memory span measures to predict comprehension results has led us to rethink the fast-mapping paradigm. The comprehension testing may simply reveal the child's knowledge that "this is the novel object that was labeled with a funny word" rather than a more complete phonological representation. If so, most of the fast-mapping research in the field needs to be re-examined for the nature of its comprehension claims, including, of course, our studies. Fast-mapping tasks are needed that provide "catch" trials in which the novel word tested differs phonologically from the target word, or has been paired with another of the novel objects, to assess comprehension more stringently.

C. Fast Mapping in Story Contexts

The learning of novel words in story contexts presents greater informational processing demands than the mapping of words in event contexts, or so we hypothesized; thus, we might expect more difficulty in fast mapping, as the listener's resources are engaged with story comprehension. When more than one novel word is embedded in stories, the tests of fast mapping of comprehension and production contain the other word, implicitly, as control. The comprehension test can then depend on the child's report of the novel word's meaning, rather than a selection among objects. Some degree of phonological representation of each word is then required to retrieve the two meanings.

Such a story fast-mapping study was carried out for 47 participants with Down syndrome and 47 typically developing children matched on nonverbal mental age (Chapman, Kay-Raining Bird, & Schwartz, 1991). Using simplified adaptations of Crais's (1987) stories, four tape-recorded stories were presented in randomized order. Each story contained three instances each of two different novel words used as nouns in the story context. The nonsense words were either monosyllabic (CVCs) or reduplicated syllables (CVCVs), with word forms counterbalanced across participants. The meaning of each novel word could be inferred from the context with high or low consensus, according to close-tests of adults. These were designated the specific and nonspecific conditions, respectively. The three instances of a word's occurrence in the story were either close (separated by only a sentence) or distant (separated by more than a sentence).

The conditions of specificity of referent and distance between instances had been previously shown to affect fast mapping of typically developing children in first, third, and fifth grade (Crais, 1987). When the instances of the novel word were close together and referred to a specific referent, the listeners were likely to choose a synonym for the meaning and to use it in production, although they performed well in recall of the novel word. When the instances of the novel word were separated by sentences and topic shifts, and the referent was nonspecific, holding on to the phonological form became more important, and listeners performed better on producing the novel word, but poorer in recalling associated propositions.

The child's task was to listen to each story, to then retell it, to define the two novel words, and to tell everything they could remember about each referent. The spontaneous occurrence of the novel words at least once in the retelling served as a production test, if at least 2/3 of the phonemes were correctly produced in order. Definitions were scored for correctness, given the story contexts, as a test of comprehension.

Our results were striking; overall story recall was poor for both groups, with the novel word produced only 10% of the time in either the DS group or the typically developing nonverbal mental age matched group. Neither specificity nor distance conditions affected responses significantly. Comprehension of the words encountered in the stories was equally poor. Approximately 10% of the novel words were defined correctly through synonyms or description, with, again no group or condition differences. Performance varied by age, with only 1–2% of the youngest age quartile fast mapping the words compared to 21–28% of the oldest quartile. The surface-level clauses of the story (text units) were also examined. Text units associated with the novel words were significantly less likely to be recalled than those that were not; and individuals with Down syndrome were significantly less likely to recall text units than the typically developing nonverbal mental age matched control group. Thus, there is evidence for a trade-off effect in comprehension: the additional resources required to process novel words apparently impaired memory for the associated content of the sentences containing them.

X. FAST MAPPING OF NOUNS VS VERBS

Most constraint theories make the assumption that the word to be learned is a noun and ascribe interpretive principles or biases to the child on that basis (e.g., the whole word principle, in which the word is to be associated with a whole object; or the mutual exclusivity principle, in which two names cannot both refer to the same object). Their extension to verbs is problematic, where actions can often be described with general pro-verb forms (*do*, *make*) or more specific ones. The later appearance of verbs vs nouns in comprehension (18 vs 12 months) in the second year of life also raises the question of whether verbs are harder to fast map than nouns in the early period of vocabulary learning (see Miller, Chapman, Branston, & Reichle, 1980). Typically developing children have been shown to fast map nouns in videotaped event and narrative contexts more easily than verbs (Rice et al., 1990). Further, individuals with Down syndrome are more likely to omit verbs in their story narratives (Hesketh & Chapman, 1998).

We assessed the ability of children and adolescents with Down syndrome to fast map action verbs, as opposed to nouns, in a study carried out with 45 participants with DS, ranging in age from 7 to 23 years, and 32 typically developing children statistically matched for nonverbal mental age and ranging in chronological age from 2 to 6 years (Chapman, Kay-Raining Bird, Sindberg, & Seung, 1994). Four brief tape-recorded stories were played to participants, two containing a single mention of a novel noun and two containing a single mention of a novel action verb. Stories were accompanied by the experimenter's story enactment with props that made story meaning clear and included the novel object and action. Each story consisted of setting statements followed by a problem—a monster appearing, boulders falling in front of a car, needing a friend, breaking one's glasses—and its resolution. The novel noun or verb occurred, in each story, near word-final position in the proposition indicating resolution of the problem. The child's production tasks (in counterbalanced orders) were to retell the story without props and to show what happened with props. Following these tasks, children were asked two comprehension questions (in counterbalanced orders), to define the novel word ("What's an X?" or "What's Xing?") and to demonstrate their understanding with props ("Show me the X" or "Show me Xing"). Novel words were monosyllabic CVCs.

Novel word production during retelling was scored correct if at least two out of three phonemes were correct in order. Fast mapping, as indicated by correct use, occurred only 5% of the time across word conditions in either group, again indicating the greater difficulty of fast mapping production forms in story contexts. Spontaneous re-enactment of novel words during pantomime recall showed no differences between the groups but a significant effect of word class: objects were included in the enactment more often (90%) than actions (66%). Comprehension, as indexed by successful definitions, was better for nouns than verbs, with the interaction of group and word class approaching significance. Participants successfully described 32% of the noun referents and 5% of the action verbs. Comprehension, as indexed by demonstration, was better for the typically developing group matched for nonverbal mental age (35%) than for participants with DS (25%), and much better for nouns (52%) than for verbs (7%). When differences in the spontaneous enactment levels are taken into account, 58% of the remembered objects are fast mapped in comprehension and 11% of the remembered actions. Thus, novel objects are inherently easier to remember than novel actions at this developmental period; and when remembered, are easier to associate with novel phonological forms. It appears that both conceptual difficulty and interpretative bias could play a role in favoring fast mapping of novel nouns occurring in story contexts.

XI. FAST MAPPING ACTION VERBS IN THE CONTEXT OF SAME OR DIFFERING OBJECTS

Individuals with Down syndrome show a split between comprehension and production in narratives at both the syntactic level and, to a lesser degree, at the lexical level, if performance on number of different words in narratives is compared to comprehension of lexical items on the PPVT-R. The number of different words is reduced, relative to the performance of typically developing children matched for nonverbal mental age; but lexical comprehension is significantly better for the DS group than the comparison group (Chapman et al., 1991, 1998). We wanted to know if the DS group ($n = 33$) showed a split between comprehension and production skills greater than that shown by the typically developing nonverbal mental age-matched comparison group ($n = 33$) early in the learning process for action verbs. We evaluated fast mapping of action verbs over two trials rather than single encounters, to compare learning of comprehension vs production forms in these two groups, as well as two other comparison groups, typically developing children matched for syntax comprehension ($n = 33$) and typically developing children matched for syntax production (MLU) ($n = 31$).

Additionally, we wished to test a prediction of the Child Talk model that contextually associated objects could serve as a prime for both the action itself and the novel word, making its comprehension and production likelier. We compared fast mapping of two novel actions on objects, one rolling a round object up an incline and letting it fall off the edge; the other making noise by moving a long thin object up and down within an open square. These were termed *meeping* and *toabing*, in counterbalanced assignment. A novel action was first demonstrated and labeled by the examiner (Trial 1). The child's ability to recall the action, label the action, and carry out the novel word was then tested. A second demonstration trial then occurred, with the same object being used for one action verb and a new object for the other. Copying the action, producing the label, and demonstrating comprehension were tested both before and after the examiner's demonstration with these materials. Trial 3 was a generalization trial in which the three tasks were repeated with new objects for both verbs. Trial 4 was a delayed assessment of generalization of each verb occurring after an hour of other activity and using yet another new object to carry out the action.

There was a context effect for all groups on assessment of comprehension before Trial 2: comprehension was better when the object was the same as Trial 1 rather than changed. No such effects occurred for the production or copying tasks. Secondly, there was a group effect for production, but not comprehension or copying, across the five tests: individuals with DS produced fewer novel verbs than the typically developing group matched on nonverbal mental age. Thus, there was a greater split in comprehension–production performance on fast-mapped verbs in DS than in the typically developing comparison group matched on nonverbal mental age, a split similar to the one that standardized assessments had suggested for lexical learning. And, although object context influences comprehension, as the Child Talk model predicted, it did not influence production in the way the model predicted. In contrast to the story contexts, performance in these event contexts, was uniformly better: approximately 90% correct across the comprehension trials, 90% correct in remembering the action, and 60% correct in production labeling of the novel actions.

XII. SUMMARY OF FAST-MAPPING FINDINGS

Fast mapping of novel nouns or verbs in event contexts is easier than their fast mapping in story contexts, where their presence also seems to impair memory for associated text. Nouns are easier than verbs to fast map in story contexts. Fast mapping of the locations and actions associated with objects in event contexts is excellent for all participants, as is comprehension of the novel words. Production of the novel words is harder than comprehension, and for novel verbs, selectively harder for the DS group compared to the mental age matched groups. Increases in the number of fast-mapped items reveal deficits for the DS group in comprehension, as well, compared to the typically developing group matched for nonverbal mental age, but better performance than the typically developing group matched for MLU. The gap between comprehension and production of verbs is greater for DS than other groups. Finally, syntax comprehension scores predict comprehension fast mapping for individuals with DS; but auditory short-term memory scores predict production. This result is replicated, with the addition of chronological age, for the typically developing children as a group. The Child Talk model's prediction that object context could prime verb learning was borne out for comprehension but not production in the fast-mapping task.

XIII. RESEARCH IMPLICATIONS: CHOOSING COMPARISON GROUPS

The questions that can be addressed in between-group comparisons depend critically on how the comparison group is chosen. In research with individuals with Down syndrome, for example, very early studies matched for chronological age—a comparison that would of little interest now, unless some additional variable, such as mental age, was also matched, yielding a comparison of groups with cognitive disability of differing etiology. When the typical pattern of skills diverges developmentally within the group studied—as is the case with Down syndrome, Williams syndrome, or fragile X syndrome, for example—then the specification of skills to match on becomes more complex.

Mental age matching, for example, was originally done by assuming that vocabulary comprehension (on the PPVT) could be taken as a proxy for general cognitive level. This is a poor choice if the group is thought to have language impairments, as it might underestimate nonverbal problem solving skills, but is quick, reliable, and correlated with performance on nonverbal cognitive tasks in typically developing children. Our work, however, has indicated that vocabulary comprehension on the PPVT actually exceeds performance on nonverbal cognitive tasks, and syntax comprehension, in adolescence (Chapman et al., 1991). Thus, to carry out mental age matching via PPVT scores would have the effect of putting individuals with DS at a disadvantage on all other measures with the comparison group. Nor are all receptive vocabulary tests equivalent. In our current studies, both PPVT-3 and TACL-3 subtest 1 are administered. The former is heavily based on picturable vocabulary of decreasing word frequency, such that the probability of encounter makes items more difficult (e.g., ball vs microscope). The latter includes a substantial number of items for spatial relations that are known to pose cognitive difficulties. And, indeed, we are finding significant differences in performance on the two tests for the DS group but not the typically developing comparison group matched for syntax comprehension (Miolo et al., submitted).

Nonverbal assessment of cognitive performance, then, is desirable; but to find tests, or tasks, that tap common dimensions across the wide span of performance (IQ 30–90) and developmental age (approximately 2–6 years) is difficult. The nonverbal performance scores of standard intelligence tests available when we began work in the 1980s were drawn from task batteries that began at differing ages in the period, thus shifting the task contribution over development. We elected to use the two visual cognition tasks on the Stanford-Binet (4th ed.) that ranged from 2 to 11 years, and assigned their mean age-equivalent score as our matching variable for mental age in the cross-sectional studies. However, the evidence in that study that scores on visual short-term memory lag the development of visual cognition led us to evaluate them as predictors of longitudinal language development separately. Further, the developmental changes in the phenotype (e.g., gains in expressive language in adolescence, but losses in receptive syntax) mean that matched groups will differ—or not—depending on the chronological age and skills of the participants with Down syndrome. We suggest that multiple regression or hierarchical linear modeling studies evaluating predictors of individual differences within the group (and within typically developing children or other groups) offer more informative analyses than the between-group comparisons.

XIV. CLINICAL IMPLICATIONS

Our research on language learning skills in individuals with Down syndrome has, we believe, important clinical implications for the recommended duration of language therapy, the selection of therapy goals, and the expectations of eventual success. We have shown that expressive language learning does not plateau with simple syntax or the onset of adolescence, but continues; that comprehension and production skills diverge; and that young adults with Down syndrome continue to learn comprehension vocabulary and complex syntax production even as they begin to show losses in syntax comprehension. These findings imply that language therapy should continue to be available during adolescence and young adulthood and that the potentially differing levels of syntax comprehension and production should be taken into account in planning goals. The fact that progress (or its lack) in syntactic comprehension predicts differences in expressive language growth trajectories suggests (as does the Child Talk model) that targeting of comprehension skills will make important contributions to continued progress in expressive language. And the significant roles of auditory and visual short-term memory in predicting performances underscores the importance of contextual support for these working memory systems in the everyday communicative tasks that individuals with Down syndrome face.

ACKNOWLEDGMENTS

This research was supported by NIH grant R01 HD23353 to the author, with additional support from the National Down Syndrome Society. We are grateful to the parents and children who participated in our studies. My thanks to the many colleagues in this research over the years, including Dr. Donna M. Boudreau, Cynthia Bridge, Christine Eisele, Dr. Linda J. Hesketh, Maura Johnson, Dr. Mina Johnson-Glenberg, Dr. Elizabeth Kay-Raining Bird, Dr. Yolanda Keller-Bell, Dr. Doris J. Kistler, Sally Miles, Dr. Suzanne Miller, Dr. Giuliana Miolo, Dorothy Ross, Dr. Robin Samlan, Dr. Scott E. Schwartz, Dr. Hye-Kyeung Seung, Heidi Sindberg, Beth Miller Swanson, Dr. Nadia Teitler, Dr. Elin Thordardottir, Dr. Laura Wagner; and many skilled transcribers. Thanks too to my colleagues Dr. Len Abbeduto and Dr. Jon Miller for helpful discussions along the way.

REFERENCES

Abbeduto, L., Pavetto, M., Kesin, E., Weissman, M., Karadottir, S., O'Brient, A., & Cawthon, S. (2001). The linguistic and cognitive profile of Down syndrome: evidence from a comparison with fragile X syndrome. *Down Syndrome Research and Practice*, *7*, 9–16.

Baddeley, A. (1992). Working memory. *Science*, *255*, 556–559.

Baddeley, A. (1998) Recent developments in working memory. *Current Opinion in Neurobiology*, *8*, 234–238.

Baddeley, A., Gathercole, S., & Papagno, C. (1998). The phonological loop as a language learning device. *Psychological Review*, *105*, 158–173.

Baddeley, A., & Hitch, G. (1974). Working memory. In G. Bower (Ed.), *The psychology of learning and motivation* (pp. 47–89). New York: Academic Press.

Baddeley, A., & Hitch, G. J. (2000). Development of working memory: Should the Pascual-Leone and the Baddeley and Hitch models be merged? *Journal of Experimental Child Psychology*, *77*, 128–137.

Bedore, L. M., & Leonard, L. B. (1998). Specific language impairment and grammatical morphology: a discriminant function analysis. *Journal of Speech, Language and Hearing Research*, *41*, 1185–1192.

Bellugi, U., Lichtenberger, L., Jones, W., Lai, Z., & St George, M. I. (2000). The neurocognitive profile of Williams syndrome: a complex pattern of strengths and weaknesses. *Journal of Cognitive Neuroscience*, *12*, 7–29.

Bellugi, U., Wang, P., & Jernigan, T. (1994). Williams syndrome: An unusual neuropsychological profile. In S. H. Broman, & J. Grafman (Eds.), *Atypical cognitive deficits in developmental disorders: Implications for brain function* (pp. 23–56). Hillsdale, NJ: Lawrence Erlbaum Associates.

Bergland, E., Eriksson, M., & Johansson, I. (2001). Parental reports of spoken language skills in children with Down syndrome. *Journal of Speech and Hearing Research*, *44*, 179–191.

Boudreau, D., & Chapman, R. S. (2000). The relationship between event representation and linguistic skill in narratives of children and adolescents with Down syndrome. *Journal of Speech, Language, and Hearing Research*, *43*, 1146–1159.

Carey, S., & Bartlett, E. (1978). Acquiring a single new word. *Papers and Reports on Child Language Development*, *15*, 17–29.

Chapman, R. S. (1995). Language development in children and adolescents with Down syndrome. In P. Fletcher, & B. MacWhinney (Eds.), *Handbook of child language* (pp. 651–663). Oxford: Blackwell.

Chapman, R. S. (1997a). Language development in adolescents with Down syndrome. In S. Pueschel, & M. Sustrova (Eds.), *Adolescents with Down syndrome* (pp. 99–110). Baltimore: Brookes.

Chapman, R. S. (1997b). Language development in children and adolescents with Down syndrome. *Mental Retardation and Developmental Disabilities Research Reviews*, *3*, 307–312.

Chapman, R. S. (1999). Language development in children and adolescents with Down syndrome. In J. F. Miller, M. Leddy, & L. A. Leavitt (Eds.), *Improving the communication of persons with Down syndrome* (pp. 41–60). Baltimore: Brookes.

Chapman, R. S. (2000). Children's language learning: an interactionist perspective. *Journal of Child Psychology and Psychiatry and Allied Disciplines*, *41*, 33–54.

Chapman, R. S., & Hesketh, L. (2000). The behavioral phenotype of Down syndrome. *Mental Retardation and Developmental Disabilities Research Review*, *6*, 84–95.

Chapman, R. S., Hesketh, L. J., & Kistler, D. J. (2002). Predicting longitudinal change in language production and comprehension in individuals with Down syndrome: Hierarchical linear modeling. *Journal of Speech, Language, and Hearing Research*, *45*, 902–915.

Chapman, R. S., Kay-Raining Bird, E., & Schwartz, S. E. (1990). Fast mapping of novel words in event contexts by children with Down syndrome. *Journal of Speech and Hearing Disorders*, *55*, 761–770.

Chapman, R. S., Kay-Raining Bird, E., & Schwartz, S. E. (1991). Fast mapping in stories: Deficits in Down syndrome. Paper presented at the American Speech–Language Hearing Association Meeting, Atlanta, GA.

Chapman, R. S., Kay-Raining Bird, E., Sindberg, H., & Seung, H.-K. (1994). Fast mapping of novel nouns and action verbs in story contexts by children and adolescents with Down syndrome. Poster presented at Wisconsin Symposium on Research in Child Language Disorders, Madison, WI.

Chapman, R. S., Miller, S., Sindberg, H., & Seung, H.-K. (1996a). Fast mapping of novel words by children and adolescents with Down syndrome. Poster presented at the Gatlinburg Research Conference on Mental Retardation, Gatlinburg, TN.

Chapman, R. S., Miller, S., Sindberg, H., & Seung, H.-K. (1996b). Fast mapping of novel words by children and adolescents with Down syndrome: Relation to auditory memory. Poster presented at the Symposium for Research on Child Language Disorders, Madison, WI.

Chapman, R. S., Schwartz, S. E., & Kay-Raining Bird, E. (1991). Language skills of children and adolescents with Down syndrome: I. Comprehension. *Journal of Speech and Hearing Research*, *34*, 1106–1120.

Chapman, R. S., Seung, H.-K., Schwartz, S. E., & Kay-Raining Bird, E. (1998). Language skills of children and adolescents with Down syndrome: II. Production deficits. *Journal of Speech, Language, and Hearing Research*, *41*, 861–873.

Chapman, R. S., Seung, H.-K., Schwartz, S. E., & Kay-Raining Bird, E. (2000). Predicting language production in children and adolescents with Down syndrome: the role of comprehension. *Journal of Speech, Language and Hearing Research*, *43*, 340–350.

Chapman, R. S., Streim, N. W., Crais, E. R., Salmon, D., Negri, N., & Strand, E. A. (1992). Child talk: implications of a developmental process model for early language learning. In R. S. Chapman (Ed.), *Processes in language acquisition and disorders* (pp. 3–19). St. Louis, MO: Mosby Year Book.

Clark, E. (1993). *The lexicon in acquisition*. Cambridge: Cambridge University Press.

Crais, E. R. (1987). Fast mapping of novel words in oral story contexts. *Dissertation Abstracts International*, *48*, 724.

Cunningham, C. C., Glenn, S. M., Wilkinson, P., & Sloper, P. (1985). Mental ability, symbolic play and receptive and expressive language of young children with Down's syndrome. *Journal of Child Psychology & Psychiatry & Allied Disciplines*, *26*, 255–265.

Dollaghan, C. (1985). Child meets word: "Fast mapping" in preschool children. *Journal of Speech and Hearing Research*, *28*, 449–454.

Dollaghan, C. (1987). Fast mapping in normal and language-impaired children. *Journal of Speech and Hearing Disorders*, *52*, 218–222.

Dykens, E. M., Hodapp, R. M., & Evans, D. W. (1994). Profiles and development of adaptive behavior in children with Down syndrome. *American Journal of Mental Retardation*, *98*, 580–587.

Eadie, P. A., Fey, M. E., Douglas, J. M., & Parsons, C. L. (2002). Profiles of grammatical morphology and sentence imitation in children with specific language impairment and Down syndrome. *Journal of Speech, Language, and Hearing Research*, *45*, 720–732.

Epstein, C. J., et al. (1991). Protocols to establish genotype–phenotype correlations in Down syndrome. *American Journal of Human Genetics*, *49*, 207–235.

Evans, J. L., & Craig, H. K. (1992). Language sample collection and analysis: interview compared to free play assessment contexts. *Journal of Speech and Hearing Research*, *35*, 343–353.
Fowler, A. E., Gelman, R., & Gleitman, L. R. (1994). The course of language learning in children with Down syndrome. In H. Tager-Flusberg (Ed.), *Constraints on language acquisition* (pp. 91–140). Mahwah, NJ: Lawrence Erlbaum Associates.
Gathercole, S. E., & Martin, A. J. (1996). Interactive processes in phonological memory. In S. Gathercole (Ed.), *Models of short-term memory* (pp. 73–100). East Sussex, UK: Psychology Press.
Hassold, T., & Sherman, S. (2000). Down syndrome: genetic recombination and the origin of the extra chromosome 21. *Clinical Genetics*, *57*, 95–100.
Hattori, M., et al. (2000). The DNA sequence of human chromsome 21. *Nature*, *405*, 311–319.
Hesketh, L. J., & Chapman, R. S. (1998). Verb use by individuals with Down syndrome. *American Journal on Mental Retardation*, *103*, 288–304.
Jarrold, C., & Baddeley, A. (1997). Short-term memory for verbal and visuo-spatial information in Down's syndrome. *Cognitive Neuropsychiatry*, *2*, 101–122.
Jarrold, C., & Baddeley, A. (2001). Short-term memory in Down syndrome: applying the working memory model. *Down Syndrome Research and Practice*, *7*, 17–23.
Jarrold, C., Baddeley, A., & Phillips, C. (2002). Verbal short-term memory in Down syndrome: a problem of memory, audition, or speech? *Journal of Speech, Language, and Hearing Research*, *45*, 531–544.
Jusczyk, P. W. (1997). *The discovery of spoken language*. Cambridge, MA: MIT Press.
Kay-Raining Bird, E., & Chapman, R. S. (1994). Sequential recall in individuals with Down syndrome. *Journal of Speech and Hearing Research*, *37*, 1369–1380.
Kay-Raining Bird, E., & Chapman, R. S. (1998). Partial representations and selectivity: the comprehension of 13- to 16-month olds. *First Language*, *18*, 105–127.
Kent, R. D. (1992). Phonological development as biology and behavior. In R. S. Chapman (Ed.), *Processes in language acquisition and disorders* (pp. 67–85). St. Louis, MO: Mosby-Year Book.
Kola, I., & Herzog, P. J. (1998). Down syndrome and mouse models. *Current Opinion in Genetic Development*, *8*, 316–321.
Korenberg, J. (1993). Toward a molecular understanding of Down syndrome. *Progress in Clinical Applied Research*, *384*, 87–115.
Korenberg, J. R., et al. (1994). Down syndrome phenotypes: the consequences of chromosomal imbalance. *Proceedings of the National Academy of Science USA*, *91*, 4997–5001.
Kumin, L. (2001). Speech intelligibility in individuals with Down syndrome: a framework for targeting specific factors for assessment and treatment. *Down Syndrome Quarterly*, *6*, 1–8.
Laws, G. (1998). The use of nonword repetition as a test of phonological memory in children with Down syndrome. *Journal of Child Psychology and Psychiatry*, *39*, 1119–1130.
Lott, I., & Head, E. (2001). Down syndrome and Alzheimer's Disease: a link between development and aging. *Mental Retardation and Developmental Disabilities Research Reviews*, *7*, 172–178.
Marcell, M., & Armstrong, V. (1982). Auditory and visual sequential memory of Down syndrome and nonretarded children. *American Journal of Mental Deficiency*, *87*, 86–95.
Marcell, M. M., & Cohen, S. (1992). Hearing abilities of Down syndrome and other mentally handicapped adolescents. *American Journal of Mental Deficiency*, *87*, 86–95.
Marcell, M. M., & Weeks, S. L. (1988). Short-term memory difficulties in Down's syndrome. *Journal of Mental Deficiency Research*, *32*, 153–162.
Mayer, M. (1969). *Frog, Where Are You?* New York: Dial Press.
Merriman, W., & Bowman, L. (1989). The mutual exclusivity bias in children's word learning. *Monographs of the Society for Research in Child Development*, *54*, Serial no. 220.

Mervis, C. B., & Bertrand, J. (1995). Acquisition of the novel name-nameless category (N3C) principle by young children who have Down syndrome. *American Journal of Mental Retardation*, *100*, 231–243.

Miles, S., & Chapman, R. S. (2002). Narrative content as described by individuals with Down syndrome and typically developing children. *Journal of Speech, Language, and Hearing Research*, *45*, 175–189.

Miles, S., Sindberg, H., Bridge, C., & Chapman, R. S. (in preparation). Context affects MLU in sampling the language of adolescents and young adults with Down syndrome.

Miller, J. F. (1995). Individual differences in vocabulary acquisition in children with Down syndrome. *Progress in Clinical Biology Research*, *393*, 93–103.

Miller, J. F. (1999). Profiles of language development in children with Down syndrome. In J. F. Miller, M. Leddy, & L. A. Leavitt (Eds.), *Improving the communication of people with Down syndrome* (pp. 11–40). Baltimore: Paul H. Brookes.

Miller, J. F., Chapman, R. S., Branston, M. B., & Reichle, J. (1980). Language comprehension in sensorimotor stages V and VI. *Journal of Speech and Hearing Research*, *23*, 384–411.

Miolo, G., Chapman, R. S., & Sindberg, H. (submitted). Sentence comprehension in adolescents with Down syndrome and typically developing children: role of sentence voice, visual context and auditory-verbal short-term memory.

Paul, R., & Alforde, S. (1994). Comment on: grammatical morpheme acquisition in 4-year-olds with normal, impaired, and late-developing language. *Journal of Speech and Hearing Research*, *37*, 1192–1194.

Pennington, B. F., Edgin, J., Moon, J., Stedron, J., & Nadel, L. (in press). The neuropsychology of Down syndrome: evidence for hippocampal dysfunction. *Child Development*.

Price, C. J., Wise, R. J. S., Warburton, E. A., Moore, C. J., Howard, D., Patterson, K., Frackowiak, R. S. J., & Friston, K. J. (1996). Hearing and saying: the functional neuroanatomy of auditory word processing. *Brain*, *119*, 919–931.

Pritchard, M., & Kola, I. (1999). The 'gene-dosage effect' hypothesis versus the 'amplified developmental instability' hypothesis in Down syndrome. *Journal of Neural Transmission*, *57* (suppl.), 293–303.

Raudenbush, S. W., & Bryk, A. S. (2002). *Hierarchical linear models: Applications and data analysis methods*. Thousand Oaks, CA: Sage.

Raudenbush, S., Bryk, A., Cheong, Y. F., & Congdon, R. (2000). *HLM-5: Hierarchical linear and nonlinear modeling*. Lincolnwood, IL: Scientific Software International.

Reeves, R., et al. (1995). A mouse model for Down syndrome exhibits learning and behaviour deficits. *Nature Genetics*, *11*, 177–183.

Reeves, R., Baxter, L., & Richtsmeier, J. (2001). Too much of a good thing: mechanisms of gene action in Down syndrome. *Trends in Genetics*, *17*, 83–88.

Rice, M. L. (1990). Preschoolers' QUIL: quick incidental learning of words. In G. Conti-Ramsden, & C. Snow (Eds.), *Children's language* (Vol. 7, pp. 171–195). Hillsdale, NJ: Lawrence Erlbaum Associates, Inc.

Rice, M. L., Buhr, J. C., & Nemeth, M. (1990). Fast mapping word-learning abilities of language delayed preschoolers. *Journal of Speech and Hearing Disorders*, *55*, 33–42.

Rondal, J. A. (1998). Cases of exceptional language in mental retardation and Down syndrome: explanatory perspectives. *Down Syndrome: Research & Practice*, *5*, 1–15.

Rosin, M. M., Swift, E., Bless, D., & Vetter, D. K. (1988). Communication profiles of adolescents with Down syndrome. *Journal of Childhood Communication Disorders*, *12*, 49–64.

Saffran, J., Aslin, R., & Newport, E. (1996). Statistical learning by 8-month-old infants. *Science*, *274*, 1926–1928.

Seung, H.-K., & Chapman, R. S. (2000). Digit span in individuals with Down syndrome and typically developing children: temporal aspects. *Journal of Speech, Language, and Hearing Research*, *43*, 609–620.

Seung, H.-K., & Chapman, R. S. (2002). Noun priming and picture descriptions in individuals with Down syndrome. Poster presented at the Joint Meeting of the International Association for the Study of Child Language and the Symposium for Research on Child Language Disorders, Madison, WI: July 16–21.

Shapiro, B. L. (1999). The Down syndrome critical region. *Journal of Neural Transmission*, *57* (Suppl.), 41–60.

Sigman, M., & Ruskin, E. (1999). Continuity and change in the social competence of children with autism, Down syndrome, and developmental delays. *Monographs of the Society for Research in Child Development*, *64*(1).

Steckol, K. F., & Leonard, L. B. (1979). The use of grammatical morphemes by normal and language-impaired children. *Journal of Communication Disorders*, *12*, 291–301.

Stein, N. L., & Glenn, C. G. (1982). Children's concept of time: the development of a story schema. In W. J. Friedman (Ed.), *The developmental psychology of time* (pp. 255–282). New York: Academic Press.

Tanenhaus, M. K., Spivey-Knowlton, M. J., Eberhard, K. M., & Sedivy, J. C. (1995). Integration of visual and linguistic information in spoken language comprehension. *Science*, *268*, 1632–1634.

Thordardottir, E., Chapman, R. S., & Wagner, L. (2002). Complex sentence production by adolescents with Down syndrome. *Applied Psycholinguistics*, *24*, 163–183.

Tomasello, M., & Barton, M. (1994). Learning words in nonostensive contexts. *Developmental Psychology*, *30*, 639–650.

Tomasello, M., & Kruger, A. C. (1992). Joint attention on actions: acquiring verbs in ostensive and nonostensive contexts. *Journal of Child Language*, *19*, 311–333.

Varnhagen, C. K., Das, J. P., & Varnhagen, S. (1987). Auditory and visual memory span: Cognitive processing by TMR individuals with Down syndrome and other etiologies. *American Journal on Mental Deficiency*, *91*, 398–405.

Vicari, S., Caselli, M. C., & Tonucci, F. (2000). Asynchrony of lexical and morphosyntactic development in children with Down syndrome. *Neuropsychologia*, *38*, 634–644.

Language Abilities of Individuals with Williams Syndrome

CAROLYN B. MERVIS

DEPARTMENT OF PSYCHOLOGICAL AND BRAIN SCIENCES,
UNIVERSITY OF LOUISVILLE, LOUISVILLE, KENTUCKY

BYRON F. ROBINSON

DEPARTMENT OF PSYCHOLOGICAL AND BRAIN SCIENCES,
GEORGIA STATE UNIVERSITY, ATLANTA, GEORGIA

MELISSA L. ROWE and ANGELA M. BECERRA

DEPARTMENT OF PSYCHOLOGICAL AND BRAIN SCIENCES,
UNIVERSITY OF LOUISVILLE, LOUISVILLE, KENTUCKY

BONITA P. KLEIN-TASMAN

DEPARTMENT OF PSYCHOLOGY, UNIVERSITY OF
WISCONSIN-MILWAUKEE, MILWAUKEE, WISCONSIN

I. INTRODUCTION

Williams syndrome is a neurodevelopmental disorder characterized by a distinctive pattern of dysmorphic facial features, cardiovascular disease, connective tissue abnormalities, delayed development leading to mental retardation or learning disabilities, a specific cognitive profile, and an unusual personality profile. The syndrome usually occurs sporadically, with an incidence of 1 in 20,000 live births in all ethnic groups. Williams syndrome is caused by a hemizygous 1.5 megabase microdeletion of chromosome 7q11.23 (Ewart et al., 1993). So far, 17 genes have been mapped to the deleted region (Osborne et al., 2001). More than 98% of individuals with

0074-7750/2003 $35.00

Williams syndrome have the same deletion breakpoints; the resulting deletion is referred to as the "classic" or "common" Williams syndrome deletion (Morris & Mervis, 2000).

The importance, from a theoretical perspective, of research on language and cognitive aspects of Williams syndrome was first made clear by Ursula Bellugi, who argued that Williams syndrome was a paradigmatic example of the independence of language and cognition. In her invited address at the International Conference on Infant Studies in 1990, Elizabeth Bates presented Bellugi's position as follows: Individuals with Williams syndrome have excellent language abilities, including correct use of complex syntax such as passives, conditionals, relative and embedded clauses, and tag questions. They also have an unusual command of vocabulary. These language abilities occur in the context of profound mental retardation, providing clear evidence of the independence of language from cognition. Upon hearing these claims, which contrasted with her own research on the relation between language and cognition for children with Down syndrome, the first author of this chapter immediately decided to expand her research program to include children with Williams syndrome. The major findings from this program regarding language abilities of individuals with Williams syndrome and the relation between language and cognition for individuals with this syndrome are presented in this chapter. We begin by describing findings from our large-sample studies of performance on standardized assessments measuring language and cognition. In the second section, we turn to early language acquisition by toddlers and preschoolers with Williams syndrome. The third section is concerned with semantic abilities of school-age children and adults with Williams syndrome. In the fourth section, we address the acquisition of grammar by children and adolescents with Williams syndrome and its relation to cognitive abilities. In the final section, we conclude by summarizing our findings concerning similarities and differences between the language acquisition patterns of children with Williams syndrome and children with typical development. Based on our findings, we consider the possibility that relative to language acquisition by children who are developing typically, language acquisition by individuals with Williams syndrome may be more dependent on verbal memory and less dependent on more conceptual aspects of cognition.

II. PERFORMANCE ON STANDARDIZED ASSESSMENTS

We begin our examination of the language and cognitive abilities of individuals with Williams syndrome by considering their performance on a variety of standardized assessments. Scores on these measures are summarized

TABLE I
DESCRIPTIVE STATISTICS FOR STANDARDIZED ASSESSMENTS[a]

Measure	*N*	Mean	*SD*	Range
DAS (School Age): GCA	50	58.14	11.44	32–88
Verbal Cluster	50	70.02	13.21	51–100
Nonverbal Cluster	50	67.56	12.09	52–98
Spatial Cluster	50	54.74	6.07	50–79
Pattern Construction T	210	23.25	5.52	20–53
Recall of Digits T	234	32.97	9.72	20–60
K-BIT: Composite IQ	250	67.38	15.39	40–108
Verbal IQ	250	71.77	15.45	40–108
Nonverbal IQ	250	68.52	17.12	40–108
Mullen: Composite	34	62.32	11.64	49–88
Visual Reception T	34	30.12	10.12	20–46
Fine Motor T	34	21.65	3.45	20–31
Receptive Language T	34	30.47	9.82	20–55
Expressive Language T	34	33.21	9.59	20–48
PPVT-III	146	77.91	15.38	40–120
EVT	119	64.14	19.18	40–106
TROG	209	73.67	12.54	55–112
Vineland: Composite	41	63.00	9.31	41–98
Socialization	41	78.71	13.71	54–110
Communication	41	71.05	12.19	51–98
Daily Living Skills	41	60.20	10.09	28–82

[a]For the general population, mean = 100 and *SD* = 15 for all measures not labeled "T." For all measures labeled "T," mean = 50 and *SD* = 10.

in Table I. Standardized assessments provide important information about these individuals' abilities relative to peers of the same chronological age (CA). Findings from more naturalistic settings also are important to a full understanding of the language and cognitive abilities of individuals with Williams syndrome; these data are considered in this section with regard to the child's adaptive behavior and later in the chapter with regard to lexical and grammatical development.

When studying a rare syndrome, it is tempting to conduct one's research on small, relatively easily obtained samples of individuals varying widely in CA. We have taken a different approach, seeking large samples across a broad age range for our studies of performance on standardized assessments and smaller but still substantial samples focused on a narrower age range for studies using observational or experimental approaches. To obtain these samples, we have sought referrals from geneticists, cardiologists, early intervention agencies, and parents of individuals with Williams syndrome in a number of states in the southeast, midwest, and southwest regions of the United States as well as from the National Williams

Syndrome Association (WSA). We also have tested as many participants as possible at regional and national family meetings of the WSA. Overall, our sample includes individuals from 42 of the 50 states in the USA.

A. Differential Ability Scales

The DAS (Elliott, 1990) is a full-scale measure of intellectual functioning designed to provide specific information about an individual's strengths and weaknesses across a wide range of intellectual activities. Two forms are available: The Preschool DAS, for use with children aged $2\frac{1}{2}$ through 6 years, and the School Age DAS, for use with children aged 5 through 17 years. Although both forms may be used with 5- and 6-year-olds, the test author recommends that the Preschool Age form be used with children in this age range who are expected to have below average abilities. The data reported in this chapter are for the performance of children aged 7 through 17 years on the School Age DAS. The six core subtests included in this form of the DAS are divided into three clusters. The Verbal Cluster measures the child's ability to define words and to perform verbal reasoning tasks. The Nonverbal Reasoning Cluster measures the child's inductive and sequential reasoning abilities. The Spatial Cluster measures visuospatial constructive abilities, spatial memory, and spatial reasoning. Visuospatial construction is known to be the area of greatest weakness for individuals with Williams syndrome (e.g., Bellugi, Wang, & Jernigan, 1994; Mervis, Morris, Bertrand, & Robinson, 1999). As indicated in Table I, mean GCA (General Conceptual Ability; similar to IQ) is 58.14 (in the range of mild mental retardation). As illustrated in Figure 1, however, the mean GCA is misleading. Mean standard scores on both the Verbal Cluster (70.02) and the Nonverbal Reasoning Cluster (67.56) are considerably higher than the GCA. In contrast, performance on the Spatial Cluster is much poorer, with 50% of the individuals tested performing at floor. Performance was best on the Recall of Digits subtest (a diagnostic subtest not included in the GCA) and worst on the Pattern Construction and Recall of Designs subtests (the two subtests in the Spatial Cluster).

B. Kaufman Brief Intelligence Test

The negative impact of the extreme weakness in visuospatial construction on IQ is well demonstrated by a comparison of the performance of individuals with Williams syndrome on the DAS and the K-BIT (Kaufman & Kaufman, 1990), an IQ test that measures only verbal ability and nonverbal (reasoning) ability. The mean verbal standard scores on the DAS and K-BIT are within 2 points of each other (70.02 and 71.77); similarly, the

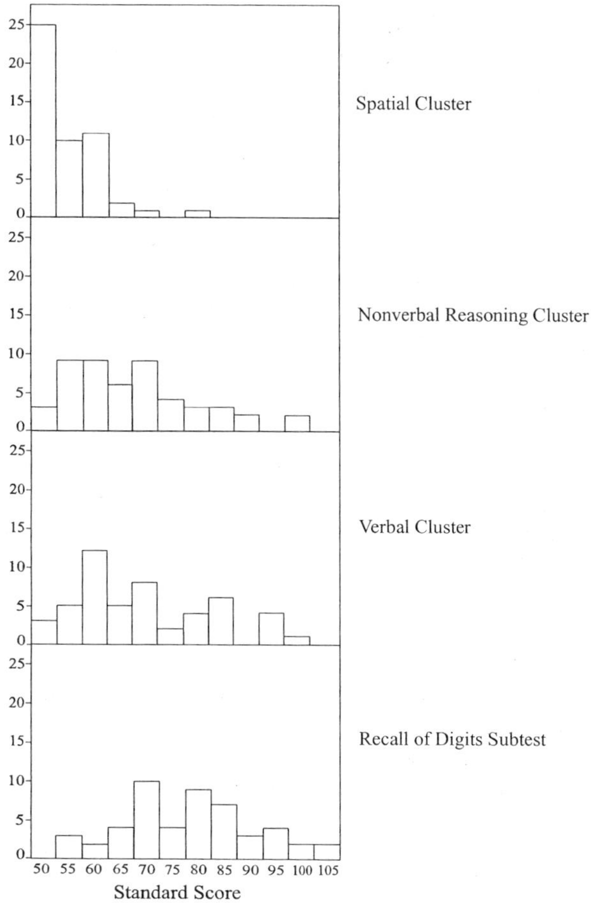

FIG. 1. Distribution of standard scores for DAS Spatial Cluster, Nonverbal Reasoning Cluster, Verbal Cluster, and Recall of Digit subtest for 50 7- to 17-year-olds with Williams syndrome. Recall of Digits T score has been converted to the same scale as the Cluster standard scores (mean = 100, *SD* = 15).

mean nonverbal reasoning standard scores are only 1 point apart (67.56 and 68.52). In contrast, mean K-BIT IQ is 9 points higher than mean DAS GCA (67.38 vs 58.14).

C. Mullen Scales of Early Learning

The Mullen (1995), like the DAS School Age assessment described above, provides a full-scale measure of intelligence, but for toddlers and preschoolers. The Mullen findings indicate that the pattern of performance evident for school-aged children with Williams syndrome (ages 7–17 years) is present by age 2 years. Performance was weakest on the Fine Motor subtest (measuring primarily visuospatial construction but also skills such as cutting with scissors); 79% of the participants scored at floor. Performance was considerably better for the two language subtests (averaging about the same as for the DAS and K-BIT verbal standard scores) and for the Visual Reception subtest (measuring many of the same types of abilities as the nonverbal reasoning sections of the DAS and K-BIT).

Thus, across the three measures of intelligence, a consistent pattern emerges, with standard scores for language abilities the highest. Language scores are similar for the three assessments even though somewhat different abilities are measured: The K-BIT focuses on picture naming and (for older children and adults) providing words based on a verbal clue plus some of the letters included in the word. The DAS requires that the participant define words and indicate how sets of words are related. The Mullen involves identifying the referent of a word provided by the researcher from a set of pictures or objects (receptive subtest) or naming pictures, providing definitions, exactly repeating utterances provided by the researcher, or answering verbal reasoning questions (expressive subtest). At one level, this pattern of performance is consistent with prior claims that language is a particular strength for individuals with Williams syndrome. However, the level of performance on these measures does not fit with the claim that language abilities are "excellent"; language standard score means are in the borderline normal to mildly impaired range. Nonverbal reasoning standard scores are only slightly lower than language standard scores. Furthermore, mean IQ is considerably higher than the profound mental retardation range. With this pattern in mind, we turn to standardized assessments that measure specific language abilities.

D. Peabody Picture Vocabulary Test (3rd edition) and Expressive Vocabulary Test

The PPVT-III (Dunn & Dunn, 1997) measures receptive single-word vocabulary knowledge. Most words are names for objects, actions, or attributes, although some label more abstract concepts. On average, individuals with Williams syndrome earn their highest standard score on this measure. Mean performance was in the borderline normal range (mean of 77.91); 9% scored at least 100 (the mean for the general population).

The Expressive Vocabulary Test (EVT; Williams, 1997) measures expressive single word vocabulary. Early items require that the participant name a picture or an attribute of a picture. Later items involve the researcher providing a word that names a picture or some aspect of a picture and the participant providing a synonym. Like the PPVT-III, most target words are labels for objects, actions, or attributes, although some refer to more abstract concepts. Although the EVT was co-normed with the PPVT-III, individuals with Williams syndrome typically have considerably more difficulty on the EVT (mean: 64.14, 13 points lower than the PPVT-III mean). This difficulty most likely is due to the conceptual requirement of providing a synonym rather than simply naming the picture.

E. Test for Reception of Grammar

The TROG (Bishop, 1989) measures receptive understanding of grammar. Constructions range in difficulty from single words for objects, actions, or attributes to simple sentences, comparatives, passives, and sentences with relative or embedded clauses. Mean performance on this measure (73.67) was in the borderline normal range, similar to that on the PPVT-III, suggesting that receptive understanding of grammar is at a similar level to receptive understanding of single-word vocabulary. The pattern of performance on the different grammatical constructions was similar to that found by Karmiloff-Smith et al. (1997) in their study of a considerably smaller British sample. In that study, particular difficulty was identified for embedded clauses. For example, if asked to choose the picture matching a sentence such as "The box the dog is jumping over is brown," the participant was likely to choose a picture of a brown dog jumping over a black box, rather than the correct picture of a black dog jumping over a brown box. Zukowski (2001, in press) reported the same difficulty in an elicited production task when individuals with Williams syndrome were prompted to describe a picture using embedded clause constructions. For example, if the target sentence was "The box (that) the dog is jumping over is brown," the participant would be likely to say "The dog that is jumping over the box is brown."

F. Vineland Adaptive Behavior Scale

The Vineland (Sparrow, Balla, & Cicchetti, 1984) measures adaptive behavior. The Communication domain focuses on the ability to understand and produce oral language and to read and write. The Daily Living Skills domain focuses on personal skills related to hygiene, eating, and dressing; household skills; and abilities related to telephone usage, time management, and money handling. The Socialization domain focuses on interpersonal interactions; use of leisure time; and responsibility and sensitivity to other people. Many of the items included in the Socialization domain assess language use (e.g., greeting, labeling emotions, conversing). We have administered the Parent Report form of this measure to the parents of 41 children between the ages of 4 and 9 years (Mervis, Klein-Tasman, & Mastin, 2001). Performance was weakest on the Daily Living Skills domain (mean: 60.20). This difficulty was expected; a large proportion of items in this domain are based on fine motor skills in general and visuospatial construction skills in particular. Examples include "zips zippers," "buttons large buttons," "ties shoelaces into a bow without assistance," "pours dry cereal and milk into a bowl," and "makes simple repairs on broken toys or possessions." Performance was best on the Socialization domain (mean: 78.13). On the Communication domain, performance was at about the same level as for the verbal subtests of the intelligence measures (mean: 71.05). The mean for the Vineland Composite, which provides an overall measure of adaptive behavior, was 63.00.

Not surprisingly, the pattern of strengths and weaknesses identified based on the performance of individuals with Williams syndrome on overall measures of intelligence holds for adaptive behavior as well, with language abilities clearly stronger than visuospatial constructive abilities. That said, the fact remains that across all of the language measures administered (IQ tests, specialized assessments of single word vocabulary or grammar, adaptive behavior), average performance is consistently in the mildly deficient to borderline normal range. This level of performance is considerably below that expected for the participants' CA, indicating that both lexical and grammatical abilities typically are well below the level expected for "excellent" language ability. It is important to note that there is a great deal of variability in language ability across the Williams syndrome population. This variability is strongly linked to both verbal short-term memory ability and verbal working memory ability (Mervis, 1999). This link will be discussed at several points throughout this chapter.

III. EARLY LANGUAGE ACQUISITION

Although people with Williams syndrome eventually have relatively good language abilities, the onset of language almost always is significantly delayed. Consider, for example, the performance of a sample of 13 children with Williams syndrome whom we have followed longitudinally from the time of their first words. Expressive vocabulary size was measured based on the 680-word vocabulary checklist included in the Words and Sentences form of the MacArthur Communicative Development Inventory (CDI; Fenson et al., 1993). The CDI is a parental report measure of language acquisition that has very high reliability and validity (Fenson et al., 1993, 1994). The age of acquisition of a 10-word expressive vocabulary was below the 5th percentile (the lowest percentile provided) for the CDI norms for all

TABLE II

MEAN CA (IN MONTHS) AND RANGE FOR AGE OF ACQUISITION OF 10-, 50-, AND 100-WORD EXPRESSIVE VOCABULARIES FOR 13 CHILDREN WITH WILLIAMS SYNDROME IN COMPARISON TO CDI NORMS

Expressive Vocabulary Size	WS mean CA	WS CA Range	CA for CDI 50th percentile	CA for CDI 5th percentile
10 words	28.19	18.84–53.95	12–13	16–17
50 words	36.59	23.80–61.25	16–17	23–24
100 words	40.90	26.24–68.05	18–20	26–28

of the children in the sample. Twelve of the 13 children scored below the 5th percentile for age of acquisition of 50-word and 100-word expressive vocabularies. Mean CA and CA range for the Williams syndrome sample at acquisition of 10-, 50-, and 100-word expressive vocabulary sizes are indicated in Table II, along with the CAs corresponding to the 50th and 5th percentiles for the CDI.

Our research group has conducted three studies of the early language acquisition of toddlers and preschoolers with Williams syndrome: (1) a cross-sectional comparison of the productive vocabulary sizes of 2-year-olds with Williams syndrome or Down syndrome; (2) a longitudinal study of early vocabulary acquisition and its relation to grammatical development and to verbal and nonverbal intelligence; and (3) a longitudinal study of developmental relations between specific aspects of language and cognition. Each of these studies is described below.

A. Expressive Vocabularies of 2-year-olds with Williams Syndrome or Down Syndrome

School-aged children with Williams syndrome repeatedly have been found to have larger expressive vocabularies than CA-matched children with Down syndrome (e.g., Bellugi, Wang, & Jernigan, 1994; Wang & Bellugi, 1993). Singer Harris, Bellugi, Bates, Jones, and Rossen (1997), however, have argued that initially young children with Down syndrome have an expressive vocabulary advantage over young children with Williams syndrome; the advantage does not shift to children with Williams syndrome until after the onset of grammar. This position is based on Singer Harris et al.'s finding that for children with fewer than 50 words in their expressive vocabulary, children with Down syndrome had significantly larger expressive vocabularies than children with Williams syndrome. This comparison is methodologically problematic, however, in that Singer

Harris et al. used the same variable (expressive vocabulary size) first as the criterion for inclusion in the sample and then as the dependent variable in the analysis. Thus, the outcome variable is confounded with the criterion for inclusion in the study in the first place, making the results uninterpretable. (See Mervis & Robinson, 2000, for a more detailed argument.)

A more methodologically sound approach to comparing the expressive vocabulary sizes of children with Williams syndrome and children with Down syndrome would be to match the two groups closely on CA and then compare their expressive vocabulary sizes. We followed this approach, tightly matching a group of 24 two-year-olds with Williams syndrome (mean CA = 2 years 6 months 18 days; $SD = 131.74$ days) to a group of 28 two-year-olds with Down syndrome (mean CA = 2 years 6 months 18 days; $SD = 120.96$ days). Two additional boys with Williams syndrome (ages 2 years 0 months and 2 years 1 month) were excluded from the analyses because their expressive vocabulary sizes were dramatically larger than any of the other children their age (more than eight standard deviations above the mean); descriptive data for these two children are provided separately. All of the children with Williams syndrome had classic deletions. Expressive vocabulary size was derived from the 680-word vocabulary checklist included in the Words and Sentences form of the CDI. Parents were told to indicate that their child "said" a word if the child produced the word spontaneously, either in verbal or signed form. For the toddlers with Williams syndrome, mean expressive vocabulary size was 132.50 words ($SD = 112.29$) with a range from 3 to 391 words. In contrast, for the toddlers with Down syndrome, mean expressive vocabulary size was 66.35 words ($SD = 79.24$) with a range from 0 to 324 words. Mean expressive vocabulary size was significantly greater for the Williams syndrome group than the Down syndrome group.

The parents of 9 of the toddlers with Down syndrome and 13 of the toddlers with Williams syndrome had filled out the vocabulary checklist for the CDI at least once when their children were between 24 and 27 months old. In order to provide a comparison for a time even closer to the onset of expressive vocabulary acquisition, a second analysis was conducted using data for these children. Mean CA was 2 years 1 month 28 days for both groups of children ($SD = 26.96$ days for the Williams syndrome group and 24.02 days for the Down syndrome group). Once again, the Williams syndrome group had a significantly larger expressive vocabulary than the Down syndrome group. Mean expressive vocabulary size for the Williams syndrome group was 55.08 words ($SD = 40.80$, range: 5–120). The two boys excluded from the analyses had expressive vocabulary sizes of 412 and 439 words. In contrast, mean expressive vocabulary size for the Down syndrome group was 19.67 words ($SD = 24.71$, range: 0–70). The results of these two sets of analyses indicate that children with Williams syndrome have, on average, a clear and significant expressive vocabulary advantage over same-CA children with Down syndrome. It is important to acknowledge, however, that almost all of the children with Williams syndrome were substantially delayed in expressive vocabulary acquisition. Other than the two boys who were excluded from the analyses (and who were at the 75th percentile for the CDI norms), none of the children in the Williams syndrome group was at even the 10th percentile for the CDI norms, and 67% were below the 5th percentile. It is also important to note that the variability in expressive vocabulary size was very high within both the Williams syndrome group and the Down syndrome group and that there was substantial overlap between the two groups. The wide range in expressive vocabulary size among toddlers with Williams syndrome presages the very large variability we described in the previous section for children and adults with Williams syndrome on standardized tests of expressive and receptive vocabulary. On these measures, although the mean for the Williams syndrome group is substantially and significantly below that for the general population, the variability is similar to that of the general population.

B. Early Vocabulary Acquisition and its Relation to Grammatical Development and to Intelligence

Children who are developing typically evidence a strong relation between productive vocabulary size and grammatical development. Bates and Goodman (1997) have argued that the onset of word combinations requires the accumulation of a "critical" mass of words in the child's expressive vocabulary. These researchers have noted that one of the strongest developmental relations is that between number of words in a young child's expressive vocabulary and the complexity of the child's spontaneous utterances. The results of our study of the expressive vocabulary size of toddlers with Williams syndrome make it clear that most children with Williams syndrome are significantly delayed in the onset of word (or sign) production. Given this finding, we would expect that the onset of grammatical development also would be delayed. If the relations between vocabulary development and grammatical development are similar for children with Williams syndrome and typically developing children, however, then both groups should evidence the same relations between productive vocabulary size and grammatical complexity.

We have been able to address these questions using data from our longitudinal study of the early language development of toddlers and preschoolers with Williams syndrome (e.g., Becerra, Thomas, Robinson, & Mervis, 2002; Mervis, 2002). Our longitudinal sample currently includes

25 children, of whom 23 are old enough to be expected to produce word combinations. The parents of the children in this study complete the CDI vocabulary checklist monthly; once their child begins to combine words, parents also complete the CDI Early Sentence Checklist monthly. This checklist consists of 37 pairs of phrases or sentences. The two phrases in a pair express the same idea, but with differing degrees of grammatical correctness or complexity. Parents are asked to indicate which of the two utterances sounds most like the way their child is currently speaking. If the simpler member of the pair is more complex than the utterances that the child is producing, then the parents are instructed not to mark either member of the pair. The child's Sentence Complexity score is the number of utterance pairs (out of 37) for which the parents have marked the more complex version. CDI data are available for an average of 40 months per child (range: 8–66 months). The mean age of the children at the time that the parents began to complete the CDI was 26 months (range: 11–40 months).

To address the question of whether the onset of grammar was delayed for children with Williams syndrome, we used the data from the Early Sentence Checklist. Only four of the 22[1] children (18%) had a Sentence Complexity score of at least 1 by age 30 months. Performance at this level corresponds to the 10th percentile for children in the general population. (Data are not available for the 5th percentile for this measure.) Based on this criterion, the onset of grammatical development is delayed for most but not all children with Williams syndrome. However, once grammatical development begins, rate of development is the same for children with Williams syndrome as for children in the general population. The relation between productive vocabulary size and grammatical ability also was the same for the children with Williams syndrome as for the general population. This relation fell between the 5th and 95th percentiles for 21 of the 22 children, with individual children's data spread fairly evenly across this percentile range, suggesting that the amount of variability in the Williams syndrome sample was similar to that for the general population. Volterra, Caselli, Capirci, Tonucci, and Vicari (2003), in a cross-sectional study of 6 children learning Italian as their native language, also have found that grammatical complexity (as measured by the Italian version of the CDI) is at the level expected for productive vocabulary size.

Vocabulary growth curves based on data from the 680-word CDI vocabulary checklist follow a logistic shape for typically developing children (e.g., Robinson & Mervis, 1999). Initially, vocabulary growth follows a linear pattern with a small slope. Eventually, however, rate of growth

[1]Sentence complexity data were not available for 1 of the 23 children.

increases rapidly for a sustained period. As the child approaches the ceiling on the CDI checklist, however, rate of growth appears to slow down, leading to a logistic shape. (This reduced rate of growth is primarily an artifact of using a checklist with a constrained number of words.) Analysis of the monthly expressive vocabulary growth data indicated that the growth curves for 20 of the 23 children with Williams syndrome were logistic in shape. Two of the remaining children evidenced slow linear growth at least until age 5 years. The final child evidenced a growth pattern that we characterized as "double linear." Until just after he turned 4 years, this child evidenced very slow linear growth. At age 49 months, however, he began to add words to his expressive vocabulary at an extremely fast pace that was maintained for several months, again yielding linear growth but this time with a very steep slope.

To determine if growth curve type was related to cognitive ability, we compared the three sets of children on their performance on the Preschool DAS at age 48 months. Results indicated that the children with logistic growth scored significantly higher on a wide range of cognitive measures. Not surprisingly, children with logistic growth curves scored significantly higher than the children with linear growth curves on other language measures such as the Preschool DAS Verbal Cluster and the PPVT-III. The logistic group also scored significantly higher on both forward digit span and overall GCA. Impressively, the logistic group scored significantly higher on the Preschool DAS Nonverbal Cluster as well. The child with a double-linear growth curve scored at a level intermediate to the other groups. There was almost no overlap in standard scores between the logistic growth and linear growth groups. This pattern of findings suggests that the shape of vocabulary growth is closely linked not only to grammatical development and to other measures of language development, but also to verbal short-term memory and to nonverbal aspects of development including visuospatial construction, the area of greatest weakness for individuals with Williams syndrome.

C. Specific Relations between Lexical Development and Cognitive Development

Based on studies of children who are developing typically and children who have Down syndrome, a number of specific relations between particular aspects of early lexical acquisition and hypothetically linked aspects of early nonverbal cognitive development have been identified (see review in Mervis & Bertrand, 1997). On average, typically developing children have equivalent levels of language abilities and nonverbal cognitive abilities (including nonverbal reasoning and spatial cognition).

Thus, findings of specific links between lexical and nonverbal cognitive development for children with typical development are not surprising. That children with Down syndrome also evidence these same links is more noteworthy, as these children's general level of nonverbal cognitive ability is usually more advanced than their general level of verbal ability. It would be even more impressive to find that these same links also hold for children whose general level of language ability is more advanced than their general level of nonverbal cognitive ability. To address this possibility, we present data from 10 children with Williams syndrome who were followed longitudinally for 3–5 years beginning at ages 4–26 months. These children participated in monthly play sessions, after which their parents completed the CDI. If children with Williams syndrome evidence the same links between specific aspects of lexical development and particular aspects of nonverbal cognitive development, then the case for the universality of these links becomes much stronger. Conversely, if these links do not hold for children with Williams syndrome but they still acquire the relevant lexical abilities, study of these children will be especially useful for identifying alternate paths to lexical competence. In this section, we briefly consider several specific links that previously had been found to hold for both children who are developing typically and children who have Down syndrome. Additional details are provided in Mervis and Bertrand (1997).

1. CANONICAL BABBLING AND RHYTHMIC BANGING

Cobo-Lewis, Oller, Lynch, & Levine (1995) have argued that rhythmic (canonical or reduplicated) babble and rhythmic hand banging should begin at about the same time because they reflect parallel manifestations of rhythmic behaviors. Canonical or reduplicated babble involves repetition of the same consonant–vowel syllable two or more times (e.g., "dada" or "mamama" but not "ga"). Both canonical babble and rhythmic hand banging appear before the onset of lexical comprehension or production. Because the rhythm of canonical babble fits the syllable patterns of mature speech, this type of babble is considered a very important step in the language acquisition process. Parents typically change the way they talk to their infants once canonical babble begins, and these changes likely facilitate the child's acquisition of an initial vocabulary.

At the time they entered the study, 8 of the 10 children with Williams syndrome already were producing both canonical babble and rhythmic hand banging. Thus, data relevant to this proposed universal were available from only two children, who entered the study at ages 4 and 5 months. Both children first produced canonical babble in the same play session in which they first produced rhythmic banging. Furthermore, the parents of both children reported that their children had begun producing both canonical babble and rhythmic hand banging in the interval between that play session and the previous one. Thus, the limited data available from this study are consistent with the putative universal link between these two abilities. More recently Masataka (2001), in a longitudinal study of eight infants with Williams syndrome acquiring Japanese as their native language, also found a strong link between the onset of canonical babble and the onset of rhythmic hand banging.

2. POINTING AND THE ONSET OF REFERENTIAL PRODUCTION OF OBJECT NAMES

The second potential universal link involves the acquisition of the ability to refer. The cognitive manifestation of this ability is referential pointing; the lexical manifestation is referential productive language (e.g., object labels). The cognitive manifestation of this link is expected to precede the lexical manifestation. This sequential ordering of referential pointing and referential labeling is one of the most robust findings regarding the transition to language. Infants express communicative intentions nonverbally, by pointing, prior to expressing them verbally, by labeling. This link, which is routinely acknowledged in textbooks on the development of language (e.g., Adamson, 1995), presumably obtains because the cognitive manifestation of reference (pointing) provides the child with an especially useful way to determine the reference of the words he or she hears. Adults use pointing gestures to indicate reference. Until the child is able to follow these gestures, he or she is likely to have difficulty determining the reference of the adult's words. At the same time, children use pointing gestures to elicit labels from adults. This link has been shown to hold for typically developing infants acquiring a wide variety of native languages and for both children with Down syndrome and children with severe mental retardation of mixed etiology.

The most delayed child in the Williams syndrome sample began to comprehend and produce referential pointing gestures approximately 3 weeks before he first produced a referential object label. Thus, this child's data are consistent with the predicted order of emergence. In contrast, the remaining nine children with Williams syndrome began to produce referential labels for objects several months (mean: 6 months) before the onset of either comprehension or production of referential pointing gestures. Apparently, referential pointing skills are not necessary for the onset of referential language. Either the knowledge that underlies comprehension and production of pointing gestures is not necessary for the onset of referential production of words or there is an alternate path to this knowledge. These possibilities are addressed at the end of this section.

3. PRIORITY OF BASIC-LEVEL CATEGORIES: LABELS AND PLAY PATTERNS

Objects can be categorized at a variety of hierarchical levels. For example, the same object can be a beach ball (subordinate level), a ball (basic level), or a toy (superordinate level). The basic level is more fundamental than the other levels (Rosch, Mervis, Gray, Johnson, & Boyes-Braem, 1976). This is the most general level at which category members have similar overall shapes and at which a person uses similar motor actions for interacting with category members. Although categories at all hierarchical levels are based on form–function correlations, these correlations are most apparent at the basic level. Because of the salience of basic level categories, they should be acquired first. Thus, children's initial functional play patterns (cognitive manifestation of categorization) and the initial extensions of the object labels that they comprehend and produce (linguistic manifestation of categorization) should converge at the (child-) basic level.[2] Longitudinal research on typically developing children and children with Down syndrome has confirmed this relation between initial play patterns and initial object labels for the two categories for which it has been addressed: *ball* and *car*. Although for many categories, nonverbal play patterns are difficult to observe, especially in the laboratory, extensive data are available concerning children's first words from diary studies of typically developing children acquiring a wide range of native languages. Results of these studies indicate that basic level labels are consistently acquired before subordinate or superordinate level labels.

Data from both the monthly play sessions and parental responses on the CDI and a specially constructed subordinate category checklist indicated

[2]Although young children are expected to use the same principles (e.g., form–function correlation) to form basic level categories, membership in these categories would not be expected to be identical to that for adult-basic level categories labeled by the same name. The actual categories formed on the basis of these principles will vary because different groups attend to different attributes of the same object, as a function of different experiences or different levels of expertise (Mervis, 1987). Because very young children may not share adults' knowledge of culturally appropriate functions of particular objects and the form attributes correlated with those functions, these children may de-emphasize attributes that are important from an adult perspective. At the same time, very young children may notice a function (and its correlated form attributes) for that object that adults ignore, leading the children to emphasize features that are unimportant to adults. In these situations, although there will be significant overlap in membership between the child-basic and adult-basic categories labeled by the same word, the child-basic category will differ systematically from the corresponding adult-basic category.

that basic level categories had the same priority for the children with Williams syndrome as for typically developing children and children with Down syndrome. The children with Williams syndrome played with all the spherical objects (e.g., balls, spherical candles, sleigh bells) in the same manner, by rolling them. In contrast, they did not try to roll any of the nonspherical objects. The children's lexical behavior also indicated that they had formed a child-basic *ball* category; "ball" was comprehended in reference to a wide range of spherical objects, whether or not an adult would have considered them to be balls, but not in relation to objects of other shapes. Eight of the 10 children also produced the word "ball." These children showed the same pattern in production as they had in comprehension. A parallel set of findings was obtained for the *car* category, with all four-wheeled vehicles (but not boats or airplanes) being pushed along, often accompanied by motor noises, and the word "car" comprehended and produced in reference to the same set of vehicles.

Examination of the data from the checklists completed by the parents indicated that in 96% of the cases, the basic level name for an object was comprehended prior to the subordinate level name; in 3% of the cases, the order of acquisition was unclear (both the basic level label and the label for a subordinate category subsumed under that basic level category were first acquired in the same month). The subordinate level name was comprehended before the basic level name in only 1% of the cases. These latter cases involved two words: "toothbrush" and "school bus," both of which are atypical of their basic level categories. Interestingly, none of the children comprehended or produced any superordinate level labels prior to comprehending at least one basic level label for an object subsumed under that superordinate.

4. SPONTANEOUS EXHAUSTIVE SORTING, THE VOCABULARY SPURT, AND FAST MAPPING

Gopnik and Meltzoff (e.g., 1987, 1992) have argued that spontaneous exhaustive sorting and the vocabulary spurt should occur at about the same time because they reflect parallel insights: all objects belong to some category (cognitive insight) and all objects have a name (linguistic insight). Mervis and Bertrand (1993, 1994) have argued that a better linguistic manifestation of this insight is the ability to fast map, that is, the ability to use the Novel Name—Nameless Category (N3C) principle. Initially, children must rely on other people to provide an explicit connection between a new word and its referent (e.g., by showing an object to a child and then labeling it, or by labeling an object to which the child was already attending). Once children acquire the N3C principle, however, they no longer need to depend on someone else to make an explicit connection between a label and its referent. According to this principle, the child should assume that novel words map to categories for which the child does not yet have a name. Within the developmental lexical principles framework (Golinkoff, Mervis, & Hirsh-Pasek, 1994; Mervis & Bertrand, 1994), the N3C principle has been interpreted as expressing the insight that all objects have a (basic level) name. Once the child has this principle, the indirect connection provided by hearing a novel word in the presence of an object for which he or she does not yet have a name is sufficient for mapping to take place. For both typically developing children and children with Down syndrome, the onsets of spontaneous exhaustive sorting, the vocabulary spurt, and fast mapping have been found to occur at about the same time.

We have found that much of this pattern does not hold for children with Williams syndrome, even though we measured the three abilities in the same way as in the studies involving typically developing children and children with Down syndrome. In particular, none of the children with Williams syndrome evidenced a temporal link between the onset of spontaneous exhaustive sorting and the vocabulary spurt, or between the onset of the vocabulary spurt and fast mapping. Nine of the 10 children had a vocabulary spurt well before the onset of spontaneous exhaustive sorting or fast mapping ability (range 6 months to more than 1 year). The remaining child evidenced spontaneous exhaustive sorting and the ability to fast map 5 months before she began her vocabulary spurt. Thus, these putatively universal links clearly do not hold for children with Williams syndrome.

The data from the children with Williams syndrome, however, did support the universality of a specific link between the onsets of spontaneous exhaustive sorting and the ability to fast map. All but two of the children demonstrated the onset of both abilities in the same session. The two remaining children demonstrated fast mapping at the session before the one at which they evidenced spontaneous exhaustive sorting.

5. SUMMARY: UNIVERSALS AND ALTERNATE PATHS TO EARLY LEXICAL COMPETENCE

In this section, we have considered a series of specific relations between particular aspects of nonverbal cognitive development and particular aspects of early lexical development. All of these specific relations already had been shown to hold for both typically developing children and children with Down syndrome and thus had been considered as putative universal links. Three of these relations were found to hold for children with Williams syndrome. First, the onset of cognitive and linguistic manifestations of rhythmic behaviors, as measured by rhythmic hand banging and canonical babble, occurred at about the same time. Second, children's initial categories, whether measured by nonverbal play patterns or verbal object label comprehension or production patterns, are basic level categories. Third, the realization that all objects belong to some category (as measured by spontaneous exhaustive sorting) and that all objects have a (basic-level) name (as measured by onset of the N3C principle; fast mapping of new object names without direct input) occurred at about the same time. The universality of this third specific link is especially impressive given the large differences between the children with Down syndrome and the children with Williams syndrome in level of general nonverbal cognitive development relative to level of language development.

The remaining two putative universal links did not hold for children with Williams syndrome. The children did acquire both the cognitive and the linguistic manifestations of these two links, however. Thus, the data from children with Williams syndrome provide critical information regarding alternate paths to two milestones of early lexical development: onset of referential production and onset of the vocabulary spurt.

In contrast to the pattern shown by typically developing children and children with Down syndrome, all but one of the children with Williams syndrome produced referential object labels several months before beginning to comprehend or produce referential pointing gestures. This finding indicates that comprehension and/or production of referential object labels is not dependent on comprehension and/or production of referential pointing gestures. Comprehension and production of referential object labels almost certainly requires that the child and adult be engaged in joint attention to an object at the time that the adult labels it. Referential pointing provides one obvious way for a person to communicate his or her focus of attention to someone else. In positing that referential pointing should precede the onset of referential productive language, researchers likely were centering on the attention-focusing function of pointing. Thus, pointing may have been intended as a proxy for participation in episodes of joint attention regarding an object. However, the data from the children with Williams syndrome serve as a reminder that there are other ways to establish joint attention to objects. Examination of the tapes of the parent–child with Williams syndrome play sessions from the longitudinal study identified three alternative methods for establishing such joint attention. (All three methods also were used by parents of typically developing children and parents of children with Down syndrome.) The first method was child-centered: The adult followed the child's focus of attention and then labeled that object. This is a method that has been shown to be especially effective, even for typically developing children (Dunham, Dunham, & Curwin, 1993;

Tomasello & Farrar, 1986). The other two methods were more adult-directed. One involved adults picking up the object to which they wanted the child to attend, putting it in the place where the child already was looking, and then labeling the object. The other involved directing a child's attention to an object by tapping it. Once the child was looking at the object, the adult labeled it. These methods apparently are successful in inducing children with Williams syndrome to comprehend and produce object labels referentially. Comprehension and production of referential pointing gestures may facilitate the onset of productive language for some children, but these abilities clearly are not necessary. What probably is necessary for the onset of referential language is the ability to participate in joint attention episodes involving object labeling.

A common explanation for the onset of the vocabulary spurt is that it is due to the child's realization that all objects have names (see Gopnik & Meltzoff, 1987). Findings from typically developing toddlers and toddlers with Down syndrome are consistent with this explanation. However, data from toddlers with Williams syndrome are not, indicating that fast-mapping abilities are not necessary for the onset of the vocabulary spurt. Some of the children with Williams syndrome had more than 500 words in their productive vocabularies before they were able to fast map. These data indicate the presence of a viable alternate path to rapid vocabulary acquisition. Although fast mapping is an excellent facilitator of rapid acquisition of new words, other ways must be possible. In many cases, the onset of the vocabulary spurt and subsequent rapid accumulation of new words probably result from the child's increasing efficiency at acquiring words using the same procedures as before the vocabulary spurt (see Bates & Carnevale, 1993). For individuals with Williams syndrome, an increase in verbal short-term memory provides a particularly likely alternate path. As indicated earlier in this chapter, individuals with Williams syndrome evidence a relative strength in verbal short-term memory. (For additional evidence of this relative strength, see Finegan, Smith, Meschino, Vallance, & Sitarenios, 1995; Mervis et al., 2000.) A large portion of children with Williams syndrome score within the normal range on the DAS Recall of Digits subtest; many score within 1 *SD* of the general population mean, and some even score above the general population mean. Good verbal short-term memory provides a solid basis for the long-term memory for words that is needed for vocabulary acquisition and retention. Thus, increases in verbal short-term memory are likely to facilitate increases in rate of vocabulary acquisition, even in the absence of fast-mapping ability. In this way, verbal short-term memory likely plays an important role in vocabulary acquisition for most individuals, not just for young children with Williams syndrome.

IV. SEMANTIC ABILITIES OF SCHOOL-AGE CHILDREN AND ADULTS

Initial studies of the semantic abilities of individuals with Williams syndrome suggested that they had an "unusual" command of vocabulary. In particular, examples were provided of the comprehension and production of words that were more sophisticated, abstract, and unusual than would be expected for someone with severe mental retardation (e.g., Bellugi, Marks, Bihrle, & Sabo, 1988; Bellugi et al., 1994). At the same time, semantic organization was argued to be deviant (e.g., Bellugi et al., 1994). To better understand the semantic abilities of individuals with Williams syndrome, our research group has conducted three studies with school-aged children and adults as participants. In this section, we order these studies by participant CA. The first study is concerned with the relation between the concrete and abstract vocabulary abilities of 5-, 6-, and 7-year-old children with Williams syndrome. The second addresses the semantic organization of 9- and 10-year-old children with Williams syndrome relative to a group of CA- and IQ-matched children with Down syndrome and two groups of typically developing children, one matched to the Williams syndrome and Down syndrome groups for CA and the other matched for MA. In the third study, we consider the ability of adolescents and adults with Williams syndrome to comprehend figurative language.

A. Relations between Concrete and Abstract Vocabulary Abilities

As indicated in the description of our standardized assessment findings, individuals with Williams syndrome perform particularly well on the PPVT-III relative to other standardized measures. Mean level of performance is only 1.5 standard deviations below that for the general population, and 73.5% of the participants scored in the normal range (70 or above), with 9.5% scoring at or above the mean of the general population (100 or above). It is important to note, however, that the PPVT-III measures primarily concrete vocabulary knowledge. It is possible that individuals with Williams syndrome have more difficulty with abstract relational vocabulary, either because of general cognitive limitations in reasoning ability and/or specific difficulties with visuospatial construction. Knowledge of abstract relational language is particularly important for success in school. Understanding of this type of language has not been considered previously for individuals with Williams syndrome.

To begin to address the question of the abstract relational vocabulary knowledge of individuals with Williams syndrome relative to their concrete vocabulary knowledge, we compared the performance of 34 5-, 6-, and 7-year-olds (mean CA = 6 years, 3 months) on the Test of Relational Concepts (TRC; Edmonston & Litchfield Thane, 1988) to their performance on the PPVT-III (Whittle, Chang, Thomas, & Mervis, 2001). A comparison group of 43 typically developing 4- to 7-year-olds (mean CA = 5 years, 1 month) matched for concrete receptive vocabulary size (as measured by raw score on the PPVT-III) also participated in the study. The TRC, which is normed for ages 3–7 years, is designed to measure the types of relational concepts that are particularly important for success in school. Five types of concepts are included: temporal (e.g., *first/last*; *before/after*), quantitative (e.g., *most/least*, *many/few*), dimensional (e.g., *tall/short*, *narrow/wide*); spatial (e.g., *back/front*, *first/last*, *under/over*, *middle*, *beginning/end*); other (*same/different*, *with/without*).

The typically developing contrast group was included in the study to provide a control for concrete receptive vocabulary size. Comparison of the raw scores of the two groups on the PPVT-III indicated that the Williams syndrome group and the contrast group were very well matched ($p = 0.66$). Despite the close match on concrete vocabulary size, the typically developing contrast group demonstrated a significantly larger abstract relational vocabulary size on the TRC (mean raw score = 30.95 for the contrast group, 21.68 for the Williams syndrome group). This pattern of results indicates that children with Williams syndrome have substantially more trouble acquiring relational vocabulary than would be expected given their concrete vocabulary knowledge. Importantly, abstract relational vocabulary size is strongly related to concrete vocabulary size for both groups, even after controlling for CA (Williams syndrome group, $r = 0.67$; contrast group, $r = 0.73$).

Not surprisingly given the raw score findings, the contrast group earned significantly higher standard scores than the Williams syndrome group on both the PPVT-III (contrast group: mean = 100.87, $SD = 13.85$; Williams syndrome group: mean = 86.35, $SD = 11.86$) and the TRC[3] (contrast group mean = 91.36, $SD = 17.68$; Williams syndrome group mean = 57.85, $SD = 17.44$). The most important comparison involved relative performance on the PPVT-III and the TRC. The typically developing contrast group earned a slightly (but significantly) higher standard score on the PPVT-III than on the TRC. For the Williams

[3]Standard scores for the TRC are expressed as T scores, with a mean of 50 and a standard deviation of 10. In order to compare standard scores on the TRC to standard scores on the PPVT-III, we converted the TRC T score to a scale with a mean of 100 and a standard deviation of 15. The lowest possible standard score on both tests was set at 40 (the actual lowest standard score for the PPVT-III).

syndrome group, the difference was much more dramatic: Mean standard score on the TRC was almost 30 points (2 standard deviations) lower than on the PPVT-III. Performance on the TRC was at floor for 32% of the children with Williams syndrome; none of these children performed at floor on the PPVT-III. The contrast in distribution of scores on the PPVT-III and the TRC for the Williams syndrome group is illustrated in Figure 2.

To determine if the relational vocabularies of children with Williams syndrome are composed of the same proportions of the different types of relational concepts as are the relational vocabularies of typically developing children, we compared subgroups of the two original groups that were matched for relational vocabulary size ($p = 0.38$). Mean TRC raw scores for the matched subgroups were 19.87 for the Williams syndrome group and 21.81 for the typically developing contrast group. An analysis of variance indicated no significant differences between the two groups for the percentage of concepts comprehended for each of the five types. Nevertheless, because other researchers (e.g., Bellugi, Lichtenberger, Jones, Lai, & St. George, 2000) have hypothesized that spatial concepts would be more difficult than other types of concepts for children with Williams syndrome, we compared the performance of the two subgroups for

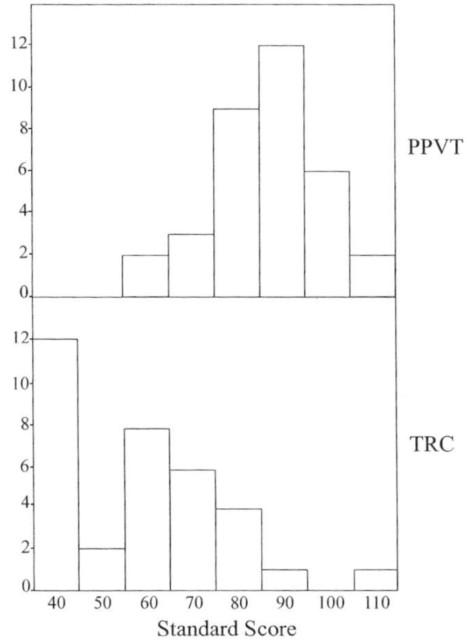

FIG. 2. Distribution of standard scores for TRC and PPVT-III for 34 five- to seven-year-olds with Williams syndrome. TRC T scores have been converted to the same scale as the PPVT-III standard scores (mean = 100, $SD = 15$).

each of the 17 spatial concepts included in the TRC. The two groups performed comparably on 14 of the concepts. On the remaining 3 (*front/back*, *middle*, *above/below*), the performance of the Williams syndrome group was significantly lower than that of the typically developing contrast group.

In summary, children with Williams syndrome have much more difficulty acquiring abstract relational vocabulary than expected, given their ability to acquire concrete vocabulary. Nonetheless, abstract relational vocabulary size is highly correlated with concrete vocabulary size. The abstract relational vocabularies of children with Williams syndrome contain the same proportions of the various types of relational concepts as typically developing children matched for relational vocabulary size. However, children with Williams syndrome find a few spatial concepts more difficult than do typically developing children matched for relational vocabulary size. To determine if the difficulty that children with Williams syndrome have in acquiring abstract relational language is, as we expect, due to mental retardation/low IQ in general, rather than to characteristics unique to Williams syndrome, comparisons with children with other etiologies of developmental delay are necessary.

B. Semantic Organization

The semantic organization of a category refers to how an individual cognitively relates the members of the category. Typically, this type of organization is measured by word fluency tests in which a person is asked to name all the items that he or she can think of that are members of the category named by the researcher (e.g., *animal*, *fruit*). The first study of the semantic organization of individuals with Williams syndrome was conducted by Bellugi and her colleagues (Bellugi, Bihrle, Neville, & Doherty, 1992; Bellugi et al., 1994), who asked 6 adolescents with Williams syndrome, 6 CA- and IQ-matched adolescents with Down syndrome, and a group of typically developing second-graders to name all the animals that they could within 1 minute. Based on the findings from this study, Bellugi et al. argued that the semantic organization of adolescents with Williams syndrome was deviant. In particular, the participants with Williams syndrome were more likely to list unusual (defined as low word frequency) animals. This finding was consistent with the researchers' statement that individuals with Williams syndrome use unusual words in their spontaneous speech.

We had also heard individuals with Williams syndrome use unusual words spontaneously. However, use of such words did not seem to be more frequent than for typically developing children of the same developmental level. Because we were surprised by Bellugi et al.'s semantic organization findings, we decided to conduct a study of the semantic organization of the *animal* domain using a larger sample and well matched control groups, as well as a wider range of measures of semantic organization (Mervis et al., 1999; Scott et al., 1995). The 48 participants included 12 9- and 10-year-olds with Williams syndrome, 12 children with Down syndrome individually matched to the children with Williams syndrome for CA and MA (as measured by raw score on the McCarthy Scales of Children's Abilities; McCarthy, 1972), 12 typically developing children individually matched to the pairs of children with Williams syndrome and Down syndrome for MA, and 12 typically developing children individually matched to the pairs for CA. Children were asked to name as many animals as they could. The researcher provided two examples: *cat* and *bear*. Although children were given as long as they wished to produce their lists, they rarely took more than 60 seconds (the time limit in Bellugi et al.'s study).

To determine participants' semantic organization for the *animal* category, we considered four types of measures of semantic fluency: fluency, representativeness, word frequency, and category composition. Fluency was measured by the number of animal names produced. Representativeness of the items produced as members of the *animal* category was determined based on goodness-of-example (GOE) ratings obtained using a procedure similar to Rosch (1973, 1975). College students were asked to use a 7-point scale to rate the animal names generated by the participants for how well each fit the student's idea or image of *animal*. Three measures of GOE were used: mean rating for all of the animal names a child produced; rating for the most representative (typical) animal name the child produced; and rating for the least representative (most atypical) animal name the child produced. Word frequency was measured in two different ways: mean frequency of the animal names the child listed in children's texts (standard frequency index or SFI; Carroll, Davies, & Richman, 1971) and proportion of items listed that had an SFI < 50 (Bellugi et al.'s criterion for classification of an animal name as low frequency). Two measures of category composition were used: percentage of animal names produced at the basic level (e.g., *dog*) and percentage of animal names produced at the subordinate level (e.g., *beagle*).

On 7 of the 8 measures used, the performance of the three groups matched for MA (Williams syndrome, Down syndrome, typically developing MA-match) was similar. The three groups performed equivalently on number of animal names produced, mean GOE rating, GOE rating for the most typical exemplar produced, mean SFI, proportion of exemplars with SFI < 50, and proportions of basic-level exemplars and subordinate-level exemplars.

For the remaining measure, GOE rating of the least typical exemplar produced, both the Williams syndrome and the Down syndrome groups performed at the same level as the typically developing CA-match group.

The least typical exemplar produced by the older groups of children was significantly less representative of the *animal* category than the least typical exemplar named by the MA-match group. Performance of the Williams syndrome group also was equivalent to that of the CA-match group on mean SFI value and proportion of basic-level animal names. However, the CA-match group named on average more than twice as many animals as the Williams syndrome group did and included a significantly higher proportion of subordinate level exemplars. In addition, mean GOE rating was significantly higher for the CA-match group, indicating that on average the exemplars listed by the Williams syndrome group were more representative of the *animal* category than were the exemplars listed by the CA-match group.

The pattern of findings we obtained indicates that in some ways the semantic organization of the *animal* category is similar for the four groups of children. The proportion of animal names listed at the basic level, the mean SFI rating, and the proportion of items for which SFI < 50 were equivalent for all four groups. The latter finding contrasts with that of Bellugi et al. (1992, 1994) who found that adolescents with Williams syndrome produced a higher proportion of items with SFI < 50 than did the Down syndrome or typically developing groups. Our finding that the least representative exemplar produced was reliably less representative for the three older groups than for the MA-match group, however, fits with Bellugi et al.'s finding that the Williams syndrome group produced more unusual animal names than the typically developing second-graders did. This component of semantic organization appears to be more dependent on amount of experience with animals (as measured by CA) than on cognitive level (as measured by MA). On all the other measures of semantic organization, however, the children with Williams syndrome performed similarly to the two groups matched for MA (Down syndrome group, typically developing MA-match group). Volterra, Capirci, Pezzini, Sabbadini, and Vicari (1996) also found that performance of children with Williams syndrome on a semantic fluency task was highly similar to that of typically developing controls matched for MA. The two groups listed equivalent numbers of animals, and most of the animals listed were of high word frequency. Thus, overall performance of individuals with Williams syndrome on semantic fluency tasks is appropriate for MA, suggesting that the development of semantic organization in Williams syndrome is delayed rather than deviant.

C. Comprehension of Figurative Language

Although individuals with Williams syndrome, on average, evidence a strength in concrete receptive vocabulary, the study we described earlier in this chapter makes it clear that this strength does not extend to more abstract vocabulary in the form of relational concepts.

Figurative language (e.g., metaphors, similes, idioms) is another form of abstract language. Two prior studies of figurative language comprehension abilities of individuals with Williams syndrome have been conducted. Karmiloff-Smith, Klima, Bellugi, Grant, and Baron-Cohen (1995), in a study focusing on comprehension of metaphor by adolescents and adults found that only about half of the participants were able to explain the meaning of the metaphors included in their study. Sullivan, Winner, and Tager-Flusberg (2003) studied the comprehension of ironic jokes by older children and adolescents with Williams syndrome. The latter study included two control groups composed of CA-, IQ-, and receptive vocabulary (PPVT-R raw score)-matched groups of individuals with either Prader-Willi syndrome or mental retardation of unknown etiology. None of the participants with Williams syndrome and only a few of the participants in the other groups were able to comprehend ironic jokes. The results of these two studies suggest that comprehension of figurative language is difficult for a large proportion of people with Williams syndrome.

To further investigate the figurative language abilities of adolescents and adults with Williams syndrome, we have conducted a study focused on comprehension of idioms and the cognitive correlates of this ability. Idioms are a common form of figurative language whose comprehension is critical for following everyday conversations among older children, adolescents, and adults in the general population. Thus, comprehension of idioms is important for successful integration of individuals with Williams syndrome with their typically developing peers. To comprehend an idiom, the listener must ignore the surface (literal) meaning of an utterance in favor of the deeper, figurative meaning. A cognitive ability which requires that surface configurations be ignored in favor of deeper underlying properties is conservation of number, liquid quantity, or substance.[4] In particular, the

[4]For example, in a conservation of number task, the researcher might first make a line of six circles and then ask the participant to construct a line containing the same number of squares. Younger typically developing participants and older children and adults with mental retardation usually construct the second line using one-to-one correspondence, resulting in two lines not only containing the same number of objects but also of the same length. Once the participant agrees that the two lines contain the same number of objects, the researcher compresses one line so that it is obviously shorter than the other. The participant is then asked if there are more circles, more squares, or the same number of each. To be considered to conserve number, the participant must both indicate that there are the same number of circles and squares and then justify this response in one of three ways: (1) Nothing was added or taken away, so the number remains the same. (2) Reversal of the transformation would make the two lines be exactly the same. (3) Change in one dimension (e.g., density) compensates for change in another (e.g., length).

ability to conserve is based on the realization that amounts remain the same regardless of what transformations are applied to the physical configurations. Because similar insights underlie both comprehension of idioms and solution of conservation problems, we hypothesized that there should be a significant correlation between performance on these two types of tasks.

To consider both the ability of individuals with Williams syndrome to comprehend idioms and the correlates of this ability, we tested 37 older adolescents and adults (mean age 25 years, range: 16–52 years) on a series of language and cognitive measures (Bertrand, Mervis, Armstrong, & Ayres, 1995). Comprehension of idioms and of the syntax underlying these idioms was assessed using the Familiar and Novel Language Comprehension Test (FANL-C; Kempler & Van Lacker, 1985). On this test, participants are asked to choose from four pictures the one that best matched the meaning of the sentence produced by the researcher. Comprehension of concrete vocabulary was measured with the Peabody Picture Vocabulary Test—Revised (PPVT-R; Dunn & Dunn, 1981). The ability to conserve number, liquid, and substance was measured using conservation tests based on Ginsburg and Opper (1979). In addition, 19 of the 37 participants also completed the K-BIT and a test of backward digit span (a measure of working memory).

Overall, the participants performed very well on the measure of comprehension of literal language, comprehending a mean of 12.95 of the 16 literal sentences ($SD = 2.37$, range: 8–16) on the FANL-C. Comprehension of idioms involving the same syntactic constructions was much weaker; participants responded correctly to a mean of 5.95 of the 16 idioms ($SD = 3.14$, range: 0–12). Nevertheless, 44% of the participants performed above chance levels (7 or more items correct) on the idiom portion of the FANL-C. Receptive concrete vocabulary ability was significantly correlated with comprehension of both literal ($r = 0.62$) and figurative ($r = 0.67$) sentences. The correlation between performance on the literal sentences and on the idioms ($r = 0.48$) also was significant.

Previous research had suggested a strong dissociation between preserved language ability and very limited cognitive ability for individuals with Williams syndrome. One oft-cited example of limited cognitive ability is the inability to solve Piagetian conservation problems despite excellent grammatical and vocabulary abilities (e.g., Bellugi et al., 1994; Bellugi, Klima, & Wang, 1996). Of the 37 participants in our study, 18 were able to solve at least some types of conservation problems: 11 were able to solve and appropriately justify their solutions to all of the conservation problems presented (*number*, *liquid*, and *substance*); 7 were able to solve and appropriately justify their solutions to number conservation problems only. This rate of success at conservation problems is considerably higher than expected based on Bellugi et al.'s findings. Performance on the figurative portion of the FANL-C was strongly and significantly related to number of conservation problems solved and justified correctly ($r = 0.74$). Even after receptive concrete vocabulary knowledge, ability to comprehend literal utterances with the same syntax as the figurative utterances, nonverbal reasoning ability (as measured by raw score on the Matrices portion of the K-BIT), and backward digit span were taken into account, the relation between comprehension of idioms and conservation ability remained significant (partial $r = 0.49$). Thus, comprehension of idioms is strongly related to a cognitive ability (conservation) that we hypothesize requires similar conceptual insights, providing a further example of a link between a specific aspect of language ability and a specific aspect of cognitive ability.

V. GRAMMATICAL ABILITY AND ITS RELATION TO COGNITIVE ABILITIES

Grammatical ability has often been considered a particular strength of individuals with Williams syndrome. In fact, the ability of individuals with Williams syndrome to comprehend and produce complex syntax was the primary basis for Bellugi et al.'s claim (e.g., Bellugi et al., 1988, 1994, 2000) that Williams syndrome provides a compelling case for the independence of language from cognition. In this section, we describe two studies of grammatical ability relative to cognitive ability that we have conducted. The first uses data from play sessions with a researcher to address relations among MLU in spontaneous speech, grammatical complexity of spontaneous utterances, and level of cognitive ability for 2- to 12-year-old children. The second is concerned with the relation between receptive grammar knowledge and verbal memory ability for school-age children and adolescents. A third study comparing the verbal and memory abilities of CA- and IQ-matched 9- and 10-year-olds with Williams syndrome and Down syndrome also is presented; this study provides further evidence that the apparent strength that individuals with Williams syndrome demonstrate for language ability is due in large part to a strength in verbal memory.

A. Relations between Level of Cognitive Ability, MLU, and Grammatical Complexity

Initial studies of the grammatical abilities of individuals with Williams syndrome all were based on very small samples of adolescents; comparison groups, when included, were composed of CA- and IQ-matched individuals with Down syndrome. Results of these studies indicated that individuals with Williams syndrome had excellent syntactic abilities; furthermore, Bellugi and her colleagues argued that the grammatical abilities evidenced were much more advanced that would be expected given the significant level of mental retardation associated with Williams syndrome (e.g., Bellugi, Bihrle, Jernigan, Trauner, &, Doherty, 1990; Bellugi et al., 1988, 1994; see Bellugi et al., 2000 for a summary including results from more recent studies). In these studies, the participants with Williams syndrome were reliably able to comprehend reversible passives (e.g., "The dog *was chased by* the squirrel"), conditionals (e.g., "*If* a bird didn't have wings, it couldn't fly"), and negatives (e.g., "The square is *not* blue"). Their spoken language was grammatically correct and included complex structures, such as embedded clauses (e.g., "The horse *that is in the field* is tired," "The boy *who has red hair* plays the drums"). The participants with Williams syndrome were able to form tag questions (e.g., "He is tall, *isn't he*?," "She can't eat peanuts, *can she*?") which requires mastery of question formation rules, the verb auxiliary system (e.g., "*can* eat," "*is* tall"), pronouns, and negation. On all these measures, the Williams syndrome group performed dramatically better than the Down syndrome group. We have compared the performance of 9- and 10-year-olds with Williams syndrome and Down syndrome (Klein & Mervis, 1999) and replicated Bellugi and her colleagues' finding that on average, the spontaneous spoken language of individuals with Williams syndrome is more complex than that of CA- and IQ-matched individuals with Down syndrome. We also have found that children with Williams syndrome are significantly more advanced at marking tense (third person singular present, regular past tense, BE) than younger children with specific language impairment (SLI) matched for MLU (Mervis & Klein-Tasman, 2000; Rice, 1999).

Individuals with Down syndrome and individuals with SLI, however, are well known to have inordinate difficulty with morphosyntax (e.g., Chapman, 1997; Leonard, 1998; Rice & Wexler, 1996). Thus, excellent performance relative to these two contrast groups does not provide convincing evidence that the grammatical abilities of individuals with Williams syndrome exceed those that would be expected for overall cognitive level of functioning or MLU. To address this issue, comparisons to other contrast groups are necessary. Studies comparing the spontaneous expressive language abilities of children with Williams syndrome to those of CA- and IQ-matched children either with mental retardation of mixed etiology or mental retardation of unknown etiology have found that MLU and syntactic abilities are equivalent for the two groups, whether the children's native language was English or German (e.g., Gosch, Städing, & Pankau, 1994; Udwin & Yule, 1990). Volterra et al. (1996) compared the spontaneous expressive language of Italian children with Williams syndrome to younger MA-matched typically developing children and found that MLU and syntactic abilities were similar for the two groups. In the only study that has considered grammatical constructions as complex as those discussed by Bellugi and her colleagues, Zukowski (2001, in press) used an elicited production task to compare the performance of a group of older children and adolescents with Williams syndrome to an MA-matched typically developing control group on tasks measuring the ability to form noun–noun compounds, embedded relative clauses, and affirmative and negative questions. For example, in the task measuring ability to produce embedded relative clauses, the participant was shown a picture on a computer screen and then asked to describe what happened when the picture changed, in such a manner that another person who did not observe the transformation could identify which object had changed. For instance, the initial picture might include two girls, one holding a cat and one chasing a different cat. When the picture changed, the latter girl might turn blue. The participant would then be asked, "Which girl turned blue?" The targeted response would be, "The girl who is chasing the cat turned blue." Consistent with Bellugi et al.'s findings, most of the participants with Williams syndrome in Zukowski's study were able to produce these constructions at least once. However, overall level of performance was similar to or somewhat weaker than that of the MA control group, suggesting that the ability to produce these grammatical constructions was what would be expected given the overall cognitive level of the participants with Williams syndrome.

A particularly extensive study of the relation between cognitive level, MLU, and grammatical ability was conducted in our laboratory (Klein, 1995; Mervis & Klein-Tasman, 2000; Mervis et al., 1999). This study included 39 children with Williams syndrome ranging in age from 2 years 6 months through 12 years, with a mean age of 7 years. All of the children produced multiword utterances. Children participated in a 30-min videotaped play session with a researcher. Analyses of the transcripts yielded a mean MLU of 3.18 morphemes ($SD = 0.73$), with a range from 1.52 to 4.82. This mean is less than that reported by Scarborough (1990) for typically developing children aged 3 years 6 months—children on average more than 3 years younger than the participants with Williams syndrome. Transcripts also were coded using the Index of Productive Syntax (IPSyn; Scarborough, 1990). The IPSyn measures the emergence of a variety of syntactic and morphological constructions. IPSyn scores ranged from 20 to 98 (out of 112 possible) with a mean of 71.77. This mean is again lower than that for Scarborough's sample of typically developing children aged 3 years 6 months, indicating a substantial delay in grammatical development. Encouragingly, however, the relation between MLU and IPSyn for the

Williams syndrome sample was virtually identical to that for Scarborough's typically developing sample, indicating that the grammatical complexity of the children with Williams syndrome was at the level expected for the length of their utterances. Further analyses taking into account the performance of the children with Williams syndrome on the DAS and the PPVT-R indicated that grammatical ability was consistent with overall cognitive ability but less advanced than expected for level of verbal short-term memory ability or receptive vocabulary ability.

The morphological abilities of this sample of children with Williams syndrome have also been compared to those of a sample of 3-year-old typically developing children matched for MLU (Morris & Mervis, 1999; Rice, 1999). Use of noun plurals, determiners, and verb aspect and tense was highly similar for the two groups, indicating that the morphological abilities of the children with Williams syndrome were at the level expected for the length of their utterances. Interestingly, the children with Williams syndrome had significantly larger receptive vocabularies (as measured by the PPVT-R) than the younger typically developing children, indicating that for the Williams syndrome sample, both utterance length and grammatical complexity were lower than expected for receptive vocabulary size.

Because the English language has relatively little morphology and the morphology that does occur is not very complex compared to the morphology of many other languages, it is important that conclusions about the morphological abilities of individuals with Williams syndrome not be based only on studies of English-speaking children. A few studies of individuals with Williams syndrome acquiring languages with more complex morphology have been conducted. The results of these studies suggest that at least some aspects of morphology may be extremely difficult for individuals with Williams syndrome, leading to performance below that expected for MA. Karmiloff-Smith et al. (1997) found that French-speaking adolescents with Williams syndrome performed considerably worse than typically developing 5-year-olds on measures of use of grammatical gender. Similarly, Volterra et al. (1996) reported that Italian children with Williams syndrome made many more grammatical gender errors than did the younger typically developing control group. Levy and Hermon (2003) found that Hebrew-speaking adolescents with Williams syndrome performed significantly worse than typically developing MA controls on measures of noun derivation and noun inflection and at MA level for verb root extraction and verb morpho-phonological alterations. Profile analyses indicated that overall, morphological ability of Hebrew-speaking adolescents was at or below MA level.

In summary, the syntactic abilities of children with Williams syndrome are delayed relative to CA-matched typically developing children and relative to both receptive vocabulary ability and verbal short-term memory ability. Syntactic abilities of children with Williams syndrome are advanced relative to matched children with Down syndrome or SLI but consistent with those of matched children with mixed etiologies of mental retardation and with expectations based on MLU. The morphological abilities of children with Williams syndrome who are learning English are at the expected level for MLU. However, children with Williams syndrome who are learning languages with more complex morphology often have weaker morphological abilities than would be expected for MA level.

B. Relations between Memory Ability and Grammatical Ability

The results of the study we just described suggested that verbal short-term memory ability (in this case, 2-item per second forward digit span as measured by the DAS) is more advanced than would be expected for syntactic ability. More generally, our research, as well as research performed in other laboratories, provides evidence that verbal short-term memory is a particular strength of individuals with Williams syndrome. For example, we (Mervis et al., 1999) found that in a sample of 104 individuals with Williams syndrome, 73% scored in the normal range on the digit-span subtest of the DAS. Similarly, individuals with Williams syndrome are proficient at repeating nonwords (Grant et al., 1997), performing at about the level expected for their MA. The ability to repeat nonwords is considered to be a better measure of verbal short-term memory than digit span because it is not confounded by how familiar an individual is with numbers (Gathercole & Baddeley, 1989). Working memory also seems to be a strength of individuals with Williams syndrome. Almost 90% of a sample of 86 individuals we tested score within the normal range on a backward-digit span task (Mervis et al., 1999). Backward-digit span requires the manipulation (i.e., reversal) of stored memory items and is therefore assumed to require processing as well as storage. This is significant because it has been suggested that the ability to manipulate verbal items in memory is related to the comprehension of complex syntax in adults and elderly individuals with normal intelligence (Kemper, Kynette, Rash, & O'Brien, 1989).

The role of short-term or working memory in the acquisition of language by children with Williams syndrome may be relatively superficial, or it may involve important general learning mechanisms. At a superficial level, the "cocktail" speech or the perception of seemingly fluent and complex language spoken by individuals with Williams syndrome may be attributed, at least in part, to excellent verbal memory. Gosch et al. (1994) and Udwin and Yule (1990) reported that individuals with Williams syndrome used an excessive number of unanalyzed stereotypical phrases and sentences. It is therefore possible that at first blush, the speech of individuals with Williams syndrome appears intact due to the rote memorization of phrases rather than the productive application of grammatical rules. The phonological memory ability of these individuals may be a factor that masks underlying weaknesses in grammatical ability that appear under standardized testing conditions (Klein & Mervis, 1999; Thal, Bates, & Bellugi, 1989).

It is also likely, however, that there is a more substantive relation between the verbal memory abilities and language skills of individuals with Williams syndrome. In typically developing populations verbal working memory is associated with the acquisition of both vocabulary (Gathercole & Baddeley, 1989, 1993) and syntax (Kemper et al., 1989; Norman, Kemper, & Kynette 1992). Similarly, the nonword repetition task has been proposed as a phenotypic marker for SLI (Bishop, North, & Dolan, 1996). These and other studies suggest that verbal working memory plays an active role in the acquisition and learning of words and grammatical structures in a number of diverse populations. We would therefore expect to find similar relations between language and working memory in individuals with Williams syndrome. Indeed, given the cognitive profile of Williams syndrome—good verbal working memory despite relatively weak reasoning skills and nonverbal abilities (especially in the area of visuospatial construction)—we hypothesized that verbal working memory may play a *more important* role in the language acquisition of these children than in language acquisition by typically developing children.

In order to examine the relations between verbal short-term memory, working memory, and language ability, we compared the receptive grammatical abilities of children with Williams syndrome to those of a matched group of typically developing children (Robinson, Mervis, & Robinson, 2003). The 39 children with Williams syndrome ranged in CA from 4.5 to 16.7 years ($M = 10.24$; $SD = 3.70$). This group was matched to a sample of 32 typically developing children based on performance on the TROG (Bishop, 1989). Given delays in the language acquisition of the children with Williams syndrome, the typically developing children were younger (range = 4.08–10.26 years; $M = 6.01$; $SD = 1.56$); importantly, both groups were able to comprehend the same kinds of grammatical constructions. In addition to the TROG we administered a memory battery including 1-item per second forward-digit span, backward-digit span, and a nonword repetition task of 48 nonwords developed by Montgomery (1996).

As expected, the correlations between the memory measures and the raw scores on the TROG (i.e., number of blocks passed) were significant for the children with Williams syndrome. Forward-digit span, nonword repetition, and backward-digit span shared partial correlations (controlling for CA) of 0.33, 0.48, and 0.52 with TROG respectively. Taken together, the memory variables accounted for 26% of the variance in the Williams syndrome TROG raw scores above and beyond CA. However, regression analysis indicated that forward-digit span alone did not uniquely contribute to variance in the scores once CA, nonword repetition, and backward-digit span were taken into account. Nonword repetition, on the other hand, did account for additional unique variance even after CA and the other memory measures were controlled. Thus, it appears that phonological memory may account, in part, for the grammatical skills of children with Williams syndrome. This finding fits with those of Grant et al. (1997), who reported that nonword repetition scores were significantly related to receptive vocabulary. We would therefore expect that the ability to encode and store small speech units, such as bound morphemes and function words, would similarly be related to grammatical ability.

The measure of verbal *working* memory (backward-digit span), however, accounted for the largest proportion of variance in TROG scores. Even after controlling for CA, forward-digit span, and nonword repetition, backward-digit span accounted for an additional 10% of variance. Thus, the ability to manipulate verbal items, not just store them, seems to be important to grammatical ability. Moreover, given that TROG items cannot be answered correctly by simply remembering previously heard sentences, it is likely that the memory ability of children with Williams syndrome plays a role in the acquisition of productive grammatical structures and not just the complexity of their speech.

Permutation tests indicated that, after controlling for CA, there were no significant differences between the Williams syndrome group and the typically developing group in the strength of relation between either forward-digit span and TROG raw scores or nonword repetition and TROG raw scores. The Williams syndrome group, however, showed a significantly stronger relation between the working memory measure and receptive grammar than did the typically developing group. Therefore, it is possible that the children with Williams syndrome may have to rely more heavily than typically developing children on verbal working memory abilities in order to puzzle out complex grammatical structures. Comprehending phrases, and, presumably, learning grammatical constructions, requires more than the storage of linguistic items in short-term memory. A child must extract the meaning of a phrase from the context of the utterance and then associate it with the linguistic item that is stored in short-term memory. The interpretation of nonlinguistic cues to meaning would involve perceptual, social, and cognitive analysis. For a typically developing child much of the process of extracting meaning from context would be effortless, and not limited by working memory capacity. For a child with deficits in one or more of the domains necessary to the processing and integration of the nonlinguistic cues, however, more effort and time would be required for the meaning extraction and therefore working memory capacity might be a much more important factor to the language learning process.

Thus, like children from other populations, children with Williams syndrome rely on verbal memory to learn language, including grammar. Additionally, however, it appears that, when learning language the children with Williams syndrome marshal a basic cognitive strength in the form of verbal working memory to overcome the difficulties posed by relative weaknesses in nonverbal ability and complex reasoning.

C. Verbal and Memory Abilities of Children with Williams Syndrome in Comparison to Children with Down Syndrome

Further support for our argument that memory ability plays an important role in grammatical ability for children with Williams syndrome comes from another study conducted in our laboratory comparing children with Williams syndrome to children with Down syndrome (Klein & Mervis, 1999). In contrast to the profile for Williams syndrome, verbal memory is a distinct weakness for individuals with Down syndrome. Bilovsky and Share (1965) found that children with Down syndrome performed relatively poorly on expressive grammar and verbal short-term memory as measured by the Illinois Test of Psycholinguistic Ability (ITPA; Kirk, McCarthy, & Kirk, 1961). Rohr and Burr (1978) reported that the verbal-verbal abilities of children with Down syndrome were significantly weaker than those of two contrast groups of children with mental retardation (children with mental retardation due to environmental circumstances and children with mental retardation of unknown etiology) matched for CA and general cognitive level. The results of several studies of digit span ability have indicated that children and adults with Down syndrome have significantly shorter digit spans than individuals matched for level of general cognitive ability (e.g., Jarrold & Baddeley, 1997).

Klein and Mervis (1999) compared the performance of 23 nine- and 10-year-olds with Williams syndrome and 25 nine- and 10-year-olds with Down syndrome on the McCarthy Scales of Children's Abilities (McCarthy, 1972). The overall level of cognitive performance was significantly higher for the Williams syndrome group, indicating that when matched for CA, children with Williams syndrome on average perform at a higher cognitive level than children with Down syndrome. The Williams syndrome group also performed significantly better than the Down syndrome group on the PPVT-R, indicating that when matched for CA but not cognitive level, children with Williams syndrome have significantly larger receptive vocabularies than children with Down syndrome. Furthermore, as expected based on previous research, the Williams syndrome group had significantly better verbal memory than the Down syndrome group.

From the original samples, Klein and Mervis were able to individually match 13 children with Williams syndrome to 13 children with Down syndrome for both CA and raw score on the McCarthy. Analysis of performance of the matched samples on the subtests of the McCarthy indicated that, as expected, the Down syndrome group performed significantly better than the Williams syndrome group on subtests measuring visuospatial construction: *Block Building*, *Draw-a-Child*, and *Draw-a-Design*. The Williams syndrome and Down syndrome groups performed virtually identically on the subtests that measured verbal ability but not memory ability: *Word Knowledge*, *Verbal Fluency*, and *Opposite Analogies*. However, there were large differences in favor of the Williams syndrome group on the subtests that measured verbal memory ability: *Numerical Memory* (forward and backward digit span) and *Verbal Memory* (memory for lists of words and for sentences). Consistent with these differences in verbal memory ability, there were large differences between the groups in the proportion of children who typically spoke in complete, grammatical sentences. Nine of the 13 children with Williams syndrome did so; in contrast, despite being closely matched on CA and overall level of cognitive ability, only 4 of the 13 children with Down syndrome typically spoke in complete grammatical sentences. Thus, despite being matched for level of overall cognitive ability and showing virtually identical verbal conceptual ability as measured by the verbal nonmemory subtests of the McCarthy, the Williams syndrome and Down syndrome groups clearly differed on productive grammatical ability. Comparisons of the original samples of children revealed an even larger difference: 19 of the 23 children with Williams syndrome but only 4 of the 25 children with Down syndrome typically spoke in complete grammatical sentences.

Klein and Mervis (1999) also compared the performance of the matched children with Williams syndrome and Down syndrome on the PPVT-R. Results indicated equivalent performance by the two groups of children. This finding that the Down syndrome group performed similarly to the Williams syndrome group on the PPVT-R despite significantly poorer performance on measures of verbal memory ability is consistent with Chapman, Schwartz, and Bird's (1991) finding that, at least by adolescence, receptive vocabulary as measured by the PPVT-R is a relative strength for individuals with Down syndrome. As indicated earlier in this chapter, concrete receptive vocabulary also is a relative strength for individuals with Williams syndrome.

VI. SUMMARY AND CONCLUSION

In 1990, when the research program described in this paper was begun, the prevailing view was that Williams syndrome provided a paradigmatic example of the independence of language from cognition. In particular, Williams syndrome was argued to provide strong evidence that excellent language abilities could exist side-by-side with severe mental retardation (e.g., Bellugi et al., 1988, 1990, 1992). Jackendoff (1994, p. 117) stated that despite significant mental retardation, the language of individuals with Williams syndrome "is if anything more fluent and advanced than that of their age-mates." The research we have conducted presents a more nuanced picture. The language abilities of individuals with Williams syndrome are indeed a relative strength. Both vocabulary (e.g., as measured by the DAS Verbal Cluster, the Mullen Verbal subtests, the PPVT-III, and the CDI) and grammar (e.g., as measured by the TROG, MLU, IPSyn, and the CDI) are considerably more advanced than would be expected for level of nonverbal cognition as measured by tests of visuospatial construction (e.g., DAS Spatial Cluster or the Mullen Fine Motor subtest). Furthermore, both receptive vocabulary and finite verb morphology are more advanced than for children with SLI matched for MLU, and both MLU and grammatical ability are more advanced than for children with Down syndrome matched for CA and MA. These findings are consistent with Bellugi et al.'s (1988, 1990, 1992, 1994) position.

However, individuals with Williams syndrome who have language abilities at the level expected for their CA are rare. No study has ever found equivalent levels of linguistic performance for individuals with Williams syndrome and CA-matched individuals with normal intelligence. Mean levels of performance by individuals with Williams syndrome on a variety of standardized assessments of language are consistently in the borderline to mild deficit range. Grammatical ability as measured by spontaneous language (MLU, IPSyn, noun and verb morphology) is below that of typically developing peers matched for CA. Instead, for individuals acquiring English as a native language, grammatical ability is at the same level as that of younger typically developing children matched for general level of cognitive ability. For individuals with Williams syndrome acquiring native languages with more complex morphology, some aspects of morphological ability are typically below the level expected for general level of cognitive ability (e.g., for French, Karmiloff-Smith et al., 1997; for Hebrew, Levy & Hermon, 2003). Language abilities are only slightly more advanced than nonverbal reasoning abilities (e.g., as measured by the DAS Nonverbal Reasoning Cluster, the K-BIT Matrices subtest, or the Mullen Visual Reception subtest). Nonconcrete language ability is considerably weaker than concrete language ability. For example, abstract relational vocabulary ability, as measured by the TRC, is considerably below the level expected for concrete vocabulary ability. Comprehension of figurative language is considerably below the level expected for both concrete vocabulary ability and receptive grammatical ability. Finally, not only are language abilities less impressive than previously claimed, IQ is considerably higher than expected based on initial reports. Mean IQ for individuals with Williams syndrome is in the range of mild mental retardation, not the severe-to-profound mental retardation range reported in Bates' (1990) presentation of Bellugi's research. Therefore, the language abilities of individuals with Williams syndrome are much more in line with what would be expected given their IQ.

In many important ways, acquisition of language by individuals with Williams syndrome is best characterized as normal but delayed. For example, although both the onset of vocabulary acquisition and the onset of grammatical acquisition are delayed, the relation between expressive vocabulary size and grammatical complexity is the same as for the general population. Grammatical ability is at the level expected for overall level of cognitive ability. Many of the specific links between particular linguistic abilities and theoretically linked cognitive abilities that hold for typically developing children and children with Down syndrome also are shown by children with Williams syndrome. For example, canonical babble, a critical step in the beginning of language acquisition, begins at the same time as rhythmic hand banging, the same pattern as found for typically developing children and children with Down syndrome. The early object labels of children with Williams syndrome name the same child-basic level categories as for typically developing children and children with Down syndrome. Basic level categories and category names are acquired before subordinate or superordinate level categories and category names. The onsets of spontaneous exhaustive sorting and the ability to fast map new words whose referents were not explicitly identified by the speaker occur at about the same time, the same pattern as for typically developing children and children with Down syndrome.

At the same time, several putative links between specific aspects of language development and particular aspects of cognitive development that are evidenced by both typically developing children and children with Down syndrome do not hold for children with Williams syndrome. In particular, unlike typically developing children, children with Down syndrome and children with severe mental retardation of a variety of etiologies, children with Williams syndrome do not comprehend and produce referential pointing gestures prior to beginning to produce referential language. Onset of referential language typically precedes onset of comprehension and production of pointing gestures by 6 months or more. Despite the delay in pointing, parents of children with Williams syndrome are able to establish joint attention by other communicative methods such as labeling the object that is already the focus of the child's attention or tapping the object on which the speaker wishes the child to focus. Such interactions allow children with Williams syndrome to begin to acquire language without the ability to comprehend or produce referential pointing gestures.

The finding that the onset of referential language usually precedes the onset of comprehension and production of pointing gestures has important implications for language intervention. The onset of referential communicative gestures often is used as an indicator that children are ready to acquire language; at this point, speech therapy and/or developmental therapy is likely to begin to focus on vocabulary acquisition. Similarly, if children do not come to the attention of intervention agencies until after acquisition of a basic vocabulary, it is assumed that these children have already mastered the referential gesture system. Both of these assumptions are incorrect for children with Williams syndrome. Children with Williams syndrome are ready for language intervention focused on vocabulary acquisition long before they begin to produce referential communicative gestures. And many young children with Williams syndrome who have 200 or more words in their productive vocabularies still have difficulty both comprehending and producing referential communicative gestures and would benefit from therapy directed at improving their nonverbal communicative abilities.

Another set of specific links that holds for typically developing children and children with Down syndrome, but not for children with Williams syndrome, involves the onset of the vocabulary spurt. For children with Williams syndrome, the onset of the vocabulary spurt precedes the onsets of both spontaneous exhaustive sorting and fast mapping, typically by 6 months or more. These three abilities, which have previously been claimed to be linked to the related conceptual realizations that all objects belong to a category and that all objects have basic-level names, are evidenced at about the same time for both typically developing children and children with Down syndrome. We have argued that the onset of the vocabulary spurt may well not indicate the realization that all objects have names. Instead, the vocabulary spurt may simply reflect increasing efficiency in applying vocabulary acquisition strategies that the child already had. Given that individuals with Williams syndrome evidence a relative strength in verbal short-term memory, and that 4-year-olds with Williams syndrome who evidence logistic vocabulary growth have considerably stronger verbal short-term memory abilities than those with slow linear vocabulary growth, it is quite possible that increases in verbal memory ability facilitate the vocabulary spurt for children with Williams syndrome. Grant et al. (1997) also have shown that phonological memory is strongly related to receptive vocabulary for older children with Williams syndrome.

Strong verbal memory abilities, however, while effective at enhancing concrete vocabulary acquisition, are not nearly as helpful for facilitating acquisition of more abstract vocabulary. Thus, although there is a strong correlation between concrete vocabulary size and abstract vocabulary size, the abstract relational vocabularies of children with Williams syndrome are considerably smaller than expected given their concrete vocabulary size. Similarly, adolescents' and adults' understanding of figurative language, although highly correlated with their understanding of concrete language using the same grammatical constructions, is much more limited. The end result is that for individuals with Williams syndrome, the acquisition of abstract language is substantially more delayed than acquisition of concrete language ability, with large discrepancies remaining even in adulthood. Most children with Williams syndrome, even if their receptive concrete vocabulary is at CA level, would benefit from speech or cognitive therapy focused on relational language and, at older ages, on figurative language. In both cases, it is important that the therapy be designed to ensure that the individual is able to generalize the language that has been taught to novel settings outside of the therapeutic context. Anecdotal reports suggest that music therapy is helpful for acquisition of relational language, especially if the therapy is structured to facilitate generalization from the original context to a wide variety of additional contexts.

The relation between vocabulary size and verbal short-term memory ability is not the only link between memory ability and language ability evidenced by individuals with Williams syndrome. At 4 years of age, the ability to produce multiword utterances also is strongly related to verbal short-term memory ability. For older children and adolescents, verbal short-term memory, phonological memory, and verbal working memory are all related to grammatical ability. This pattern of relations between memory abilities and grammatical ability also is shown by typically developing children. However, the strength of the relation between verbal working memory and grammatical ability is significantly greater for children with Williams syndrome than for typically developing children matched for receptive grammatical level. This finding suggests that individuals with Williams syndrome may need to depend more than typically developing individuals on verbal working memory to figure out complex grammatical structures. In particular, typically developing children may rely on more advanced conceptual abilities to learn grammar that place fewer demands on verbal working memory, whereas children with Williams syndrome, who are not able to apply some of these strategies, place a higher demand on verbal working memory to acquire the same grammatical constructions.

In conclusion, language ability is a relative strength for individuals with Williams syndrome. In many important ways, the acquisition of language by these individuals proceeds in the same manner as for individuals in the general population. There is increasing evidence, however, that verbal memory—usually the strongest ability of individuals with Williams syndrome—is more important for the acquisition of language by these individuals than for their typically developing peers. The importance of verbal short-term memory to the acquisition of vocabulary by children with Williams syndrome and the importance of verbal working memory to their grammatical development highlight basic differences between how children with Williams syndrome and typically developing children acquire language. It is an open question as to whether these differences are a matter of extremes, or if children with Williams syndrome acquire language using significantly different mechanisms from typically developing children.

ACKNOWLEDGMENTS

This research was supported by Grant No. HD29957 from the National Institute of Child Health and Human Development and by Grant No. NS35102 from the National Institute of Neurological Disorders and Stroke. We thank all of the participants and their families. We are grateful to the geneticists, cardiologists, and early intervention agencies who referred individuals with Williams syndrome to our research, as well as to Terry Monkaba, executive director of the National Williams Syndrome Association, who has encouraged and facilitated the conduct of research at regional and national meetings of the Williams Syndrome Association. Portions of this chapter are based on Mervis & Bertrand (1997), Mervis & Klein-Tasman (2000) and Mervis et al. (1999).

REFERENCES

Adamson, L. B. (1995). *Communication development during infancy*. Madison, WI: Brown & Benchmark.

Bates, E. (1990, April). Early language development: *How things come together and how they come apart*. International Conference on Infant Studies, Montreal, Quebec.

Bates, E., & Carnevale, G. F. (1993). New directions in research on language development. *Developmental Review*, *13*, 446–470.

Bates, E., & Goodman, J. C. (1997). On the inseparability of grammar and the lexicon: evidence from acquisition, aphasia and real-time processing. *Language and Cognitive Processes*, *12*, 507–586.

Becerra, A. M., Thomas, M. L., Robinson, B. F., & Mervis, C. B. (2002, July). *Patterns of early language acquisition of children with Williams syndrome*. International Association for the Study of Child Language/Society for Research on Child Language Disorders, Madison, WI.

Bellugi, U., Bihrle, A., Jernigan, T., Trauner, D., & Doherty, S. (1990). Neuropsychological and neuroanatomical profile of Williams syndrome. *American Journal of Medical Genetics*, *6*, 115–125.

Bellugi, U., Bihrle, A., Neville, H., & Doherty, S. (1992). Language, cognition, and brain organization in a neurodevelopmental disorder. In M. Gunnar, & C. Nelson (Eds.), *Developmental behavioral neuroscience: The Minnesota symposium* (pp. 201–232). Hillsdale, NJ: Lawrence Erlbaum Associates.

Bellugi, U., Klima, E. S., & Wang, P. P. (1996). Cognitive and neural development: clues from genetically based syndromes. In D. Magnusson (Ed.), *The lifespan development of individuals: behavioral, neurobiological, and psychosocial perspectives* (pp. 223–243). Cambridge, UK: Cambridge University Press.

Bellugi, U., Lichtenberger, L., Jones, W., Lai, Z., & St. George, M. (2000). The neurocognitive profile of Williams syndrome: a complex pattern of strengths and weaknesses. *Journal of Cognitive Neuroscience*, *12*(Supplement 1), 7–29.

Bellugi, U., Marks, S., Bihrle, A., & Sabo, H. (1988). Dissociation between language and cognitive functions in Williams syndrome. In D. Bishop, & K. Mogford (Eds.), *Language development in exceptional circumstances* (pp. 177–189). London: Churchill Livingstone.

Bellugi, U., Wang, P., & Jernigan, T. L. (1994). Williams syndrome: an unusual neuropsychological profile. In S. H. Broman, & J. Grafman (Eds.), *Atypical cognitive deficits in developmental disorders: Implications for brain function* (pp. 23–56). Hillsdale, NJ: Erlbaum.

Bertrand, J., Mervis, C. B., Armstrong, S. C., & Ayres, J. (1995). Figurative language and cognitive abilities of adults with Williams syndrome. *Genetic Counseling*, *6*, 135–137.

Bilovsky, D., & Share, J. (1965). The ITPA and Down's syndrome: an exploratory study. *American Journal of Mental Deficiency*, *70*, 78–82.

Bishop, D. V. M. (1989). *Test for the reception of grammar* (2nd ed.). Manchester, UK: Chapel Press.

Bishop, D. V. M., North, T., & Dolan, C. (1996). Nonword repetition as a behavioural marker for inherited language impairment: evidence from a twin study. *Journal of Child Psychology and Psychiatry*, *37*, 391–403.

Carroll, J. B., Davies, P., & Richman, B. (1971). *Word frequency book*. New York: American Heritage.

Chapman, R. (1997). Language development in children and adolescents with Down syndrome. *Mental Retardation & Developmental Disabilities Research Reviews*, *3*, 307–312.

Chapman, R., Schwartz, S., & Bird, E. K. (1991). Language skills of children and adolescents with Down syndrome: I. Comprehension. *Journal of Speech and Hearing Research*, *34*, 1106–1120.

Cobo-Lewis, A. B., Oller, D. K., Lynch, M. P., & Levine, S. L. (1995, March). *Relationships among motor and vocal milestones in normally developing infants and infants with Down syndrome*. Gatlinburg Conference on Research and Theory in Mental Retardation and Developmental Disabilities, Gatlinburg, TN.

Dunham, P. J., Dunham, F., & Curwin, A. (1993). Joint-attentional states and lexical acquisition at 18 months. *Developmental Psychology*, *29*, 827–831.

Dunn, L. M., & Dunn, L. M. (1981). *Peabody picture vocabulary test—revised*. Circle Pines, MN: American Guidance Service.

Dunn, L. M., & Dunn, L. M. (1997). *Peabody picture vocabulary test* (3rd ed.). Circle Pines, MN: American Guidance Service.

Edmonston, N. K., & Litchfield Thane, N. (1988). *TRC: Test of relational concepts*. Austin, TX: PRO-ED.

Elliott, C. D. (1990). *Differential ability scales*. San Antonio, TX: Psychological Corporation.

Ewart, A. K., Morris, C. A., Atkinson, D., Jin, W., Sternes, K., Spallone, P., Stock, A. D., Leppert, M., & Keating, M. T. (1993). Hemizygosity at the elastin locus in a developmental disorder, Williams syndrome. *Nature Genetics*, *5*, 11–16.

Fenson, L., Dale, P. S., Reznick, J. S., Bates, E., Thal, D., & Pethick, S. (1994). Variability in early communicative development. *Monographs of the Society for Research in Child Development*, *59*, Serial no. 242.

Fenson, L., Dale, P. S., Reznick, J. S., Thal, D., Bates, E., Hartung, J. P., Pethick, S., & Reilly, J. S. (1993). *MacArthur communicative development inventories: User's guide and technical manual*. San Diego, CA: Singular.

Finegan, J.-A., Smith, M. L., Meschino, W. S., Vallance, P. L., & Sitarenios, G. (1995, March). *Verbal memory in children with Williams syndrome*. Society for Research in Child Development, Indianapolis, IN.

Gathercole, S. E., & Baddeley, A. D. (1989). Evaluation of the role of phonological STM in the development of vocabulary in children: a longitudinal study. *Journal of Memory and Language*, *28*, 200–213.

Gathercole, S. E., & Baddeley, A. D. (1993). *Working memory and language*. Hillsdale, NJ: Erlbaum.

Ginsburg, H., & Opper, S. (1979). *Piaget's theory of intellectual development* (2nd ed.). Englewood Cliffs, NJ: Prentice Hall.

Golinkoff, R. M., Mervis, C. B., & Hirsh-Pasek, K. (1994). Early object labels: the case for a developmental lexical principles framework. *Journal of Child Language*, *21*, 125–155.

Gopnik, A., & Meltzoff, A. N. (1987). The development of categorization in the second year and its relation to other cognitive and linguistic developments. *Child Development*, *58*, 1523–1531.

Gopnik, A., & Meltzoff, A. N. (1992). Categorization and naming: basic level sorting in eighteen-month-olds and its relation to language. *Child Development*, *63*, 1091–1103.

Gosch, A., Städing, G., & Pankau, R. (1994). Linguistic abilities in children with Williams-Beuren syndrome. *American Journal of Medical Genetics*, *52*, 291–296.

Grant, J., Karmiloff-Smith, A., Gathercole, S. A., Paterson, S., Howlin, P., Davies, M., & Udwin, O. (1997). Phonological short-term memory and its relationship to language in Williams syndrome. *Cognitive Neuropsychiatry*, *2*, 81–99.

Jackendoff, R. (1994). *Patterns in the mind: Language and human nature*. New York: Basic.

Jarrold, C., & Baddeley, A. D. (1997). Short-term memory for verbal and visuospatial information in Down's syndrome. *Cognitive Neuropsychiatry*, *2*, 101–122.

Karmiloff-Smith, A., Grant, J., Berthoud, I., Davies, M., Howlin, P., & Udwin, O. (1997). Language and Williams syndrome: How intact is "intact." *Child Development*, *68*, 274–290.

Karmiloff-Smith, A., Klima, E., Bellugi, U., Grant, J., & Baron-Cohen, S. (1995). Is there a social module? Language face processing and theory of mind in individuals with Williams syndrome. *Journal of Cognitive Neuroscience*, *7*, 196–208.

Kaufman, A. S., & Kaufman, N. L. (1990). *Kaufman brief intelligence test*. Pines, MN: American Guidance Services.

Kemper, S., Kynette, D., Rash, S., & O'Brien, K. (1989). Life span changes to adults' language: effects of memory and genre. *Applied Psycholinguistics*, *10*, 49–66.

Kempler, D., & Van Lacker, D. (1985). *Familiar phrases and novel language comprehension test.* Unpublished: copyright.

Kirk, S. A., McCarthy, J. J., & Kirk, W. D. (1961). *Illinois test of psycholinguistic abilites.* Urbana: University of Illinois Press.

Klein, B. P. (1995). *Grammatical abilities of children with Williams syndrome.* Unpublished master's thesis, Emory University.

Klein, B. P., & Mervis, C. B. (1999). Cognitive strengths and weaknesses of 9- and 10-year-olds with Williams syndrome or Down syndrome. *Developmental Neuropsychology, 16,* 177–196.

Leonard, L. B. (1998). *Children with specific language impairment.* Cambridge, MA: MIT Press.

Levy, Y., & Hermon, S. (2003). Morphological abilities of Hebrew-speaking adolescents. *Developmental Neuropsychology, 23,* 61–85 (special issue on Williams syndrome).

Masataka, N. (2001). Why early linguistic milestones are delayed in children with Williams syndrome: late onset of hand banging as a possible rate-limiting constraint on the emergence of canonical babbling. *Developmental Science, 4,* 158–164.

McCarthy, D. (1972). *McCarthy scales of children's abilities.* New York: Psychological Corporation.

Mervis, C. B. (1987). Child-basic object categories and early lexical development. In U. Neisser (Ed.), *Concepts and conceptual development: Ecological and intellectual factors in categorization* (pp. 201–233). Cambridge: Cambridge University Press.

Mervis, C. B. (1999). The Williams syndrome cognitive profile: strengths, weaknesses, and interrelations among auditory short-term memory, language, and visuospatial constructive cognition. In E. Winograd, R. Fivush, & W. Hirst (Eds.), *Ecological approaches to cognition: Essays in honor of Ulric Neisser* (pp. 193–227). Mahwah, NJ: Erlbaum.

Mervis, C. B. (2002, July). *Language and cognitive development in Williams syndrome.* International Association for the Study of Child Language/Society for Research on Child Language Disorders, Madison, WI.

Mervis, C. B., & Bertrand, J. (1993). Acquisition of early object labels: The roles of operating principles and input. In A. P. Kaiser, & D. B. Gray (Eds.), *Enhancing children's communication: Research foundations for intervention* (pp. 281–316). Baltimore: Brookes.

Mervis, C. B., & Bertrand, J. (1994). Acquisition of the Novel Name–Nameless Category (N3C) principle. *Child Development, 65,* 1646–1662.

Mervis, C. B., & Bertrand, J. (1997). Developmental relations between cognition and language: evidence from Williams syndrome. In L. B. Adamson, & M. A. Romski (Eds.), *Communication and language acquisition: Discoveries from atypical development* (pp. 75–106). New York: Brookes.

Mervis, C. B., & Klein-Tasman, B. P. (2000). Williams syndrome: cognition, personality and adaptive behavior. *Mental Retardation and Developmental Disabilities Research Reviews, 6,* 148–158.

Mervis, C. B., Klein-Tasman, B. P., & Mastin, M. E. (2001). Adaptive behavior of 4- through 8-year-old children with Williams syndrome. *American Journal on Mental Retardation, 106,* 82–93 (special issue on Behavioral Phenotypes).

Mervis, C. B., Morris, C. A., Bertrand, J., & Robinson, B. F. (1999). Williams syndrome: findings from an integrated program of research. In H. Tager-Flusberg (Ed.), *Neurodevelopmental disorders* (pp. 65–110). Cambridge, MA: MIT Press.

Mervis, C. B., & Robinson, B. F. (2000). Expressive vocabulary of toddlers with Williams syndrome or Down syndrome: a comparison. *Developmental Neuropsychology, 17,* 111–126.

Mervis, C. B., Robinson, B. F., Bertrand, J., Morris, C. A., Klein-Tasman, B. P., & Armstrong, S. C. (2000). The Williams syndrome cognitive profile. *Brain and Cognition*, *44*, 604–628.

Montgomery, J. A. (1996). Examination of phonological working memory in specifically language-impaired children. *Applied Psycholinguistics*, *16*, 355–378.

Morris, C. A., & Mervis, C. B. (1999). Williams syndrome. In S. Goldstein, & C. Reynolds (Eds.), *Handbook of neurodevelopmental and genetic disorders in children* (pp. 555–590). New York: Guilford.

Morris, C. A., & Mervis, C. B. (2000). Williams syndrome and related disorders. *Annual Review of Genomics and Human Genetics*, *1*, 461–484.

Mullen, E. M. (1995). *Mullen scales of early learning*. Circle Pines, MN: American Guidance Service.

Norman, S., Kemper, S., & Kynette, D. (1992). Adult reading comprehension: effects of syntactic complexity and working memory. *Journals of Gerontology*, *47*, 258–265.

Osborne, L. R., Li, M., Pober, B., Chitayat, D., Bodurtha, J., Mandel, A., Costa, T., Grebe, T., Cox, S., Tsui, L. C., Scherer, S. W. (2001). A 1.5 million-base pair inversion polymorphism in families with Williams-Beuren syndrome. *Nature Genetics*, *29*, 321–325.

Rice, M. L. (1999). Specific grammatical limitations in children with specific language impairment. In H. Tager-Flusberg (Ed.), *Neurodevelopmental disorders* (pp. 331–359). Cambridge, MA: MIT Press.

Rice, M. L., & Wexler, K. (1996). A phenotype of specific language impairment: Extended optional infinitives. In M. L. Rice (Ed.), *Toward a genetics of language* (pp. 215–237). Mahwah, NJ: Erlbaum.

Robinson, B. F., & Mervis, C. B. (1999). Comparing productive vocabulary measures from the CDI and a systematic diary study. *Journal of Child Language*, *26*, 177–185.

Robinson, B. F., Mervis, C. B., & Robinson, B. W. (2003). Roles of verbal short-term memory and working memory in the acquisition of grammar by children with Williams syndrome. *Developmental Neuropsychology*, *23*, 13–31 (special issue on Williams syndrome).

Rohr, A., & Burr, D. B. (1978). Etiological differences in patterns of psycholinguistic development of children of IQ 30 to 60. *American Journal of Mental Deficiency*, *82*, 549–553.

Rosch, E. (1973). On the internal structure of perceptual and semantic categories. In T. E. Moore (Ed.), *Cognitive development and the acquisition of language* (pp. 111–144). New York: Academic Press.

Rosch, E. (1975). Cognitive representation of semantic categories. *Journal of Experimental Psychology: General*, *104*, 192–233.

Rosch, E., Mervis, C. B., Gray, W. D., Johnson, D. M., & Boyes-Braem, P. (1976). Basic objects in natural categories. *Cognitive Psychology*, *8*, 382–439.

Scarborough, H. S. (1990). Index of productive syntax. *Applied Psycholinguistics*, *11*, 1–22.

Scott, P., Mervis, C. B., Bertrand, J., Klein, B. P., Armstrong, S. C., & Ford, A. L. (1995). Semantic organization and word fluency in 9- and 10-year-old children with Williams syndrome. *Genetic Counseling*, *6*, 172–173.

Singer Harris, N. G., Bellugi, U., Bates, E., Jones, W., & Rossen, M. (1997). Contrasting profiles of language development in children with Williams and Down syndromes. *Developmental Neuropsychology*, *13*, 345–370.

Sparrow, S. S., Balla, D. A., & Cicchetti, D. V. (1984). *Vineland adaptive behavior scales-interview edition*. Circle Pines, MN: American Guidance Service.

Sullivan, K., Winner, E., & Tager-Flusberg, H. (2003). Can adolescents with Williams syndrome tell the difference between lies and jokes? *Developmental Neuropsychology*, *23*, 87–105 (special issue on Williams syndrome).

Thal, D., Bates, E., & Bellugi, U. (1989). Language and cognition in two children with Williams syndrome. *Journal of Speech and Hearing Research*, *32*, 489–500.

Tomasello, M., & Farrar, M. J. (1986). Joint attention and early language. *Child Development*, *57*, 1454–1463.

Udwin, O., & Yule, W. (1990). Expressive language of children with Williams syndrome. *American Journal of Medical Genetics Supplement*, *6*, 108–114.

Volterra, V., Capirci, O., Pezzini, G., Sabbadini, L., & Vicari, S. (1996). Linguistic abilities in Italian children with Williams syndrome. *Cortex*, *32*, 663–677.

Volterra, V., Caselli, M. C., Capirci, O., Tonucci, F., & Vicari, S. (2003). Early linguistic abilities of Italian children with Williams syndrome. *Developmental Neuropsychology*, *23*, 33–59 (special issue on Williams syndrome).

Wang, P. P., & Bellugi, U. (1993). Williams syndrome, Down syndrome, and cognitive neuroscience. *American Journal of Diseases of Children*, *147*, 1246–1251.

Whittle, M. B., Chang, F., Thomas, M. L., & Mervis, C. B. (2001, April). *Acquisition of concrete and relational vocabulary by children with Williams syndrome*. Society for Research on Child Development, Minneapolis, MN.

Williams, K. T. (1997). *Expressive vocabulary test*. Circle Pines, MN: American Guidance Service.

Zukowski, A. (2001). *Uncovering grammatical competence in children with Williams syndrome*. Unpublished doctoral dissertation, Boston University.

Zukowski, A. (in press). Investigating knowledge of complex syntax: Insights from experimental studies of Williams syndrome. In M. Rice, & S. Warren (Eds.), *Developmental language disorders: From phenotypes to etiologies*. Mahwah, NJ: Erlbaum.

Language and Communication in Fragile X Syndrome

MELISSA M. MURPHY and LEONARD ABBEDUTO

WAISMAN CENTER AND DEPARTMENT OF EDUCATIONAL PSYCHOLOGY, UNIVERSITY OF WISCONSIN-MADISON, MADISON, WISCONSIN

I. INTRODUCTION

Fragile X syndrome (FXS) is the leading inherited cause of mental retardation and is second only to Down syndrome as a genetic cause of mental retardation. FXS is an X-linked disorder, affecting approximately one in 4000 males and one in 8000 females (Hagerman, 1999). The syndrome results from an expansion of a trinucleotide sequence (CGG) in a gene (FMR1) located on the X chromosome at Xq27.3 (Brown, 2002). This expansion leads to methylation that, in turn, inhibits production of the protein that is typically produced by the gene (FMRP; Oostra, 1996). FMRP has been shown to play a role in neural development, affecting both the maturation of synapses and neuronal pruning (Greenough et al., 2001). There are a variety of physical and behavioral sequelae that are associated with the syndrome. Physical sequelae include large ears, prominent forehead, high-arched palate, and, for males, machroorchidism (Dykens, Hodapp, & Finucane, 2000; Hagerman, 1999). Behavioral sequelae include cognitive impairments, ranging from mental retardation in most males and roughly half of all females to mild learning disabilities or even normal IQs in many females (Mazzocco, 2000). Many individuals with FXS also have difficulty with attention or manifest autistic-like behaviors. In fact, it is not uncommon for individuals with FXS to receive a concurrent diagnosis of Attention Deficit-Hyperactivity Disorder (ADHD; Hagerman, 1999, 2002) and estimates indicate that 10–35% of individuals with FXS meet diagnostic criteria for autism (Feinstein & Reiss, 2001). Moreover, many individuals with FXS, even those with relatively mild cognitive and physical impairments, also display behaviors suggesting high levels of anxiety, or hyperarousal, particularly in social situations (Hagerman, 1999).

0074-7750/2003 $35.00

Physiological measures support this picture of high levels of arousal (Belser & Sudhalter, 1995; Hessl, 2002; Miller et al., 1999; Wisbeck et al., 2000). With regard to language learning and use, clinical observations and research have documented problems in many areas. These include difficulties with speech, such as problems in intelligibility, omission or distortion of certain consonant or vowel sounds, a variable rate of production; high rates of perseverative language; difficulties with topic maintenance, including the production of tangential utterances; and delays in syntax and semantics relative to age-matched typically developing peers (Abbeduto & Hagerman, 1997; Dykens et al., 2000; Sudhalter, Cohen, Silverman, & Wolf-Schein, 1990). The occurrence of these physical and behavioral sequelae is often assumed to be simply the result of the reduced levels of FMRP. It is important to note, however, that these sequelae are variable across individuals and ages, with many emerging, or becoming more pronounced, in adolescence and others attenuating with age (Dykens et al., 2000; Hagerman, 1999, 2002). Little is known about the factors that account for this variability, particularly variability with age, or about the ways in which the environment contributes to the emergence and variable expression of the FXS phenotype. The purpose of this chapter is to provide an overview of current research on language learning and use in FXS, as well as to highlight gaps in the research to date and propose an agenda for future behavioral research on FXS.

II. RESEARCH ON THE LANGUAGE CHARACTERISTICS ASSOCIATED WITH FRAGILE X SYNDROME

In studying language, it is useful to decompose language into several components, each of which involves knowledge of different types of linguistic elements, forms, or rules as well as different skills for acquiring and using that knowledge. It is important to recognize, however, that these components interact in the learning and real-time use of language (Abbeduto & Hesketh, 1997). In this chapter, we focus largely on knowledge and use of words (lexical development), rules for combining words into sentences (syntactic development), and using spoken language to communicate effectively with others (communication development). Where possible, we also distinguish between expression and reception within each component because there is considerable evidence that the two involve different, albeit overlapping, performance systems that pose different challenges to language learners (see, e.g., Chapman, this volume). To date, researchers have typically examined language ability separately for males and females. In keeping with this tradition, the following sections present the literature on males followed by the literature on females. In a third section, we consider the few studies that have included both males and females, which are critical for understanding the extent and nature of gender differences and achieving an integrated picture of language development in FXS.

A. Language Characteristics of Males with Fragile X Syndrome

1. LEXICAL DEVELOPMENT

Lexical learning (i.e., vocabulary acquisition) is a lifelong process that both depends on, and facilitates, achievements in other domains of language (e.g., syntax; Gleitman & Gillette, 1995) and cognition (e.g., working memory; Ellis Weismer, in press). Moreover, the sound–meaning mappings that constitute lexical knowledge are learned within the context of social interactions. As a result, acquiring meaning is dependent on the learner's ability to participate fully in social interactions and attend to the behavior and mental states of other people (Baldwin & Tomasello, 1998). The limitations that characterize males with FXS in the domains of cognition and social functioning suggest that lexical learning will be a serious challenge for them. It is surprising, therefore, how few studies have focused on lexical learning in these individuals. Moreover, the existing research has been designed only to characterize the extent of the delay rather than the processes by which words are learned (Abbeduto & Hagerman, 1997), despite the fact that many aspects of this process are well documented for typically developing children (Barrett, 1995; Clark, 1995).

The data that do exist indicate that males with FXS achieve well below chronological age expectations on receptive and expressive measures of lexical knowledge (Madison, George, & Moeschler, 1986; Paul et al., 1987; Sudhalter, Maranion, & Brooks, 1992). In contrast, the data are inconsistent as to whether achievements in the lexical domain keep pace with, exceed, or lag behind those in the nonlinguistic cognitive domain or those in other domains of language (e.g., syntax). Although inferential statistical tests were not conducted, Madison et al. (1986), for example, found that the adult males in the single family that they studied generally scored higher on standardized tests of vocabulary than on more general tests of cognitive ability. In contrast, Sudhalter et al. (1992) found that their male participants, who ranged in age from 6 to 41 years and had a mean Communication Age Equivalent on the Vineland Adaptive Behavior Scales (Sparrow, Balla, & Cicchetti, 1984) near 4 years, supplied more semantically incorrect words in a sentence-completion task than did a comparison group of typically developing 4-year-olds. Whether the Sudhalter et al. finding reflects a deficit in lexical knowledge or in sentence-level comprehension processes, however, cannot be determined from the task used. In a study that focused on institutionalized adult males, Paul et al. (1987) found that their participants did not differ in the scores they achieved on a standardized test of vocabulary from two other groups of age- and cognitive level-matched males: males with nonspecific mental retardation and males with autism. Without an appropriately matched typically developing comparison group, however, it is impossible to know whether the three groups in the Paul et al. study were at, above, or below mental age levels as regards their lexical achievements (Abbeduto et al., 2003). Differences in sample characteristics (e.g., age range of participants, history of institutionalization), measures, and methodological limitations (e.g., a failure to include appropriately matched comparison groups) make it difficult to reconcile these contradictory findings concerning lexical development.

Recently, we (Abbeduto et al., 2003) examined lexical comprehension in adolescents and young adults with FXS by administering the Test for Auditory Comprehension of Language—Revised (TACL-R; Carrow-Woolfolk, 1985). The TACL-R includes several subtests, one of which focuses largely on vocabulary (i.e., Word Classes and Relations). Two findings are relevant here. First, the participants with FXS, who included both males and females, did not differ in lexical knowledge, as reflected in their age-equivalent scores, from either of two nonverbal MA-matched comparison groups: adolescents and young adults with Down syndrome and typically developing children. Second, the participants with FXS, like the typically developing comparison children, achieved similar age-equivalent scores on the lexical and syntactically oriented subtests of the TACL-R. Importantly, this finding of a synchrony between lexical and syntactic development and between lexical and nonverbal cognitive development held for both males and females with FXS, despite the fact that males achieved lower scores overall than did females. Although these findings suggest that lexical development keeps pace with both syntactic development and cognitive development in males (and females) with FXS, it is important to be cautious in generalizing this finding to younger or older individuals than those we tested or to other aspects of lexical development not measured by the TACL-R. Indeed, we believe that one of the most glaring gaps in our knowledge of language learning and use by individuals with FXS is a lack of data, particularly longitudinal data, on the trajectory of development. This lack of data on age-related change is especially troubling in light of the fact that there is evidence that IQ declines with age beginning in late childhood or early adolescence (Fisch et al., 1996). Among other things, this decline in IQ may reflect a slowing of cognitive development, which is closely tied to lexical development (Abbeduto et al., 2003).

We also have little understanding of whether receptive and expressive vocabularies are delayed to a similar extent in males with FXS. Although Madison et al. (1986) and Sudhalter (2002) have reported finding higher scores on expressive than on receptive measures of vocabulary for males with FXS, Paul et al. (1987) found no differences between the scores for these domains in their sample of institutionalized adult males with FXS. Again, the varying results may reflect across-study differences in the types of words included in the measure (e.g., concrete vs abstract words), the way in which knowledge of these words was measured, or the ages of the participants studied.

Examining the relative difficulty of expressive and receptive vocabulary is important in light of recent studies employing gross measures of language (i.e., measures that collapse across the many domains of language) that suggest that expression poses a greater challenge than does reception for males with FXS (Roberts, Mirrett, & Burchinal, 2001). Whether this asynchrony characterizes the lexical domain per se, however, remains to be determined. Moreover, future studies of expressive and receptive vocabulary in males with FXS will need to consider the possibility of variations in their relative difficulty with age. This is suggested by the finding that differences between gross measures of expressive and receptive language increase with age, at least in males with FXS during the preschool and early school years (Roberts et al., 2001). Indeed, there is even some evidence that language development, again assessed through gross measures, shows a decreasing rate during later childhood and into adolescence (Fisch et al., 1999; Freund, Peebles, Aylward, & Reiss, 1995; Prouty et al., 1988). It is unclear, however, whether there is also variation in the magnitude of this decrease in rate across vocabulary and the other domains of language.

In addition, data are lacking on the processes underlying new word learning by males with FXS. This is problematic not only because it represents a gap in our description of the behavioral phenotype, but also because such data are essential for creating effective therapeutic interventions. Research on typically developing children has demonstrated that from very early in life children bring to bear on word learning a powerful capacity to detect regularities in the linguistic input (Saffran, Newport, & Aslin, 1996), a set of reasonable simplifying assumptions that drastically reduce the number of candidate meanings that need to be considered for novel sound patterns (Barrett, 1995; Clark, 1995), and a sensitivity to the intentions and mental states of other speakers that are relevant to determining reference (Akhtar, 2002; Baldwin & Tomasello, 1998). Moreover, research on typical development has documented the roles played by specific cognitive functions (e.g., auditory memory; Ellis Weismer, in press) and caregiver behaviors (Tomasello & Todd, 1983) in children's lexical learning. At present, the ways in which lexical learning is affected by the profile of cognitive strengths and weaknesses that characterizes the phenotype of males with FXS is not known. Additionally, the nature of the interactions that occur between care providers and males with FXS have rarely been studied, especially from the perspective of evaluating the extent and nature of their contributions to lexical learning. Future research on lexical learning and use in males with FXS, therefore, should focus on examining the ways in which the syndrome affects these capacities, assumptions, sensitivities, functions, and caregiver behaviors.

2. SYNTACTIC DEVELOPMENT

As a group, males with FXS consistently perform below chronological age expectations on receptive and expressive measures of syntax (Abbeduto & Hagerman, 1997). The weight of the evidence thus far, however, indicates that receptive syntax generally keeps pace with nonverbal cognition in affected males (Abbeduto et al., 2002; Paul et al., 1987). In the Abbeduto et al. (2003) study discussed previously, the TACL-R provided insights into the receptive language skills of the three groups studied (i.e., adolescents and young adults with FXS, adolescents and young adults with Down syndrome, and typically developing 3- to 6-year-olds, all matched groupwise on a nonverbal measure of mental age). The TACL-R includes two syntactically oriented subtests, one focused on mastery of grammatical morphemes (e.g., the *s* for marking plurality and the *ed* for marking past tense in English) and the other on mastery of phrase- and sentence-level rules and patterns (e.g., the interrogative form, multi-clause sentences). The participants with FXS, who included males and females, did not differ from the typically developing matches on either of the two syntactic subtests. This finding suggests that achievements in both domains are on a timetable that parallels, or is perhaps driven by, cognitive development. These data are consistent with those obtained by Paul et al. (1987) for institutionalized adult males. Importantly, however, one must use caution in applying these findings to younger males with FXS. Indeed, the receptive syntax of children with FXS (separate from other dimensions of language) has been examined in only two studies (Madison et al., 1986; Paul, Cohen, Breg, Watson, & Herman, 1984), and their results have been inconsistent. Madison et al. (1986) reported that the young males they studied, all of whom were from a single family, had receptive syntax that was commensurate with their mental age scores. In contrast, Paul et al. (1984) studied three 10- to 14-year-old males and found that receptive syntax slightly exceeded nonverbal mental age for two of the three participants and exceeded expressive syntax for all three. There is a need, therefore, for longitudinal data, particularly on the development of early syntax comprehension.

The evidence for expressive syntax is less clear than that for receptive syntax. Madison et al. (1986) examined the conversation of the males in their study and found that they generally displayed a mean length of utterance (MLU), which is a measure of syntactic complexity, that was at or above expectations based on their nonverbal mental ages. In contrast, Paul et al. (1984) reported delays in expressive syntax relative to nonverbal mental age. Complicating the picture further, Paul et al. (1987) found no differences on several measures of expressive syntax in conversational language between institutionalized adult males with FXS and age- and IQ-matched groups of individuals with nonFXS mental retardation or autism. Similarly, Ferrier, Bashir, Meryash, Johnston, and Wolff (1991) found that the males with FXS that they studied did not, as a group, differ from cognitively matched individuals with Down syndrome or typically developing children on syntactic measures derived from an analysis of conversational samples.

There are several possible explanations for these inconsistent findings across studies as regards syntax. First, the ages of the participants vary across studies and thus, the differences may well reflect differences that are attributable to development. Future research should evaluate this possibility, particularly through the collection of longitudinal data. Second, the sample sizes in these studies were generally quite small. This is particularly problematic in light of the extensive variability of affectedness in the syndrome. Moreover, the possibility of ascertainment bias (i.e., selective recruitment of participants into a study) is especially serious with small sample sizes because it limits the generalizability of the results and can lead to descriptions and prevalence estimates of behaviors that are not reflective of the syndrome group as a whole. Third, it is important to note that the studies cited were all conducted in advance of the availability of DNA testing to confirm the diagnosis of FXS. This raises the possibility that some of the participants actually did not have FXS—a fact that is also especially problematic in light of the small samples typically employed. Fourth, there are differences across studies as regards whether and how the participants with FXS were evaluated for the possibility that they met diagnostic criteria for autism. The methods of evaluation for autism are especially important given the recent data that many aspects of behavioral functioning, including linguistic aspects, may vary substantially with autism status (Feinstein & Reiss, 1998; Philofsky, Hepburn, Hayes, Rogers, & Hagerman, 2002; Rogers, Whener, & Hagerman, 2002). Fifth, interpretive difficulties arise because of the failure to include appropriate comparison groups. In particular, questions about the relative rates of development in language and cognition require the inclusion of a cognitively matched group of typically developing children unless the tests used to measure these domains have been standardized on the same sample of people (Mervis & Robinson, 1999). Matching should also be done on the basis of a nonverbal measure of mental age. Using a verbal measure of cognitive ability to match the groups, as was done in several studies (e.g., Ferrier et al., 1991), may lead to an underestimation of the difference between syntax and cognitive ability in the diagnostic groups (Rosenberg & Abbeduto, 1993).

It is also important to recognize that although nearly all of the studies of expressive syntax have indexed syntactic maturity by calculating MLU, or other similar measures, from conversational language samples, unfortunately, the ways in which those samples were collected have generally been poorly described. More importantly, there is typically no indication that steps were taken to ensure standardization of the language sampling contexts across participants within a study. This is troubling in light of the fact that there is abundant evidence that variations in context can have a substantial impact on the nature of the language produced by young typically developing children (Dollaghan, Campbell, & Tomlin, 1990), as well as by individuals with mental retardation (Abbeduto, Benson, Short, & Dolish, 1995; Johnson-Glenberg & Chapman, in press). Moreover, there is evidence that diagnostic group differences in syntactic capabilities are typically underestimated in conversation, which does not generally fully tax those capabilities (Abbeduto et al., 1995). In fact, recent evidence from our lab (Abbeduto et al., 2001) suggests that differences in syntactic capabilities between individuals with FXS and individuals with Down syndrome are not apparent in conversation but are in narration (i.e., story telling), with the narrative data showing a significant advantage on MLU for individuals with FXS. Furthermore, comparisons with a cognitively matched typically developing group indicated that the syntactic capabilities of the adolescents and young adults with FXS that we studied were commensurate with their nonverbal mental ages. When taken together, our findings suggest that there is a need to investigate the language capabilities of individuals with FXS via a multi-method approach so as to ensure that limitations on the generalization of the findings are understood. Moreover, the methods should be selected so as to tax the syntactic capabilities of the participants, thereby ensuring that the failure to find diagnostic group differences does not simply reflect a context sensitive ceiling effect.

In closing this section, it is important to note that research to date has been limited to a concern with evaluating the level of achievements of affected individuals in the syntactic realm. Just as with lexical development, this limited focus has led to a dearth of data and hypotheses as regards the underlying processes involved in mastering syntax. Are those processes similar to or different from those characterizing typically developing children or others with mental retardation? Why are those processes less effective? Can the processes that are used be facilitated? What role, if any, does the linguistic environment, particularly care provider talk and interactional behaviors, play in the syntactic development of males with FXS? Unfortunately, progress in developing language interventions for the syntactic delays that characterize males with FXS cannot proceed very far without answers to these and other questions about how development occurs (or does not occur) in affected individuals.

3. COMMUNICATION DEVELOPMENT

An analysis of the requirements of communication suggest that it will be an area of great challenge for males with FXS. Communication obviously requires some facility with language. As described in preceding sections, males with FXS have fewer lexical and syntactic "tools" compared to their typically developing peers, which all but ensures below age-level performance. Moreover, communication draws on a variety of cognitive and social-cognitive skills, all of which are likely to be areas of challenge for any individual with mental retardation (Abbeduto & Hesketh, 1997). Communication also requires knowledge and skills specific to the task of communication (i.e., pragmatic skills; McTear & Conti-Ramsden, 1992; Ninio & Snow, 1996). Included here would be knowledge of the procedures governing turn-taking (e.g., points at which changes in speakership are allowed), knowledge of the politeness or intrusiveness of various forms of requesting (e.g., the knowledge that "Sign this" is less polite, on average, than is "Would you sign this?"), the ability to monitor comprehension and solicit clarification as needed (e.g., by asking, "Which one?"), and knowledge of the need to formulate utterances that are appropriately informative in light of the listener's needs and the context (Abbeduto, 2003). Limitations in linguistic knowledge, social skills, and cognitive abilities are likely to hinder acquisition of such pragmatic skills and knowledge. Additionally, communication requires the coordinated use of linguistic and pragmatic knowledge to meet the real-time demands of goal-directed social interaction (Abbeduto & Short-Meyerson, 2002). Lacking the cognitive and other resources needed to meet these demands in a flexible manner may also be difficult for males with FXS, as it is for many individuals with mental retardation (Rosenberg & Abbeduto, 1993); however, this may be especially challenging for males with FXS because of their difficulties with social anxiety and hyperarousal.

Much of what we know about the communication development of males with FXS comes from studies that have relied on informant reports of adaptive behavior. Dykens, Leckman, Paul, and Watson (1988) found that the scores of males with FXS on the Vineland Adaptive Behavior Scales (Sparrow et al., 1984), including those for the Communication domain, are closer to mental age than chronological age expectations. Further, Dykens et al. found that Communication domain scores begin to lag behind those in the Daily Living domain during adolescence. This raises the possibility that communication is not only an area of relative weakness, but also one that becomes increasingly challenging for the individual with age (Dykens, Hodapp, & Leckman, 1994; Dykens, Hodapp, Ort, & Finucane, 1989; Dykens et al., 1996). It is, therefore, an important task for future research to determine the causes that underlie this decline. It is possible, for example, that the decline is linguistic in nature, reflecting a slowing of achievements in the lexical or syntactic domains that support communication. It might also reflect, however, a failure to acquire pragmatic knowledge and skills or the inhibitory effects of social anxiety and arousal on their use. In light of the decline in IQ with age, the results for communication might also reflect a failure to acquire the cognitive skills needed to coordinate and access the various sources of knowledge to meet the real-time demands of communicating with others. Another possibility is that the declining rate of development in communication reflects a change in the nature of the requirements of communication in adolescence (i.e., a shift in the type of "item" included on adaptive measures in adolescence). More specifically, during adolescence communication increasingly requires interactions with unfamiliar people in unfamiliar settings and a consideration of topics that are increasingly abstract and removed in time. Such demands may be particularly challenging for males with FXS because of the linguistic, cognitive, and social demands of these tasks.

A similar picture, at least as regards the special challenges posed by communication, emerges from studies that have observed communication directly rather than relying on informant report. In these studies, males with FXS have been found to do poorly compared to age-matched typically developing individuals on every dimension of communication examined. Males with FXS even do more poorly than developmentally matched individuals with other neurodevelopmental disorders (e.g., autism, Down syndrome) in some domains of communication.

This is illustrated in the findings of a series of studies we recently conducted. We worked from a conceptualization of communication developed by Clark (1996), which we call the *Collaborative Model*. In this model, language use is seen to entail collaboration between people working toward shared goals over the course of extended sequences of talk. This contrasts with the "traditional" model, in which the participants in a communicative interaction are seen to work independently, motivated by a desire to follow principles of internal coherence, such as "each utterance should be on topic" (Abbeduto & Short-Meyerson, 2002). As it relates to persons with neurodevelopmental disorders, the Collaborative Model requires studying the extent to which affected individuals engage in effective collaboration and the ways in which collaboration is constrained by limitations in other domains, such as cognition and mastery of language forms.

In one study, we examined the use of collaborative behaviors in making clear the referents of one's talk when in the role of speaker. Referential talk is critical to linguistic interaction because listeners use the speaker's intended referents as the foundation upon which they construct their representation of the meaning of the talk (Graesser, Millis, & Zwaan, 1997). The task we used was a variant of the *barrier task* pioneered by Glucksberg and Krauss (Glucksberg, Krauss, & Higgins, 1975). In our task, the participant played the role of speaker, and a researcher, whose behavior was highly scripted, played the role of listener. The participant and listener were separated by an opaque partition. Each had an identical set of four novel shapes. The participant's task on each trial was to describe a shape (i.e., target) so that the listener could select the same shape from his or her set. To encourage collaboration, no shape had a universally agreed upon description and the listener feigned noncomprehension on some trials. Each shape recurred several times across trials, making it possible to examine the ways in which the participant's collaborative behaviors changed or did not change as shared knowledge accrued.

Three groups of participants were tested: adolescents and young adults with FXS, adolescents and young adults with Down syndrome, and typically developing, preschool children. The three groups were matched groupwise on a nonverbal measure of MA, and the participants with FXS were matched on nonverbal IQ and chronological age to those with Down syndrome. Although females and males with FXS were included, there were few differences between them, a point to which we return in a subsequent section.

We conducted several analyses of the talk that the participants generated during the task, the results of which suggested that some aspects of collaboration are more challenging than others for individuals with FXS. In one analysis, we focused on whether the participants created unique (i.e., one-to-one) mappings between their descriptions and the shapes (e.g., referred to a specific shape as "house" every time it appeared). Unique mappings are required to meet the listener's informational needs. It was found that the participants with FXS were less likely than the typically developing children to rely on unique mappings; however, the participants with FXS were similar to those with Down syndrome in this regard. These findings suggest that the individuals with FXS find it especially difficult to create unique mappings, but that this is not a problem that is unique to the syndrome.

In a second analysis, we focused on whether the participants used the same description for a shape every time it occurred. The alternative to such consistency would be to use a new description each time a particular shape was talked about, which would violate the listener's expectations and increase his or her processing burden. The participants with FXS were proportionally less likely than either the Down syndrome or typically developing participants to use consistent descriptions as a shape recurred. Interestingly, the use of consistent descriptions was negatively correlated with parent-reported attentional problems for the participants with FXS, suggesting that an inability to direct attention might be causing them to unnecessarily change their referential descriptions. More generally, these findings demonstrate the impact on communication of the profile of strengths and weaknesses that define the broader behavioral phenotype of the syndrome.

In a third analysis, we examined whether participants shifted from indefinite descriptions (e.g., "It's *a* house") on early trials to definite descriptions (e.g., "It's *the* house") on later trials, which reflects the degree to which participants recognized that shared knowledge increased as the interaction progressed. It was found that participants with FXS were as likely as those in the other two groups to switch from indefinite to definite descriptions. Thus, despite their difficulties creating and consistently using unique mappings, adolescents and young adults with FXS have a developmental level-appropriate appreciation of the fact that accumulation of shared knowledge has consequences for language.

In a second study, we focused on noncomprehension signaling, which is a fundamental requirement of collaboration when in the role of listener. Such signaling requires monitoring one's own comprehension, determining the source of any problem, and formulating a linguistic signal that will elicit the information needed for clarification (e.g., "Which one?"). Failure to signal noncomprehension can seriously disrupt an interaction, especially because early misunderstandings can have a "snowball" effect. We used a task in which the participant was the listener and responded to simple directions from an adult speaker. The directions required moving one of several potential referents into a scene in a book. The challenge for the participant arose from the fact that some directions were designed to create noncomprehension. Three types of problematic directions were included. In *incompatible* directions, the speaker referred to an item that was not present (e.g., "Put the red lamp on the desk" when the referents were a yellow lamp and a green lamp). In *novel* directions, the speaker used an unfamiliar word to refer to the item (e.g., "Put the azure balloon in the sky" when the referents were a blue balloon and a red balloon). In *ambiguous* directions, there were multiple exemplars of the category named (e.g., "Put the hat on the man" when the referents were a brown hat and a gray hat). Nonverbal MA-matched groups of adolescents and young adults with FXS or Down syndrome and typically developing children again participated. Males and females were again included in all three groups, but there were few differences of note between males and females.

Although the participants with FXS signaled noncomprehension of the problematic directions more often than did the participants with Down syndrome, they were less likely to do so than were the typically developing comparison children. The relative difficulty of the different problem types, however, was similar across diagnostic groups: noncomprehension signals were more likely for incompatible directions than for ambiguous or novel directions. These results suggest that the development of the collaborative behaviors entailed in noncomprehension signaling is severely delayed in individuals with FXS, but not qualitatively different from that seen in typically developing individuals. Interestingly, the appropriate use of noncomprehension signals was related to a measure of theory of mind (i.e., understanding of how people mentally represent the world) for the participants with FXS. This finding demonstrates again that communication is shaped by the broader behavioral FXS phenotype.

In addition to the challenges already described, males with FXS display especially high rates of self-repetition and off topic or tangential utterances (Belser & Sudhalter, 2001; Ferrier et al., 1991; Sudhalter et al., 1990). These language characteristics are often seen to collectively constitute a tendency to perseverate (i.e., excessive self-repetition of words, phrases, sentences, or topics; Ferrier et al., 1991; Sudhalter et al., 1990). In fact, some researchers have suggested that perseveration is a unique and defining characteristic of individuals with FXS (Abbeduto & Hagerman, 1997; Bennetto & Pennington, 1996). Several studies have examined perseveration in males with FXS (Belser & Sudhalter, 1995; Ferrier et al., 1991; Sudhalter et al., 1990, 1992; Sudhalter, Scarborough, & Cohen, 1991). For the most part, the results have suggested that males with FXS produce more perseverative language (i.e., self-repetition) than do males with Down syndrome or autism (Ferrier et al., 1991; Sudhalter et al., 1990). In contrast, Paul et al. (1987) failed to find differences in topic perseveration or echolalia (i.e., repetition of others) among their three diagnostic groups: males with FXS, males with autism, and males with nonspecific mental retardation. The inconsistent findings on perseveration may be attributable, in part, to the fact that, unlike participants in the other studies, the participants in the Paul et al. study had been institutionalized (Ferrier et al., 1991).

Interpreting the results on repetition and tangential language is also complicated, however, by a number of methodological and conceptual limitations. First, perseveration has been operationalized inconsistently across studies. Moreover, different types of self-repetition (e.g., word and topic), which could reflect different underlying problems, have typically not been distinguished. Second, standardized procedures for eliciting language samples have not been used. Standardization of the materials and especially the examiner's behavior across participants is critical for making meaningful comparisons across participant groups and across studies. Third, studies to date have typically relied only on analyses of language samples collected in conversational contexts, which as noted previously, limits the generalizability of the findings and in some cases may lead to an underestimate of the magnitude of diagnostic group differences. Finally, studies to date have all but ignored the developmental origins of perseveration and whether this presumably "universal" characteristic of the syndrome actually occurs regularly among females with FXS.

We have attempted to overcome some of these limitations in our investigations of self-repetition in language (Pavetto & Abbeduto, 2002b). The results thus far indicate that the occurrence of different types of repetition depend on the language sampling context (i.e., narration vs conversation). In a group of male and female adolescents and young adults with FXS, we found that more topic repetition occurred in a conversational context than in a narrative context; a finding that further highlights the importance of measuring language characteristics in multiple language contexts. We also found that males were more likely to produce repetitions of conversational devices than were females. Conversational devices were defined as utterances that performed the mechanics of the interaction but did not necessarily have any semantic content or convey specific meaning (e.g., "that's a wrap" or "that's interesting" as a transition between topics). Interestingly, however, gender differences were not found for the other types of repetition measured (i.e., repetition of topics, words, phrases, sentences). These results suggest the possibility that different mechanisms may underlie different types of repetition, thereby necessitating a more detailed look at the type of repetitions occurring in the language of individuals with FXS than has been the case in previous studies.

Several investigators have argued that perseveration and, perhaps, other language problems associated with FXS are manifestations of problems with social anxiety and hyperarousal, which, in turn, are reflective of impaired regulation in the autonomic nervous system (Belser & Sudhalter, 2001; Cohen, 1995). More specifically, this "hyperarousal" hypothesis attributes excessive repetition to a heightened state of arousal; thus, the more aroused (e.g., excited, anxious, nervous) an individual becomes the more likely he is to perseverate. In support of this hypothesis, work by Allan Reiss and colleagues (Hessl, 2002; Wisbeck et al., 2000) has demonstrated that levels of the stress hormone, cortisol, take longer to return to baseline after a stressful situation among individuals with FXS, particularly males, compared to control groups. In addition, Miller et al. (1999) found that males with the syndrome have more difficulty habituating to sensory stimuli (for all senses) than a control group of age- and gender-matched typically developing individuals. In a preliminary study, Belser and Sudhalter (1995) reported an increase in skin conductance among males with FXS in conversations that were especially demanding (i.e., required eye gaze). When taken together, these results suggest that arousal state may be an important influence on the behavior of individuals with FXS, including their language behavior; however, the data have not yet clearly established a causal role for hyperarousal in perseveration or why arousal would necessarily manifest itself in repetitive language.

A second, perhaps, complementary hypothesis, suggests that abnormalities in the frontal lobe of the brain result in a difficulty inhibiting high strength, salient, or previously activated responses (Abbeduto & Hagerman, 1997). According to this hypothesis, it is difficult for individuals with FXS to inhibit high strength responses, which results in repetitions of previously uttered forms and content or the intrusion of idiosyncratic material. In support of this hypothesis, deficits have been documented in executive function among females (Mazzocco, Pennington, & Hagerman, 1993; Sobesky et al., 1996) and are suspected among males (Abbeduto & Hagerman, 1997). Additionally, individuals with FXS also tend to have difficulty with attention and impulsively that makes it difficult for them to focus or direct their behavior for extended periods of time (Baumgardner & Reiss, 1994; Baumgardner, Reiss, & Freund, 1995; Cohen, 1995; Hagerman, 1996; Hatton, Bailey, Hargett-Beck, Skinner, & Clark, 1999; Lachiewicz, Spiridigliozzi, Gullion, Ransford, & Rao, 1994; Miller et al., 1999). Unfortunately, there is insufficient evidence of a link between behaviors reflective of frontal lobe impairments and perseverative language. Future research would do well to explore this hypothesis and its theoretical and empirical implications for language development in FXS more generally.

A third hypothesis is that self-repetition and tangential language are the result of limited expressive language ability. According to this hypothesis, these maladaptive language behaviors function as place holding devices or strategies for maintaining engagement in discourse in the absence of sufficient language skills (Ferrier et al., 1991; Sudhalter et al., 1992). Even less information is available to confirm or disconfirm this hypothesis compared to the other two. Indeed, Sudhalter et al. (1992) failed to find a significant relationship between the occurrence of perseveration and the extent of deficits in expressive semantics. It may be, however, that self-repetition and tangential language compensate for limitations in other domains of language not measured by Sudhalter et al. More information is needed with regard to the language competencies of those with FXS, the contexts in which repetition occurs, and the factors influencing its occurrence before a determination can be made about the compensatory role (if any) it may have in discourse.

Although the causes of the perseverative and topic-related difficulties that are associated with FXS are unclear, the hypotheses offered thus far are helpful for formulating predictions about how development should proceed, the profile of strengths and challenges that should be observed, and the types of intervention that may have the greatest impact. More generally, these hypotheses emphasize the need to contextualize problems with language learning and use relative to the broader behavioral phenotype of the syndrome.

B. Language Characteristics of Females with Fragile X Syndrome

There are surprisingly few data on the language of females with FXS. Overall, the existing data indicate a relative strength in verbal ability, at least when measured by broad, summary measures of language ability (Freund & Reiss, 1991; Hagerman, 1996; Madison et al., 1986): females with FXS display higher verbal IQs than nonverbal IQs on standardized tests of intelligence. This finding, however, reflects a relative strength within the individual and not a strength relative to age-matched peers (Mazzocco, 2000). More importantly, there have been few attempts to examine the profile of development in females across the various domains of language (e.g., the lexical and syntactic). With regard to expressive and receptive language performance, no discrepancy has been observed between the two domains to date (Abbeduto & Hagerman, 1997); however, there have been only a few studies of this issue, and the sample sizes have generally been quite small, which means that the power to detect such differences, even if they do exist, has been limited. There have been even fewer attempts to learn about variations in development across the lexical, syntactic, and pragmatic skills of females with FXS (Abbeduto & Hagerman, 1997). In this section, we review in some detail the few studies that do exist and try to reach some tentative conclusions.

In a descriptive group case study, Canales (1994) examined the expressive language characteristics of adult women with FXS (i.e., they carried the full mutation) compared to women with the permutation, who are generally cognitively unaffected (Keysor & Mazzocco, 2002) and an age-matched comparison group of typically developing women without FXS. Canales collected language samples using pictures from the Thematic Apperception Test (TAT) and then coded "deviant language" using six categories based on the "TAT Communication Deviance" model of Jones and Doane (1979): long-windedness, distorted perceptions of reality; flighty attention; excessive use of personal experience; over intellectualizing the task (i.e., inappropriate use of "large" words); and difficulty reaching a conclusion. Canales found that the performance of the women with FXS seemed to be characterized by long-windedness and a lack of story coherence as evidenced by a difficulty attending to the task; however, no inferential statistical analyses were performed and the sample size was small ($n = 5$ in each of the three groups); thus, these results are in need of replication.

With regard to receptive language, two studies have been conducted. First, Madison et al. (1986) reported on the receptive language skills of several females from a single extended family; however, the small sample size and wide variability in age and level of functioning of the participants make generalization impossible. Second, Simon, Keenan, Pennington, Taylor, and Hagerman (2001) investigated the discourse comprehension of high functioning females with FXS. They were interested in determining whether the communicative problems observed clinically among females with FXS are a reflection of an inability to follow and make connections between the elements and propositions of a discourse (i.e., establish coherence). These investigators found that females with the full mutation had difficulty selecting appropriate humorous endings for stories that they read relative to IQ-matched women without FXS: the women with FXS tended to select endings that did not complete the story in a coherent manner. In the Simon et al. study, however, the participants did not have access to the story when selecting answer choices and thus, had to recall the story while attempting to select an ending. As a result, it is possible that the performance of the women with FXS had less to do with their language skills than with their ability to remember the story.

It is also important to recognize that the Simon et al. (2001) study did not measure "on line" language performance, but rather judgments about linguistic "events" after they had occurred. This raises questions about the generalizability of their results. Engaging in discourse requires the use of many skills under severe temporal constraints (Clark, 1996; Rosenberg & Abbeduto, 1993) and in a variety of contexts with a variety of different partners (Rosenberg & Abbeduto, 1993). In order to formulate a more complete picture of the language characteristics of females with FXS, it will be necessary to follow up the findings presented by Simon et al. with studies of specific aspects of discourse using on-line language tasks (i.e., taking turns in conversation, telling a coherent narrative) in a variety of contexts, with varying partners (i.e., parents, peers, teachers), and in tasks in which the individual with FXS is a participant rather than an uninvolved judge or evaluator. Nevertheless, the Simon et al. study is noteworthy because the women with FXS who participated displayed relatively poor language performance despite functioning in the range of normal intelligence. It is possible, therefore, that females with FXS, who meet the criteria for mental retardation, may have more serious language problems, and with more "basic" facets of language (e.g., vocabulary and syntax).

Taken together these studies represent only the beginning of the research needed to develop an understanding of the language characteristics of females with FXS and how those characteristics are related to, and affected by, FXS. These studies provide descriptive information about the nature of the behavioral phenotype for adult females with FXS, but they are also only static representations of language ability. Future research must address the development of language skills among females in order to understand how adult language characteristics arise. Direct comparison with males will be needed as well.

C. Gender Differences in Language Characteristics

Direct comparisons of males and females with FXS within the same study or under similar task conditions have been virtually nonexistent. As a result, it is difficult to understand the role that gender plays in shaping the language characteristics of FXS (Pavetto & Abbeduto, 2002a). Dykens et al. (2000) have suggested that, despite differences in the severity of affectedness, the profile of strengths and weaknesses associated with the syndrome does not vary based on gender; however, this conclusion is based largely on a synthesis of results from studies employing widely differing methodologies. Nevertheless, data from direct comparisons we have conducted, also supports this conclusion. In our study of receptive language involving the TACL-R, we conducted preliminary analyses to examine gender differences in receptive vocabulary and syntax. We found that although females with FXS had higher receptive language scores than males, on average, there were no differences in scores across the three subtests of the TACL-R for males or for females. In addition, males and females both displayed synchrony between their mental ages and TACL-R scores. These results are consistent with a pattern of quantitative rather than qualitative differences between males and females; that is, differences in the degree of affectedness rather than in the mechanisms involved in acquiring or using the linguistic skills and knowledge of interest.

With regard to gender differences in expressive language performance, we (Pavetto & Abbeduto, 2002a) compared the language produced by males and females in conversation and narration on the following dimensions: talkativeness (i.e., number of communication units attempted per minute), fluency (i.e., percent of communication units containing mazes), lexical diversity (i.e., number of different word roots), and syntactic complexity (i.e., MLU). We found that only talkativeness and syntactic complexity were influenced by gender: males were more talkative (i.e., had a higher number of communication units attempted per minute) than females, whereas females produced utterances of greater syntactic complexity (i.e., had a higher MLU, which is not surprising given their higher level of performance overall). The interesting point to note about our results, in addition to the lack of gender differences on fluency and lexical diversity, is that we also found differences based on the context in which the expressive language sample was taken. We found that although an effect of gender on syntactic complexity (i.e., MLU) was significant for both contexts, and MLU was higher in narration than conversation for both males and females, the magnitude of the gender effect was greater in narration than in conversation. This finding is likely to reflect the different demands of the narration vs conversation task and is consistent with previous research suggesting that narration elicits language with greater syntactic complexity than conversation (Abbeduto et al., 1995). Moreover, it suggests that the language characteristics of both males and females are influenced in fairly similar ways by the sampling context, again suggesting quantitative rather than qualitative differences in the language of males and females with FXS.

As mentioned previously, we have also examined gender differences in our studies on communication, although the small sample sizes in our studies to date require caution in the conclusions drawn. In those studies, the differences that emerged between males and females with FXS were generally quantitative rather than qualitative. Interestingly, however, the differences between males and females with FXS have been relatively small in our studies on communication, and generally of lesser magnitude than those in our studies of lexical and syntactic skills. Although we must be cautious because of the small sample sizes in our studies, these results suggest an interesting hypothesis: not only is communication one area of special challenge, it is an area in which gender differences may be minimized despite large differences in performance on indicies of affectedness (e.g., IQ).

D. General Limitations

Although the research conducted to date has contributed greatly to our understanding of the linguistic challenges facing those with FXS, there are many gaps in our knowledge and methodological limitations that need to be addressed before it will be possible to fully describe and explain the impact of the syndrome on the behavioral phenotype (Abbeduto & Hagerman, 1997). First, most of the research on language has focused on males. Apart from the studies presented in the preceding sections, clinical reports and anecdotal statements are the primary source of information with regard to the language characteristics of females. Thus, it is unclear whether features like perseveration, variable speaking rates, and sound omissions are also characteristic of the language of females and, if so, whether their expression in females is similar to or different from their expression in males not only in severity but in their essential nature.

Second, the FXS and comparison groups are often matched on broad measures of ability, such as IQ (Ferrier et al., 1991) or Vineland Communication age (Belser & Sudhalter, 2001), that are likely to include precisely those aspects of language on which the investigators expect to find diagnostic group differences (Abbeduto & Murphy, in press). Of course, this reduces the likelihood of finding differences on the dependent variables, even when they do exist. Moreover, the failure of most studies to include an appropriately matched, typically developing comparison group makes it difficult to determine whether the characteristics observed in the participants with FXS are consistent with age and cognitive level expectations or whether they present an area of particular challenge or strength for those with the syndrome (Mervis & Robinson, 1999).

Third, there has been a lack of longitudinal data available on the development of specific aspects of language (e.g., the lexicon, syntax). Thus, little is known about the developmental course or causal factors underlying language acquisition and use. As a result, it is unclear whether problematic language characteristics such as perseveration are learned behaviors (i.e., a strategy for maintaining engagement), the result of an additional, nonlinguistic, problem (i.e., arousal or social anxiety), or the cause of other social deficits (e.g., perseveration makes talk difficult for the listener to follow thereby limiting opportunities to engage in discourse and thus practice existing language skills and acquire new ones).

Fourth, sample size has typically been quite small. Small sample sizes lead to limited statistical power for detecting group differences, limit the generalizability of findings, and make comparisons across studies difficult. They also exacerbate design limitations (e.g., wide age ranges and limited comparison groups). Indeed, most studies in this area have involved comparisons between FXS and other groups (e.g., autism), but have included small samples of participants of widely varying ages (e.g., children through older adults). A large age range is particularly problematic because few studies have treated age as a variable of interest, despite at least some evidence that there are important changes with age in domains of functioning likely to impact language learning and use (e.g., Cohen, Vietze, Sudhalter, Jenkins, & Brown, 1989, 1991; Fisch et al., 1996; Fisch et al., 1999; Roberts et al., 2001). In fact, the inconsistent results that plague research on language in FXS are likely due, at least in part, to the failure to seriously consider age-related differences in the linguistic challenges that face individuals with FXS.

Fifth, much of the existing literature on language has used gross measures of language and behavior (Dykens et al., 2000), which do not take into account the possibility of variable delays and limitations across the components of language (i.e., syntax, semantics) or distinguish between problems related to the acquisition of linguistic forms and contents and their use in social interaction. For example, several investigations have relied on the Vineland Adaptive Behavior Scales, which yields only a single communication score that summarizes performance across numerous domains of communication. These studies have suggested that, at least for males, communication is a strength compared to individuals with Down syndrome (Burack et al., 1999). However, this obscures the fact that the differences relative to Down syndrome likely reflect differences in syntactic skill rather than lexical or communicative skills. Indeed, our own research, described in the preceding sections, has demonstrated that, on average, communication is actually more impaired than are lexical and syntactic skills in individuals with FXS. Moreover, within communication, some skills may be more challenging than others (e.g., attending to the needs of the listener vs recognizing that shared knowledge increases during an interaction).

Sixth, research on child language has demonstrated the importance of measuring language in multiple contexts in order to obtain a more representative sample of the child's language ability and to be maximally sensitive to diagnostic group differences in various language capabilities (Abbeduto et al., 1995). As mentioned previously, there is considerable evidence that narration, or story telling, places greater demands on expressive syntax than does conversation (Dollaghan et al., 1990). As a result, diagnostic group differences in syntactic capabilities are more apparent in narration than in conversation (Abbeduto et al., 1995; Abbeduto et al., 2002; Abbeduto et al., 2003; Pavetto, 2001; Pavetto & Abbeduto, 2002a). At the same time, diagnostic group and gender differences in lexical skill and in talkativeness are, as discussed previously, more pronounced in conversation than in narration. The fact that previous studies of expressive language in FXS have relied almost exclusively on conversation as the context for assessment means that they have failed to provide a complete picture of the language profiles of affected individuals. Moreover, reliance on conversation suggests that these studies have probably underestimated differences between individuals with FXS and comparison participants on some dimensions of language (e.g., syntax). In addition, the failure to standardize the procedures and contexts in which expressive language samples are collected, make diagnostic group comparisons difficult to interpret.

When taken together, the data available on language and FXS suggest that future research must make comparisons across syndromes in a variety of contexts in order to assess the specificity of language challenges to FXS syndrome. Also, males and females need to be compared under similar task conditions in order to understand the role of gender in the development of the linguistic profile of the syndrome. In addition, it is important to examine the developmental course of more narrowly defined and conceptually justified domains of language, as well as the environmental factors (e.g., context, task demands, environmental stimuli), individual psychological factors, and biological factors that impact behavioral and linguistic outcomes. Taking such a developmental perspective will yield important clinical data about the ways in which the behavioral phenotype varies with the gender and age (i.e., childhood, adolescence, adulthood) that is being considered and will lead to a better understanding of the factors operating to produce the phenotype of FXS characteristic of each gender and age period.

III. NEW DIRECTIONS IN RESEARCH ON FRAGILE X SYNDROME

In order to understand the pathways that produce the behavioral phenotype, it is important to consider that the phenotype emerges over time and reflects the complex interactions of genotype and environment (Hodapp & Dykens, 2001). Without a clear understanding of the developmental course of the phenotype, it is difficult to formulate hypotheses about causal mechanisms, determine the syndrome specificity of the phenotype, or gain insight into behavioral interventions that might provide a means of remediation for particular behavioral limitations. In addition, current theory has conceptualized the behavioral phenotype as a probabilistic pattern; that is, a pattern that is more likely to be found in one syndrome than another but not necessarily among all individuals with the syndrome in question (Dykens et al., 2000). As a result, there is a need to determine the degree of adherence to the prototypical behavioral phenotype and determine the causes of individual differences in adherence and to do so within the context of a developmental approach that attends to both genetic and environmental differences among individuals (Hodapp & Dykens, 2001).

Until recently, a static, single-factor model has dominated much of the work on FXS as well as work on other genetic syndromes. Under this model, it has been assumed that all of the characteristics associated with a particular syndrome are the "direct" result of the genetic anomaly; that is, the behaviors defining the phenotype are thought to be the inexorable result of the anomaly and will emerge in more or less the same form, or to the same degree, no matter what the environment or context. In addition, the model has been concerned largely with the "final" outcome of what has been essentially seen as a disease process; thus, researchers have been content to determine whether a particular linguistic skill or behavior is present or absent in individuals with FXS. Individual differences in adherence to the "final" phenotype are assumed to be largely, if not solely, the result of genetically conditioned biological variations (e.g., in levels of FMRP). This model is limited because it ignores changes with age in the phenotype, as well as the possibility that learning, broadly defined as change occasioned by the interaction of environments with individual characteristics and capacities, has contributed to the emergence of the phenotype.

Recently, however, there has been a promising increase in the number of studies designed to document age-related changes in the behavioral phenotype of FXS. Examples of age-related changes documented thus far include the attenuation of autistic symptomatology with age in FXS (Kau, Meyer & Kaufmann, 2002; Kau, Reider, Payne, Meyer, & Freund, 2000); the emergence of other potentially syndrome-specific characteristics, such as eye gaze aversion and repetitive language, in late childhood and early adolescence (Cohen et al., 1989; Wolf, Gardner, Paccia, & Lappen, 1989); changes in the stability of IQ among males, with stability between 16 and 24 months (Freund et al., 1995) and declines in later childhood and adolescence (Dyer-Freidman et al., 2002); and declines with age in the extent of communication delays (as measured by the Vineland) that may begin as early as the preschool years (Freund et al., 1995) or as late as around 10 years of age (Bailey, Hatton, & Skinner, 1998; Dykens, Hodapp, Ort, & Leckman, 1993). These examples provide compelling evidence of the need to study the developmental trajectory of behavior in FXS, especially the relative trajectories across different domains of behavior, as well as the factors that shape that trajectory. We encourage such an approach in studies of language in FXS.

A. Accounting for Individual Variability in the Behavioral Phenotype

FXS is characterized by considerable variability across individuals. Understanding the nature and causes of this variability is of critical importance, both clinically and theoretically. To this end, investigators have examined the relationship between individual variability in behavior and biologically conditioned genetic variability, such as the number of CGG repetitions and FMRP level (Abrams et al., 1994; Bailey, Hatton, Tassone, Skinner, & Taylor, 2001). This research has provided evidence that at least some dimensions of language and communication are related to such biological variations; however, the findings are not always straightforward or easy to interpret. Interestingly, these studies have actually demonstrated the importance of environmental variations on phenotypic expression.

Bailey et al. (2001) found in their sample of young boys with FXS that FMRP levels were positively correlated with measures of overall development and with Communication domain scores on the Vineland Adaptive Behavior Scales. Among females, variability in affectedness has been found to be explained, in part, by the ratio of activated X chromosomes containing a healthy allele rather than the unhealthy FMR1 allele (i.e., the activation ratio), which is itself an approximation of FMRP level (Abrams et al., 1994). Kuo et al. (2002) found that the activation ratio predicted various composite measures of IQ, including verbal IQ, in girls with FXS. Furthermore, in a study of adult females with FXS, most of whom had IQs in the normal range, Simon et al. (2001) found a positive correlation between activation ratio and a measure of the ability to construct a coherent representation of nonliteral stories during language comprehension.

Not all aspects of behavior, however, are highly correlated with FMRP levels or other biological markers of the disorder. Indeed, several recent studies have offered evidence of the impact of the environment on producing variations in behavioral development (Bailey, 2002; Bailey et al., 2001; Hessl, 2002; Van Lieshout, De Meyer, Curfs, & Fryns, 1998). Glaser et al. (2003), for example, found that FMRP levels were unrelated to adaptive behavior as measured by the Vineland, including the Communication domain, in male and female children and adolescents with FXS. Moreover, looking longitudinally, Bailey et al. (2001) found that although FMRP levels predicted level of communication functioning as measured by the Vineland scales, it did not predict rate of development in this domain (or other domains of adaptive behavior). Similarly, Dyer-Friedman et al. (2002) found that FMRP levels predicted scores on an index of distractibility for females with FXS, but not their verbal or performance IQs or various other indices of cognitive functioning. In addition, activation ratios have not been related to a host of important developmental milestones and behavioral characteristics (e.g., age of first walk and first talk, parent rating of attention problems, adaptive behavior) even though evidence links the activation ratio to overall affectedness (as measured by IQ; Abrams et al., 1994).

Even when FMRP has been found to be correlated with behavioral measures, it often accounts only for a small portion of the variance (Bailey et al., 2001; Dyer-Friedman et al., 2002). Bailey et al. (2001), for example, found that "... FMRP expression accounts for a small but statistically significant difference in developmental outcomes for young children" (p. 24) on the Battelle Developmental Inventory and the Vineland Adaptive Behavior Scales. Further, Kwon et al. (2001) and Menon, Kwon, Eliez, Taylor, and Reiss (2000) have suggested that FMRP and other biological markers are highly correlated with brain function, but less highly correlated with behavioral measures because of the multiple determinants (including environmental) of behavior. In fact, there is evidence that much of the variability in the behavioral phenotype is related to other gene effects and the environment: "... many behaviors are strongly influenced by the remainder of the individual's genome and environment, not just by the genetic disorder per se" (Hodapp, 1997; p. 68). Thus, adaptive behavior in the study by Glaser et al. (2003) was predicted only by child IQ (for females) or by both child IQ and environmental responsiveness (for males) as opposed to levels of FMRP. These results are not surprising given what is known about typical development. Indeed, in the literature on typical development, both biological and environmental factors influence development in complex ways within virtually every other domain of behavior examined, including the domains of language learning and use. Thus, it is clear that there is a need for research that examines changes in behavior and biology longitudinally, and that considers the multiple determinants of behavior. Longitudinal studies that can examine change over time in well-defined domains of language in relation, not only to FMRP levels, but also the environments in which that behavior is occurring will be essential in this regard. In the remaining sections of this chapter, we sketch in some detail a set of guidelines for this research agenda.

B. Examining the Factors that Shape the Behavioral Phenotype

1. GENES: DIRECT AND INDIRECT EFFECTS

Hodapp (1997) and others (Abbeduto, Evans, & Dolan, 2001; Dykens et al., 2000; Hodapp & Zigler, 1997) have drawn attention to the distinction between the direct and indirect effects that genes have on the individual with FXS or other genetic syndrome. According to Hodapp, genes can act directly to affect the behaviors and characteristics that a child brings into the world (Abbeduto et al., 2001; Hodapp, 1997; Scarr, 1992, 1993). They can also, however, indirectly influence development by changing the child's environment. Further, there are three primary ways in which genes exert their influence indirectly on development. First, the child is born into an environment that is partly comprised of, and shaped by, the behaviors and characteristics of the parents, which themselves reflect the parental genotype. This represents the *passive effects* of genes on development because the child has no role in shaping these initial dimensions of the environment. In the case of FXS, for example, a mother who passes the mutation on to her child might also show effects of carrying the mutation in her own behavior, which could then affect the child's development. Second, the child, by virtue of his or her characteristics, which are themselves determined in part by his or her genotype, will evoke a different response from the environment than would a child with different characteristics. In the case of FXS, for example, a child with FXS who produces language that is highly perseverative and thus is nonresponsive to the goals and needs of others may discourage others from interacting with him or her, thereby reducing the number of opportunities to engage in discourse or other social interactions that could facilitate language development. The third type of effect, an *active effect*, refers to those effects occasioned by the child actively seeking out environments that are the most consistent or compatible with his or her characteristics, including the characteristics that have a genetic component, while avoiding those that are inconsistent with those characteristics. In the case of FXS, social anxiety may lead an affected individual to actively avoid or withdraw from social situations (e.g., family gatherings, group projects, friends), which are precisely those that would provide the child with developmentally valuable social and linguistic experiences. Understanding language development, and behavioral development more generally, in FXS will require examining both the direct and indirect effects of genes, with the latter entailing a consideration of the complex ways in which genes and environments interact.

2. CHARACTERIZING THE ENVIRONMENT

In addition to considering the direct and indirect effects of genes, there are a variety of ways in which the environment can be characterized and many levels on which to consider its influence (e.g., home, school, community, culture; Bronfenbrenner & Morris, 1998). These levels will interact with the individual's characteristics and behaviors in different ways to shape the phenotype. A handful of studies in the field of FXS research have begun to consider environmental influences on behavioral outcomes, although few have focused on environmental influences on language learning and use except through the use of gross measures (e.g., verbal IQ). Dyer-Friedman et al. (2002), for example, used the Home Observation for Measurement of the Environment (HOME), Revised Edition (Caldwell & Bradley, 1984) to assess environmental influences on behavior. The HOME is a combination observation and parent interview measure that characterizes the quality of the environment in which the adolescent lives (e.g., aspects of the physical environment, emotional responsiveness of the parent, enrichment opportunities available to the adolescent). Dyer-Friedman et al. found that the HOME was predictive of IQ for both males and females with FXS and that it contributed to prediction even after controlling for the effects of parental IQ and child FMRP levels. Interestingly, responsiveness of the home environment was especially strongly related to verbal IQ for girls and boys (Dyer-Friedman et al., 2002). The finding that verbal IQ is predicted by HOME scores for both males and females with FXS is important because it demonstrates that such skills are open to environmental intervention. From a clinical perspective, therefore, it is important to understand more precisely which language skills can benefit from which types of environmental contingencies. There is no evidence, for example, that being raised in a family in which one or more siblings have FXS in and of itself confers any increased risk for negative developmental outcomes for girls and adolescent females without FXS (Mazzocco, Baumgardner, Freund, & Reiss, 1998); however, this does not rule out the possibility of such effects for individuals with fewer personal "resources" (e.g., lower IQs) for dealing with stressful or otherwise adverse environmental circumstances due to possession of the FMR1 gene.

There is evidence that not only the home, but also other environmental contexts, may be less than optimal for individuals with FXS. For example, special educators have less experience with, and knowledge of, FXS than Down syndrome and feel poorly prepared to deal with students with FXS (York, von Fraunhofer, Turk, & Sedgwick, 1999). Although it is premature to draw conclusions about the impact on the quality of the educational programs for individuals with FXS, such research draws attention to the importance of considering the ways in which the person with FXS may experience and interact with different levels of his or her environment (e.g., school, home), and the impact those environments may have on him or her. Future research should consider the mechanisms by which the environment impacts well-defined domains of language, such as vocabulary. In addition, it will be important to consider how those mechanisms change over time, how their interaction with the environment changes, and how they impact the individual's developmental trajectory.

3. APPLYING DEVELOPMENTAL MODELS

Understanding typical language development has required models that address the relationship between the emergence of language and achievements in other domains of functioning, as well as the interactions between environmental and genetic causal factors. Indeed, several models (e.g., social interactionist, sociocognitive, information processing) have proved fruitful in generating research and providing insights into at least some strands of language learning and use (Chapman, 2000). By applying the basic concepts and frameworks of such models to the study of FXS and other genetic syndromes, it will be possible to enhance the present understanding of syndrome-specific phenotypes by providing insight into the processes and mechanisms of change in the behavioral phenotype and potential end-states.

More specifically, there have been a variety of claims advanced to account for the acquisition of language under typical circumstances. At the extremes are the behaviorist views that emphasize the role of input from the environment (Skinner, 1957) and the nativist views that emphasize innate processes internal to the child (Chomsky, 1959; Pinker, 1994). These theories are challenged by more "moderate" positions that focus on the interactions between biology and environment (i.e., the sociocognitive, information processing, social interactionist, and connectionist, or emergentist, approaches). Rather than considering language to be independent of other cognitive domains, these interactionist theories emphasize the multiple skills required for language learning and use (i.e., cognitive processing, working memory, attention). They also consider the biological origins of such skills and their dependence on complex environmental inputs. For example, the skills that are required to engage in discourse (e.g., turn taking, initiating and maintaining conversation, establishing common ground, signaling that a message has been understood, verifying that the listener is following the conversation) require more than knowledge of words and sentences; rather, they also require, among other things, cognitive skills, social skills, and interpersonal understanding (Clark, 1996; Rosenberg & Abbeduto, 1993). In order to fully comprehend how the syndrome impacts the developing individual, it is necessary to examine the separate components of language, the relationships among them, and the ways in which skills and deficits in other domains of behavioral and psychological functioning impact language learning and use over time. This is particularly important in the case of FXS because social deficits, problems with attention, and anxiety, all of which may impact language acquisition and use, are relatively common in affected individuals, but may be more important in some components of language than in others (Belser & Sudhalter, 2001).

Social interactionist theory is one example of a developmental model that can be of particular value in generating hypotheses about the mechanisms underlying development in genetic syndromes. This theory focuses attention on the reciprocal influences of child and caregiver during interaction and how those influences shape language acquisition. For example, research conducted by Peter Mundy, Connie Kasari, and others has demonstrated that, for typically developing children, the ability to engage in joint attention to an object or event with an adult is positively related to the child's acquisition of vocabulary and perhaps other components of language as well (Baldwin & Tomasello, 1998; Markus, Mundy, Morales, Delgado, & Yale, 2000; Mundy & Gomes, 1998; Mundy, Kasari, Sigman, & Ruskin, 1995). Similar relationships have been documented for Down syndrome (Harris, Kasari, & Sigman, 1996; Landry & Chapieski, 1989; Mundy et al., 1995) and autism (Kasari, Sigman, Mundy, & Yirmiya, 1990; Leekam, & Moore, 2001; Loveland & Landry, 1986; Mundy & Neal, 2001). Little is known about the early language and communication behavior of individuals with FXS, including early prelinguistic nonverbal communicative behaviors, such as pointing and gesturing, which are so crucial in establishing joint attention. How do delays in prelinguistic communication impact acquisition of more complex language skills (e.g., formulating sentences, navigating conversation, narrating a story)? Are delays in vocabulary acquisition (relative to chronological age expectations) related to differences in joint attention skills? How do characteristics such as hyperarousal and hypersensitivity to environmental stimulation, so prevalent in FXS, impact the infant's ability to sustain attention and subsequent joint attention with parent and object? What implications do difficulties in these areas have across development?

In addition to these questions, social interactionist theory considers the capacities and characteristics that both the child and caregiver bring to the interaction. In FXS in particular, it is possible that not only the child, but also the mother, who as a carrier, may show some effects (Keysor & Mazzocco, 2002). As a result, the expression of the syndrome phenotype manifested in the mother (e.g., her success with and comfort in engaging in social interaction) may well impact the linguistic experiences of her child. As a result, the nature of their interactions may unfold in such a way as to create an atypical environment that has important consequences for language outcomes. Based on what is known about joint attention and the early behavioral characteristics of infants and children with FXS, it is possible to hypothesize ways in which the syndrome might impact the frequency and quality of the joint attentional interaction between caregiver and child, which would ultimately lead to predictable language outcomes that could be measured over time.

IV. CONCLUSION

Although great strides have been made in understanding the behavioral phenotype associated with FXS, much work remains to be done particularly in the areas of language acquisition and use. Language is a critical area on which to focus attention because it provides the foundation for most social interaction and often mediates the interaction between the individual and the world. As a result, research in this area will inform our understanding of the ways in which impairments across domains influence the broader behavioral phenotype associated with FXS. It is essential, however, that future research on language learning and use in FXS apply a developmental approach to describing and explaining changes with age within the individual and differences across individuals. Such an approach is particularly important because it will allow researchers and clinicians to chart the origins and developmental trajectories of the behavioral phenotype associated with specific syndromes and provide insights into the indirect effects that genes have on development through interactions with the environment (Hodapp, 1997). Moreover, it is important that future research continue to make comparisons across syndromes and with appropriate typically developing groups in standardized and methodologically sound research programs. Comparisons of this nature are valuable for elucidating the multiple pathways by which development occurs as well as for clarifying the similarities and differences across syndromes.

A second point of note is that the study of language acquisition and use has important clinical implications. Results from our lab, for example, suggest that essential communication skills (e.g., noncomprehension signaling and establishing referents) are areas of special challenge for individuals with FXS and that broader phenotypic characteristics (e.g., inability to direct attention) may influence successful acquisition and use of these skills. Practitioners would do well, then, to consider how these phenotypic characteristics influence, and are influenced by, treatment and intervention; it may be necessary to simultaneously target intervention at improving the skill as well as addressing the behavioral factors that underlie its use. In addition, understanding areas of relative strength (or at least developmental-level appropriate skills) for males and females with FXS (e.g., appreciation of the accumulation of shared knowledge and its consequences for language and theory of mind) may provide valuable insights for directing intervention and facilitating acquisition of more advanced skills. In this regard, there is much to gain from research that considers the similarities and differences between syndromes. Doing so will provide clinicians and practitioners data upon which to customize interventions, educational environments, and strategies. Note, however, it is important to recognize that there are more commonalities than differences between most genetic syndromes associated with mental retardation, at least at the level of behavior. As a result, it will be essential to place behavioral differences between syndromes in proper perspective by using the data on syndrome differences to tailor existing programs, interventions, and strategies rather than creating them anew according to a syndrome-specific profile.

ACKNOWLEDGMENTS

Preparation of this article was supported by grant R01 HD24356 to the second author, fellowships awarded to the first author through the John H. Merck Scholars II program and the Jeanette Anderson Hoffman Memorial Wisconsin Distinguished Graduate Fellowship, and by NIH grant P30 HD03352 awarded to the Waisman Center. We thank Mina Johnson Glenberg, Ph.D. for her insightful comments on the chapter. We also are deeply indebted to all of the families who have volunteered their time in support of our research and who have taught us so much about fragile X syndrome.

REFERENCES

Abbeduto, L. (2003). Speaking and listening. In L. Nadel (Ed.), *Encyclopedia of cognitive science* [CD-ROM]. London: Macmillan.

Abbeduto, L., Benson, G., Short, K., & Dolish, J. (1995). Effects of sampling context on the expressive language of children and adolescents with mental retardation. *Mental Retardation, 33*, 279–288.

Abbeduto, L., Evans, J., & Dolan, T. (2001). Theoretical perspectives on language and communication problems in mental retardation and developmental disabilities. *Mental Retardation and Developmental Disabilities Research Reviews, 7*, 45–55.

Abbeduto, L., & Hagerman, R. (1997). Language and communication in fragile X syndrome. *Mental Retardation and Developmental Disabilities Research Reviews, 3*, 313–322.

Abbeduto, L., & Hesketh, L. J. (1997). Pragmatic development in individuals with mental retardation: learning to use language in social interactions. *Mental Retardation and Developmental Disabilities Research Reviews, 3*, 323–334.

Abbeduto, L. & Murphy, M. M. (in press). Language, social cognition, maladaptive behavior, and communication in Down syndrome and fragile X syndrome. In M. Rice, & S. Warren (Eds.), *Developmental Language Disorders: From Phenotypes to Etiologies*. Mahwah, NJ: Lawrence Erlbaum Associates, Inc.

Abbeduto, L., Murphy, M. M., Cawthon, S. C., Kesin, E., Weissman, M. D., & Karadottir, S. (2002, July). *Expressive language and contextual influences in fragile X syndrome*. Paper presented at the biennial international conference of the National Fragile X Foundation, Chicago, IL.

Abbeduto, L., Murphy, M. M., Cawthon, S. W., Richmond, E. K., Weissman, M. D., Karadottir, S., & O'Brien, A. (2003). Receptive language skills of adolescents and young adults with Down syndrome or fragile X syndrome. *American Journal on Mental Retardation, 108*, 149–160.

Abbeduto, L., Pavetto, M., Kesin, E., Weissman, M. D., Karadottir, S., O'Brien, A., & Cawthon, S. (2001). The linguistic and cognitive profile of Down syndrome: Evidence from a comparison with fragile X syndrome. *Down Syndrome Research and Practice, 7*, 9–15.

Abbeduto, L., & Short-Meyerson, K. (2002). Linguistic influences on social interaction. In H. Goldstein, L. Kaczmarek, & K. M. English (Eds.), *Promoting social communication in children and youth with developmental disabilities* (pp. 27–54). Baltimore: Brookes.

Abrams, M. T., Reiss, A. L., Freund, L. S., Baumgardner, T. L., Chase, G. A., & Denckla, M. B. (1994). Molecular–neurobehavioral associations in females with the fragile X full mutation. *American Journal of Medical Genetics, 51*, 317–327.

Akhtar, N. (2002). Relevance and early word learning. *Journal of Child Language, 29*, 677–686.

Bailey, D. B. (2002, July). Association between fragile X and autism. Symposium conducted at the 8th International Fragile X Conference, Chicago, IL.

Bailey, D. B., Jr., Hatton, D. D., & Skinner, M. (1998). Early developmental trajectories of males with fragile X syndrome. *American Journal on Mental Retardation, 103*, 29–39.

Bailey, D. B., Hatton, D. D., Tassone, F., Skinner, M., & Taylor, A. K. (2001). Variability in FMRP and early development in males with fragile X syndrome. *American Journal on Mental Retardation, 106*, 16–27.

Baldwin, D. A., & Tomasello, M. (1998). Word learning: A window on early pragmatic understanding. In E. V. Clark (Ed.), *The proceedings of the twenty-ninth annual child language research forum* (pp. 3–23). Chicago, IL, US: Center for the Study of Language and Information.

Barrett, M. (1995). Early lexical development. In P. Fletcher, & B. MacWhinney (Eds.), *The handbook of child language* (pp. 362–392). Oxford: Blackwell.

Baumgardner, T., & Reiss, A. L. (1994). Fragile X syndrome: a behavioral genetics' window into understanding social emotional learning disability. In A. J. Capute, P. J. Accardo, & B. K. Shapiro (Eds.), *Learning disabilities spectrum: ADD, ADHD, & LD* (pp. 67–84). Baltimore, MD: York Press, Inc.

Baumgardner, T., Reiss, A. L., & Freund, L. (1995). Specification of the neurobehavioral phenotype of males with fragile X syndrome. *Pediatrics, 95*, 744–752.

Belser, R. C., & Sudhalter, V. (1995). Arousal difficulties in males with fragile X syndrome: a preliminary report. *Developmental Brain Dysfunction, 8*, 270–279.

Belser, R. C., & Sudhalter, V. (2001). Conversational characteristics of children with fragile X syndrome: repetitive speech. *American Journal on Mental Retardation, 106*, 28–38.

Bennetto, L., & Pennington, B. F. (1996). The neuropsychology of fragile X syndrome. In R. J. Hagerman, & A. C. Cronister (Eds.), *Fragile X syndrome: Diagnosis, treatment, and research* (2nd ed., pp. 210–248). Baltimore, MD: Johns Hopkins University Press.

Bronfenbrenner, U. & Morris, P. A. (1998). The ecology of developmental processes. In W. Damon (Editor-in-Chief) & R. M. Lerner (Vol. Ed.), *Handbook of child psychology: Vol. 1. Theoretical models of human development* (5th ed., pp. 993–1028). New York: Wiley.

Brown, W. T. (2002). The molecular biology of the fragile X mutation. In R. J. Hagerman & P. J. Hagerman (Eds.), *Fragile X syndrome: Diagnosis, treatment and research* (3rd ed., pp. 110–135). Baltimore: Johns Hopkins University Press.

Burack, J. A., Shulman, C., Katzir, E., Schaap, T., Brennan, J. M., Iarocci, G., Wilansky, P., & Amir, N. (1999). Cognitive and behavioural development of Israeli males with fragile X and Down syndrome. *International Journal of Behavioral Development, 23*, 519–531.

Caldwell, B., & Bradley, R. (1984). *Home Observation for Measurement of the Environment.* Little Rock, AR: University of Arkansas at Little Rock.

Canales, D. N. (1994). *Communication Deviance in Females with Fragile X Syndrome.* Unpublished master's thesis, Trinity University, Pennsylvania.

Carrow-Woolfolk, E. (1985). *Test for Auditory Comprehension of Language, Revised.* Austin, TX: DLM Teaching Resources.

Chapman, R. S. (2000). Children's language learning: an interactionist perspective. *Journal of Child Psychology and Psychiatry, and Allied Disciplines*, *41*, 33–54.

Chomsky, N. (1959). Review of B. F. Skinner's verbal behavior. *Language*, *35*, 26–58.

Clark, E. V. (1995). Later lexical development and word formation. In P. Fletcher, & B. MacWhinney (Eds.), *The handbook of child language* (pp. 393–412). Cambridge, MA: Blackwell Publishers Ltd.

Clark, H. H. (1996). *Using language*. New York: Cambridge University Press.

Cohen, I. L. (1995). A theoretical analysis of the role of hyperarousal in the learning and behavior of fragile X males. *Mental Retardation and Developmental Disabilities Research Reviews*, *1*, 286–291.

Cohen, I. L., Vietze, P. M., Sudhalter, V., Jenkins, E. C., & Brown, W. T. (1989). Parent–child dyadic gaze patterns in fragile X males and in non-fragile X males with autistic disorder. *Journal of Child Psychology and Psychiatry*, *30*, 845–856.

Cohen, I. L., Vietze, P., Sudhalter, V., Jenkins, E. C., & Brown, W. T. (1991). Effects of age and communication level on eye contact in fragile X males and non-fragile X autistic males. *American Journal of Medical Genetics*, *38*, 498–502.

Dollaghan, C. A., Campbell, T. F., & Tomlin, R. (1990). Video narration as a language sampling context. *Journal of Speech and Hearing Research*, *55*, 582–590.

Dyer-Friedman, J., Glaser, B., Hessl, D., Johnston, C., Huffman, L. C., Taylor, A., Wisbeck, J., & Reiss, A. L. (2002). Genetic and environmental influences on the cognitive outcomes of children with fragile X syndrome. *Journal of the American Academy of Child and Adolescent Psychiatry*, *41*, 237–244.

Dykens, E. M., Hodapp, R. M., & Finucane, B. M. (2000). *Genetics and mental retardation syndromes: A new look at behavior and interventions*. Baltimore: Brookes.

Dykens, E. M., Hodapp, R. M., & Leckman, J. F. (1994). *Behavior and development in fragile X syndrome*. Thousand Oaks: Sage Publications.

Dykens, E. M., Hodapp, R. M., Ort, S., & Finucane, B. M. (1989). The trajectory of cognitive development in males with fragile X syndrome. *Journal of the American Academy of Child and Adolescent Psychiatry*, *28*, 422–426.

Dykens, E. M., Hodapp, R. M., Ort, S. I., & Leckman, J. F. (1993). Trajectory of adaptive behaviour in males with fragile X syndrome. *Journal of Autism and Developmental Disorders*, *23*, 135–145.

Dykens, E. M., Leckman, J., Paul, R., & Watson, M. (1988). Cognitive, behavioral, and adaptive functioning in fragile X and non-fragile X retarded men. *Journal of Autism and Developmental Disorders*, *18*, 41–52.

Dykens, E. M., Ort, S., Cohen, I. L., Finucane, B. M., Spiridigliozzi, G., Lachiewicz, A., Reiss, A., et al. (1996). Trajectories and profiles of adaptive behavior in males with fragile X syndrome: multicenter studies. *Journal of Autism and Developmental Disorders*, *26*, 287–301.

Ellis Weismer, S. (in press). Memory and processing capacity. In R. D. Kent (Ed.), *MIT Encyclopedia of Communication Disorders*. Boston: MIT Press.

Feinstein, C., & Reiss, A. L. (2001). Autism: the point of view from fragile X studies. *Journal of Autism and Developmental Disorders*, *28*, 393–405.

Ferrier, L. J., Bashir, A. S., Meryash, D. L., Johnston, J., & Wolff, P. (1991). Conversational skills of individuals with fragile-X syndrome: a comparison with autism and Down syndrome. *Developmental Medicine and Child Neurology*, *33*, 776–788.

Fisch, G. S., Carpenter, N., Holden, J. J. A., Howard-Peebles, P. N., Simensen, R., Maddalena, A., et al. (1999). Longitudinal assessment of adaptive and maladaptive behaviors in fragile X males: Growth, development, and profiles. *American Journal of Medical Genetics*, *83*, 257–263.

Fisch, G. S., Holden, J. J. A., Carpenter, N. J., Howard-Peebles, P. N., Maddalena, A., Pandya, A., & Nance, W. (1999). Age-related language characteristics of children and adolescents with fragile X syndrome. *American Journal of Medical Genetics, 83*, 253–256.

Fisch, G. S., Simensen, R., Tarleton, J., Chalifoux, M., Holden, J. J. A., Carpenter, N., Howard-Peebles, P. N., & Maddalena, A. (1996). Longitudinal study of cognitive abilities and adaptive behavior levels in fragile X males: a prospective multicenter analysis. *American Journal of Medical Genetics, 64*, 356–361.

Freund, L. S., Peebles, C. D., Aylward, E., & Reiss, A. L. (1995). Preliminary report on cognitive and adaptive behaviours of preschool-aged males with fragile X. *Developmental Brain Dysfunction, 8*, 242–251.

Freund, L. S., & Reiss, A. L. (1991). Cognitive profiles associated with the fra(X) syndrome in males and females. *American Journal of Medical Genetics, 38*, 542–547.

Glaser, B., Hessl, D., Dyer-Friedman, J., Johnstone, C., Wisbeck, J., Taylor, A., & Reiss, A. (2003). Biological and environmental contributions to adaptive behaviour in fragile X syndrome. *American Journal of Medical Genetics, 117A*, 21–29.

Gleitman, L. R., & Gillette, J. (1995). The role of syntax in verb learning. In P. Fletcher, & B. MacWhinney (Eds.), *The handbook of child language* (pp. 413–427). Oxford: Blackwell.

Glucksberg, S., Krauss, R., & Higgins, E. T. (1975). The development of referential communication skills. In F. D. Horowitz (Ed.), *Review of child development research* (Vol. 4, pp. 305–346). Chicago: University of Chicago Press.

Graesser, A. C., Millis, K. K., & Zwaan, R. A. (1997). Discourse comprehension. In J. T. Spence, J. M. Darley, & D. J. Foss (Eds.), *Annual review of psychology* (pp. 163–189). Palo Alto, CA: The Annual Reviews, Inc.

Greenough, W. T., Klintsova, A. Y., Irwin, S. A., Galvez, R., Bates, K. E., & Weiler, I. J. (2001). Synaptic regulation of protein synthesis and the fragile X protein. *Proceedings of the National Academy of Sciences of the United States of America, 98*, 7101–7106.

Hagerman, R. J. (1996). Physical and behavioral phenotype. In R. J. Hagerman, & A. Cronister (Eds.), *Fragile X Syndrome: Diagnosis, treatment, and research* (pp. 3–87). Baltimore, MD: The Johns Hopkins University Press.

Hagerman, R. J. (1999). *Neurodevelopmental disorders*. Oxford: Oxford University Press.

Hagerman, R. J. (2002). The physical and behavioral phenotype. In R. J. Hagerman & P. J. Hagerman (Eds.), *Fragile X syndrome: Diagnosis, treatment, and research* (3rd ed.). Baltimore, MD: Johns Hopkins University Press.

Harris, S., Kasari, C., & Sigman, M. D. (1996). Joint attention and language gains in children with Down syndrome. *American Journal on Mental Retardation, 100*, 608–619.

Hatton, D. D., Bailey, D. B., Hargett-Beck, M. Q., Skinner, M., & Clark, R. D. (1999). Behavioral style of young boys with fragile X syndrome. *Developmental Medicine and Child Neurology, 41*, 625–632.

Hessl, D. (2002, July). *Is it all genes? The impact of environmental and neurohormonal variables on outcome in children with fragile X*. Paper presented at the 8th International Fragile X Conference, Chicago, IL.

Hodapp, R. M. (1997). Direct and indirect behavioral effects on different genetic disorders of mental retardation. *American Journal on Mental Retardation, 102*, 67–79.

Hodapp, R. M., & Dykens, E. M. (2001). Strengthening behavioral research on genetic mental retardation syndromes. *American Journal on Mental Retardation, 106*, 4–15.

Hodapp, R. M., & Zigler, E. (1997). New issues in the developmental approach to mental retardation. In Williams E. MacLean (Ed.), *Ellis' Handbook of Mental Deficiency, Psychological Theory, and Research* (pp. 115–136). Mahwah, NJ: Lawrence Erlbaum Associates.

Johnson-Glenberg, M., & Chapman, R. S. (in press). Predictors of parent–child language during novel task play: a comparison between children who are typically developing and individuals with Down syndrome. *Journal of Intellectual Disability Research.*

Jones, J. E., & Doane, J. A. (1979). Communication deviance scoring manual. Unpublished manuscript.

Kasari, C., Sigman, M. D., Mundy, P., & Yirmiya, N. (1990). Affective sharing in the context of joint attention interactions of normal, autistic, and mentally retarded children. *Journal of Autism and Developmental Disorders, 20*, 87–100.

Kau, A. S., Meyer, W. A., & Kaufmann, W. E. (2002). Early development in males with fragile X syndrome: a review of the literature. *Microscopy Research & Technique, 57*, 174–178.

Kau, S. M. A., Reider, E. E., Payne, L., Meyer, A. W., & Freund, L. (2000). Early behaviour signs of Miller, J. F. (1991). Quantifying productive language disorders. In J. F. Miller (Ed.), *New directions in research in child language disorders*. Austin, TX: Pro-Ed.

Keysor, C. S., & Mazzocco, M. M. M. (2002). A developmental approach to understanding Fragile X syndrome in females. *Microscopy Research and Technique, 57*, 179–186.

Kuo, A. Y., Reiss, A. L., Freund, L. S., & Huffman, L. C. (2002). Family environment and cognitive abilities in girls with fragile X syndrome. *Journal of Intellectual Disabilities Research, 46*, 328–339.

Kwon, H., Menon, V., Eliez, S., Warsofsky, I. S., White, C. D., Dyer-Friedman, J., Taylor, A. K., Glover, G. H., & Reiss, A. L. (2001). Functional neuroanatomy of visuospatial working memory in fragile X syndrome: relation to behavioral and molecular measures. *American Journal of Psychiatry, 158*, 1040–1051.

Lachiewicz, A. M., Spiridigliozzi, G. A., Gullion, C. M., Ransford, S. N., & Rao, K. (1994). Aberrant behaviors of young boys with fragile X syndrome. *American Journal of Mental Retardation, 98*, 567–579.

Landry, S. H., & Chapieski, M. L. (1989). Joint attention and infant toy exploration: Effects of Down syndrome and prematurity. *Child Development, 60*, 103–118.

Leekam, S., & Moore, C. (2001). The development of attention and joint attention in children with autism. In J. A. Burack & T. Charman (Eds.), *The development of autism: Perspectives from theory and research* (pp. 105–129). Mahwah, NJ: Lawrence Erlbaum Associates.

Loveland, K. A., & Landry, S. H. (1986). Joint attention and language in autism and developmental language delay. *Journal of Autism and Developmental Disorders, 16*, 335–349.

Madison, L. S., George, C., & Moeschler, J. B. (1986). Cognitive functioning in the fragile X syndrome: a study of intellectual, memory, and communication skills. *Journal of Mental Deficiency Research, 30*, 129–148.

Markus, J., Mundy, P., Morales, M., Delgado, C. E. F., & Yale, M. (2000). Individual differences in infant skills as predictors of child–caregiver joint attention and language. *Social Development, 9*, 302–315.

Mazzocco, M. M. M. (2000). Advances in research on the fragile X syndrome. *Mental Retardation and Developmental Disabilities Research Reviews, 6*, 96–106.

Mazzocco, M. M. M., Baumgardner, T., Freund, L. S., & Reiss, A. L. (1998). Social functioning among girls with fragile X or Turner syndrome and their sisters. *Journal of Autism and Developmental Disorders, 28*, 509–517.

Mazzocco, M. M., Pennington, B. F., & Hagerman, R. J. (1993). The neurocognitive phenotype of female carriers of fragile X: additional evidence for specificity. *Journal of Developmental & Behavioral Pediatrics, 14*, 328–335.

Mc Tear, M., & Conti-Ramsden, G. (1992). *Pragmatic disability in children*. London: Whurr Publishers.

Menon, V., Kwon, H., Eliez, S., Taylor, A. K., & Reiss, A. L. (2000). Functional brain activation during cognition is related to FMR1 gene expression. *Brain Research, 877*, 367–370.

Mervis, C. B., & Robinson, B. F. (1999). Methodological issues in cross-syndrome comparisons: matching procedures, sensitivity (Se) and specificity (Sp). *Monographs of the Society for Research in Child Development, 64*, 115–130.

Miller, L. J., McIntosh, D. N., McGrath, J., Shyu, V., Lampe, M., Taylor, A. K., et al. (1999). Electrodermal responses to sensory stimuli in individuals with fragile X syndrome: A preliminary report. *American Journal of Medical Genetics, 83*, 268–279.

Mundy, P., & Gomes, A. (1998). Individual differences in joint attention skill development in the second year. *Infant Behavior and Development, 21*, 469–482.

Mundy, P., Kasari, C., Sigman, M. D., & Ruskin, E. (1995). Nonverbal communication and early language acquisition in children with Down syndrome and in normally developing children. *Journal of Speech and Hearing Research, 38*, 157–167.

Mundy, P., & Neal, R. (2001). Neural plasticity, joint attention, and a transactional social-orienting model of autism. *International Review of Research in Mental Retardation, 23*, 139–168.

Ninio, A., & Snow, C. E. (1996). *Pragmatic development*. Boulder, Colorado: Westview Press.

Oostra, B. A. (1996). FMR1 protein studies and animal model for fragile X syndrome. In R. J. Hagerman & A. C. Cronister (Eds.), *Fragile X syndrome: Diagnosis, treatment, and research* (2nd ed., pp. 193–209). Baltimore: Johns Hopkins University Press.

Paul, R., Cohen, D. J., Breg, R., Watson, M., & Herman, S. (1984). Fragile X syndrome: its relations to speech and language disorders. *Journal of Speech and Hearing Disorders, 49*, 326–336.

Paul, R., Dykens, E., Leckman, F., Watson, M., Breg, W. R., & Cohen, D. J. (1987). A comparison of language characteristics of mentally retarded adults with fragile X syndrome and those with nonspecific mental retardation and autism. *Journal of Autism and Developmental Disorders, 17*, 457–468.

Pavetto, M. M. (2001). *Gender differences in repetitive language among males and females with fragile X syndrome*. Unpublished master's thesis, University of Wisconsin-Madison, Wisconsin.

Pavetto, M. M., & Abbeduto, L. (2002a). *Characteristics of expressive language among males and females with fragile X syndrome*. Poster presented at the Annual Meeting of the Academy of Mental Retardation, Orlando, FL.

Pavetto, M. M., & Abbeduto, L. (2002b). *Gender differences in repetitive talk among adolescents with fragile X syndrome*. Paper presented at the 126th Annual Meeting of the American Association on Mental Retardation, San Diego, CA.

Philofsky, A., Hepburn, S. L., Hayes, A., Rogers, S. J., & Hagerman, R. J. (2002, July). *Language profiles in young children with fragile X: Comparisons with autism and Down syndrome*. Paper presented at the 8th International Fragile X Conference, Chicago, IL.

Pinker, S. (1994). *The language instinct*. New York: Harper Collins.

Prouty, L. A., Rogers, R. C., Stevenson, R. E., Dean, J. H., Palmer, K. K., Simensen, R. J., et al. (1988). Fragile X syndrome: growth, development, and intellectual function. *American Journal of Medical Genetics, 30*, 123–142.

Roberts, J. E., Mirrett, P., & Burchinal, M. (2001). Receptive and expressive communication development of young males with fragile X syndrome. *American Journal on Mental Retardation, 106*, 216–230.

Rogers, S. J., Whener, E. A., & Hagerman, R. (2002). The behavioural phenotype of fragile X: symptoms of autism in very young children with fragile X syndrome, idiopathic autism and other developmental disorders. *Developmental and Behavioral Pediatrics, 6*, 409–417.

Rosenberg, S., & Abbeduto, L. (1993). *Language and communication in mental retardation: development, processes, and intervention*. Hillsdale, NJ: Lawrence Erlbaum Associates.

Saffran, J., Newport, A., & Aslin, R. (1996). Statistical learning by 8-month-old infants. *Science, 274*, 1926–1928.

Scarr, S. (1992). Developmental theories for the 1990s: development and individual differences. *Child Development, 63*, 1–19.

Scarr, S. (1993). Biological and cultural diversity: the legacy of Darwin for development. *Child Development, 64*, 1333–1353.

Simon, J. A., Keenan, J. M., Pennington, B. F., Taylor, A. K., & Hagerman, R. J. (2001). Discourse processing in women with fragile X syndrome: evidence for a deficit establishing coherence. *Cognitive Neuropsychology, 18*, 1–18.

Skinner, B. F. (1957). *Verbal behavior*. Englewood Cliffs, NJ: Prentice-Hall.

Sobesky, W. E., Taylor, A. K., Pennington, B. F., Bennetto, L., Porter, D., Riddle, J., & Hagerman, R. J. (1996). Molecular/clinical correlations in females with fragile X. *American Journal of Medical Genetics, 64*(2), 340–345.

Sparrow, S. S., Balla, D. A., & Cicchetti, D. V. (1984). *Vineland adaptive behavior scales*. Circle Pines, MN: American Guidance Co.

Sudhalter, V. (2002, July). *The role of hyperarousal and inhibitory control deficits in the speech and language difficulties of individuals with fragile X*. Symposium conducted at the 8th International Fragile X Conference, Chicago, IL.

Sudhalter, V., Cohen, I. L., Silverman, W., & Wolf-Schein, E. G. (1990). Conversational analyses of males with fragile X, Down syndrome, and autism: comparison of the emergence of deviant language. *American Journal on Mental Retardation, 94*, 431–441.

Sudhalter, V., Maranion, M., & Brooks, P. (1992). Expressive semantic deficit in the productive language of males with fragile X syndrome. *American Journal of Medical Genetics, 43*, 65–71.

Sudhalter, V., Scarborough, H. S., & Cohen, I. L. (1991). Syntactic delay and pragmatic deviance in the language of fragile X males. *American Journal of Medical Genetics, 38*, 493–497.

Tomasello, M., & Todd, J. (1983). Joint attention and lexical acquisition style. *First Language, 4*, 197–212.

Van Lieshout, C. F. M., De Meyer, R. E., Curfs, L. M., & Fryns, J. P. (1998). Family contexts, parental behaviour, and personality profiles of children and adolescents with Prader-Willi, fragile-X, or Williams syndrome. *Journal of Child Psychology and Psychiatry, 39*, 699–710.

Wisbeck, J. M., Huffman, L. C., Freund, L., Gunnar, M., Davis, E. P., & Reiss, A. L. (2000). Cortisol and social stressors in children with fragile X: a pilot study. *Developmental and Behavioral Pediatrics, 21*, 279–282.

Wolf, P. H., Gardner, J., Paccia, J., & Lappen, J. (1989). The greeting behavior of fragile X males. *American Journal on Mental Retardation, 93*, 406–411.

York, A., von Fraunhofer, N., Turk, J., & Sedgwick, P. (1999). Fragile X syndrome, Down's syndrome and autism: awareness and knowledge amongst special educators. *Journal of Intellectual Disabilities Research, 43*, 314–324.

On Becoming Socially Competent Communicators: The Challenge for Children with Fetal Alcohol Exposure

TRUMAN E. COGGINS

CENTER ON HUMAN DEVELOPMENT AND DISABILITY
UNIVERSITY OF WASHINGTON, SEATTLE, WASHINGTON

LESLEY B. OLSWANG

SPEECH AND HEARING SCIENCES
UNIVERSITY OF WASHINGTON, SEATTLE, WASHINGTON

HEATHER CARMICHAEL OLSON

PSYCHIATRY AND BEHAVIORAL SCIENCES
UNIVERSITY OF WASHINGTON, SEATTLE, WASHINGTON

GERALYN R. TIMLER

DEPARTMENT OF COMMUNICATIVE DISORDERS
SUNY AT BUFFALO, NEW YORK

I. INTRODUCTION

More than a generation has passed since fetal alcohol syndrome (FAS) was formally identified as a birth defect (Jones & Smith, 1973). Much of the information that has accumulated over the past 30 years has focused on

0074-7750/2003 $35.00

describing characteristic features of the syndrome and demonstrating the teratogenic effects that prenatal alcohol exposure can have on fetal development (see Carmichael Olson, Morse, & Huffine, 1998; Mattson & Riley, 1998; Thomas, Kelly, Mattson, & Riley, 1998; Streissguth, 1997). Clinical and epidemiology data in humans (see Driscoll, Streissguth, & Riley, 1990), paralleling a large body of experimental animal research (see Astley, Magnuson, Omnell, & Clarren, 1999), reveal that alcohol exposure has a broad range of deleterious effects on growth and development. High levels of prenatal alcohol exposure can interfere with the developing brain at multiple levels and cause lifelong disabilities (Streissguth, Barr, Kogan, & Bookstein, 1997).

Clinical researchers have explored developmental outcomes of fetal alcohol exposed children. The results reveal a population of children who seem less adept than their age peers at benefiting from experience, who struggle to keep track of important pieces of information, who have difficulty understanding logical consequences and, not surprisingly, experience remarkable difficulty during social interactions (Kleinfeld & Wescott, 1993; Spohr, Willms, & Steinhausen, 1993a, 1993b; Thomas et al., 1998). The social and behavioral problems appear to become more pronounced during the school years and coincide with problems in adaptive behavior and secondary disabilities, such as mental health problems and educational failures (Streissguth, 1997).

Investigators, clinicians and parents have identified a variety of language problems in fetal alcohol exposed children (see Carmichael Olson et al., 1998). The findings from several recent studies at the University of Washington suggest that children with significant prenatal alcohol exposure have limitations in their interpersonal uses of language, particularly when confronted with the demands associated with more sophisticated social interactions (Coggins, Friet, & Morgan, 1998; Olswang, Coggins, & Timler, 2001; Timler, 2000; Timler & Olswang, 2001). These findings add further support to the notion that children with social problems often present with co-occurring conditions that include language problems (Guralnick, 1999; Redmond & Rice, 1998, 2002). The findings also suggest that the social communicative performance of children with high levels of prenatal alcohol exposure may vary as a function of environmental demands.

The ability to use language appropriately in different contexts is critical for social success. To date, research with children who have been exposed to high levels of prenatal alcohol has largely ignored this basic tenet of language acquisition. The purpose of this paper is to present a social communicative framework for understanding and examining why these children have such difficulty using language interpersonally. To create this framework, we first present demographic and descriptive data. We also briefly consider the challenges that clinicians and researchers have routinely encountered diagnosing children who have been exposed to alcohol in utero. We then summarize the findings from a variety of studies that have focused on the cognitive, social and language abilities of this clinical population. Building on this information, we then argue that deficits in these areas create special problems in the way children communicate during social interactions. Based on this argument, we present the reader with a conceptual framework for considering social communication competence. The framework provides the basis for research and clinical practice focused on the social communicative competence of children with prenatal alcohol exposure.

II. INCIDENCE, IDENTIFICATION AND INCLUSION

A. Incidence

Alcohol is the most frequently ingested teratogen in the world (Streissguth, 1997). In the United States, data from the National Co-morbidity Study indicate that one in four people between the ages of 15 and 54 have a substance abuse disorder at some point in life. Of all individuals with a substance abuse disorder, a striking 88% have an alcohol disorder with or without other drug involvement. Moreover, men and women in their peak childbearing years (i.e., ages 18–34) are two to four times more likely to have a DSM-IV alcohol dependence diagnosis than are individuals in other age ranges (Zucker et al., 2000). Because so many women drink alcohol during pregnancy, disabilities associated with alcohol have been estimated to occur in as many as six per thousand live births (Institute of Medicine [IOM], 1996). Using this estimate, 2000–12,000 of the projected four million children born each year in the United States are likely to have an alcohol spectrum disorder. The incidence of disorders linked to alcohol is greater than that of children born with chromosomal disorders, metabolic or exocrine disorders, or specific neurological disorders (Plumridge, Bennett, Dinno, & Branson, 1993; Streissguth, 1997).

B. Identification

Alcohol is a neurobehavioral teratogen that can cause permanent defects in the structure and/or function of the central nervous system (CNS). The timing, quantity and/or pattern of maternal drinking can determine the impact on CNS development (Astley et al., 1999). Sampson et al. (1997) demonstrated that maternal drinking patterns associated with the highest risk to the developing fetus are those in which drinking occurs early in pregnancy and in which "binge" drinking occurs. Prenatal alcohol exposure can interfere with the developing brain at multiple levels and alter the coordinated developmental schedule of the entire central nervous system (Carmichael Olson et al., 1998).

Teratogenic alcohol exposure has a broad range of individually variable effects. For example, while virtually all children exposed to teratogenic doses of alcohol have alterations in brain functioning (Astley & Clarren, 2000), a sizable majority have IQ scores within the normal range (Carmichael Olson et al., 1998). Further, the interpersonal interactions of children with FAS and associated clinical conditions range from mildly impaired (e.g., difficulty interacting with peers) to severely abnormal (e.g., physical aggression against others) (Roebuck, Mattson, & Riley, 1999; Streissguth et al., 1997; Thomas et al., 1998; Timler, 2000). Finally, notable variability occurs in the linguistic performance of these children and their use of language for communicative purposes (Coggins et al., 1998). This means that children with high levels of prenatal alcohol-exposure are a heterogeneous group, not unlike other clinical populations, with varying levels of compromise that create a variety of outcomes.

The effects of prenatal alcohol exposure fall on a continuum with fetal alcohol syndrome (FAS) at one end and relative normal growth and development at the other. Interestingly, most children exposed to alcohol during gestation do not present with the complete fetal alcohol syndrome. The National Institute on Alcohol Abuse and Alcoholism (1997) has estimated that even among children with significant prenatal exposure histories, there are approximately three times as many children who manifest a partial expression of the FAS condition as there are children with the complete syndrome. Over the years, a variety of diagnostic terms have been introduced to characterize children with prenatal alcohol exposure who do not meet the complete FAS criteria. These terms have included "fetal alcohol effects" (FAE) (Clarren & Smith 1978), "alcohol-related neurodevelopmental disorders" (ARND) (IOM, 1996), "alcohol-related birth defects" (ARBD) (Sampson, Kerr, Carmichael Olson et al., 1997) and, most recently, "fetal alcohol spectrum disorders" (O'Malley & Hagerman, 1998).

Numerous behavioral characteristics and associated physical features occur between the ends of this alcohol continuum. Mattson and Riley (1998) aptly note that the impressive range of clinical conditions is "representative of the continuous nature of alcohol's behavioral teratogenicity" (p. 279). Because FAS represents only one discrete point on this continuum, it is imperative for researchers and clinicians to evaluate the impact of prenatal alcohol on all exposed children.

C. Inclusion

FAS is widely regarded as the most recognizable teratogenic effect of prenatal alcohol exposure. This birth defect syndrome is characterized by abnormalities in three areas (Rosett & Weiner, 1984):

1. Prenatal and/or postnatal growth retardation—Below the 10th percentile for weight and/or length when corrected for gestational age.
2. A set of minor facial anomalies—Specifically, short palpebral fissures, a long and flattened philtrum and thin upper lip.
3. Brain dysfunction—Alterations include neurological abnormality, developmental delay, structural abnormalities or brain malformation (found through brain imaging).

Trained clinicians, dysmorphologists or clinical geneticists have little difficulty in making the diagnosis of FAS when "anomalies in growth, face and brain are extreme and the alcohol exposure is conclusive and substantial" (Astley & Clarren, 2000, p. 400). However, as noted earlier, the clinical features associated with prenatal alcohol exposure are rarely "fully" present or "altogether" absent. Nominal scales have traditionally been used to capture differences in the growth, facial morphology and brain functioning. In fact, virtually all of the investigations reviewed in the following section have used nominal scales. Unfortunately, the terms that investigators and clinicians have used to identify children with prenatal alcohol histories, particularly FAE, ARND and ARBD, lack precision and equivalence.

In an attempt to reliably diagnose this clinical population, an interdisciplinary research team at the University of Washington has introduced a new methodology for examining the spectrum of disabilities present among children with fetal alcohol exposure (Clarren, Carmichael Olson, Clarren, & Astley, 2000). The "4-Digit Diagnostic Code" is a descriptive, case-defined approach that uses quantitative scales to measure and report outcomes (Astley & Clarren, 2000, 2001; Clarren et al., 2000). The 4-Digit Diagnostic Code is presented in Figure 1.

The four digits of the diagnostic code reflect the magnitude of expression of key FAS features. These features include: (1) growth deficiency; (2) facial phenotype; (3) brain dysfunction or damage; and (4) teratogenic exposure to alcohol. A "1" on any scale characteristic signals a finding within the normal range. In contrast, a "4" reveals a finding consistent with confirmed cases of FAS. Scores of "2" or "3" represent intermediate steps between average and atypical. Each four-point scale thus reflects the degree of confidence "that the sought FAS characteristic is present" (Clarren et al., 2000).

Significant	Severe	Definite	4			
Moderate	Moderate	Probable	3			
Mild	Mild	Possible	2			
None	Absent	Unlikely	1			
Growth Deficiency	**Facial Phenotype**	**Brain Dysfunction**	**Numeric Code**	Growth	Face	Brain

:

High Risk	High Risk	High Risk	4			
Some Risk	Some Risk	Some Risk	3			
Unknown	Unknown	Unknown	2			
No Risk	No Risk	No Risk	1			
Prenatal Alcohol	**Pre-Natal Conditions**	**Post-Natal Conditions**	**Numeric Code**	Alcohol	Pre Natal	Post Natal

FIG. 1. A diagnostic code grid for quantifying the spectrum of disabilities among children with fetal alcohol exposure (following Astley & Clarren, 2000, 2001).

The alcohol exposure scale is based on dose exposure patterns that cause fetal damage in animal models. An example of a "4" on this scale would be a woman who consumed enough alcohol to cause drunkenness on a weekly basis throughout the first trimester of pregnancy. The system also includes ratings for prenatal (e.g., nutrition, prescription and non-prescription medications) and postnatal (e.g., physical or sexual abuse) co-morbidities in order to account for other developmental influences.

Although FAS is a recognizable syndrome, the diagnosis cannot be reliably established by one professional on the basis of a single distinctive feature or laboratory test (Carmichael Olson et al., 1998). The spectrum of individuals with fetal alcohol exposure has made differential diagnosis a challenging proposition, and one that is most likely accomplished in the context of an interdisciplinary team assessment (Clarren et al., 2000). To increase the accuracy of characterizing the full spectrum of disabilities associated with prenatal alcohol exposure, several research teams at the University of Washington have used the quantitative measurement scales and specific case definitions of the 4-Digit Diagnostic Code (Astley, Clarren, Stachowiak, & Clausen, 2001; Carmichael Olson et al., under review; Timler, Olswang, & Coggins, under review). However, most investigators have yet to consider this approach for studying children who show some, but not all, of the features of the full FAS syndrome. Future investigations will establish the clinical utility of using quantitative scales in measuring and reporting different behavioral outcomes as well as designing differential interventions.

III. BEHAVIORAL PHENOTYPE

Abnormal brain development is regarded as the most debilitating outcome associated with high prenatal alcohol exposure (Carmichael Olson et al., 1998; Carmichael Olson, Feldman, Streissguth, Sampson, & Bookstein, 1998). Children with conditions associated with fetal alcohol exposure exhibit diminished cognitive capacity, atypical neuropsychological functioning, and remarkable social problems (Coles et al., 1997; Mattson & Riley, 1998; Streissguth Barr, Kogan, & Bookstein, 1996). The difficulty in reasoning and problem-solving has led some to characterize these children as "living in a new world each day" (Kleinfeld & Wescott, 1993).

IV. COGNITION

A. Intellectual Functioning

Interestingly, mental retardation is not a defining feature of an alcohol spectrum disability. Although overall intelligence can be compromised, the majority of individuals with full or partial expression of FAS have intellectual functioning broadly within the normal range. Streissguth et al. (1996) examined the cognitive abilities of 473 individuals with FAS and clinical conditions associated with prenatal alcohol exposure. Primary disabilities were documented with an age-appropriate *Wechsler* intelligence scale. The investigators found that 73% of individuals with the full expression of FAS and 91% of individuals with high levels of prenatal alcohol exposure performed broadly within the average range. Mean IQ for the former group was 79 (range 29–120) whereas the latter group attained a mean IQ of 90 (range 42–142).

B. Neuropsychological Functioning

A growing number of neuropsychological investigations have provided more specific descriptions of FAS and clinical conditions associated with heavy prenatal alcohol exposure (Coles et al., 1997; Conry, 1990; Janzen, Nanson, & Block, 1995; Nanson, 1990). Virtually all individuals exposed to teratogenic levels of alcohol show specific cognitive deficits, even those with IQs in the normal range (Kerns, Don, Mateer, & Streissguth, 1997). Findings from executive function testing have revealed some commonalties in neuropsychological profiles. Limitations in concept formation and planning, response inhibition and self-regulation have been documented (Jacobson & Jacobson, 1997; Kodituwakku, Handmaker, Cutler, Weathersby, & Handmaker, 1995; Kopara-Frye, Dehaene, & Streissguth, 1996; Mattson, Goodman, Caine, Delis, & Riley, 1999). Researchers have also identified deficits in attention, memory and learning (Coles et al., 1997; Mattson & Riley, 1998; Uecker & Nadel, 1996). Mattson and Riley (1998) have argued that not only are attention deficits frequently observed, they do not resolve over time. Hyperactivity, frequently reported in younger alcohol exposed children, appears to manifest itself in adolescence as problematic social behavior (National Institute on Alcohol Abuse & Alcoholism, 1997).

Several investigators have reported that processing limitations constrain the amount of information fetal alcohol exposed children can manipulate when solving complex problems. Kodituwakku et al. (1995) investigated the performance of 10 school-age children and adolescents with high prenatal alcohol exposure and 10 control peers, on difficult puzzles that involved manipulating information in memory. The two groups of participants were matched on receptive vocabulary. The participants with alcohol exposure demonstrated "severely impaired performances" on tasks that required them to retain, manipulate, and manage more complex amounts of information. In a related study, Carmichael Olson et al. (1998) also found difficulties in processing speed and accuracy in nine adolescents with FAS. Kerns et al. (1997) administered a battery of intellectual and neuropsychological tests to 16 young adults with clinical conditions associated with prenatal alcohol exposure. Half the participants had full scale IQs well within the normal range of intellectual functioning (range 90–118). Nevertheless, these eight participants had remarkably lower performance levels than expected on tasks that required higher levels of processing. Collectively, these findings suggest that processing constraints may compromise planning and decision-making of children with high prenatal alcohol exposure.

Processing limitations may also interfere with social performance and language performance. Timler et al. (under review) assessed the social and neuropsychological development of three school-aged children with FAS. To document social competence and adaptive functioning, the investigators had the parents of these children complete the *Social Skills Rating System* (*SSRS*) (Gresham & Elliot, 1990). The *SSRS* is "a broad assessment of social behaviors that can affect teacher–student relations, peer acceptance and academic performance" (p. 1). The parents rated their respective children as having remarkable difficulty interacting effectively; for example, asking permission before using another person's property or controlling one's temper in conflict situations. As a result, the three children were enrolled in a treatment project designed to improve their effectiveness in solving social conflicts. As part of the pre-intervention assessment, the *Developmental Neuropsychological Assessment* (*NEPSY*) (Korkman, Kirk, & Kemp, 1998) was administered to each child. The *NEPSY* examines processing abilities considered critical for learning. The results for the *SSRS* and *NEPSY* are presented in Figure 2.

C# CHILD #	*CA*	*Social Skills Rating Scale* Problem Behaviors Domain (PBDSS) - (Scores > 1 SD above the mean are viewed as "clinical concern") - (Mean = 100; SD = 15)	*A Developmental Neuropsychological Assessment (NEPSY)* - Clinical Interpretation of performance
# 1	9;8	PBDSS 133	Difficulties in immediate and delayed visual memory, memory for visual–verbal paired-associate learning and retrieval. Problems in visual-motor precision; tendency to impulsively and rapidly complete tasks, trading reduced accuracy for increased speed in performance.
# 2	12;3	PBDSS 138	Loss of information from memory after a time delay, difficulties in processing speed.
# 3	10;1	PBDSS 133	Considerable scatter in individual subtest scores. Difficulty with auditory attention, narrative memory, comprehension of spoken and complex instructions, verbal fluency.

FIG. 2. Results (quantitative and descriptive) of the Social Skills Rating System (*SSRS*) and Developmental Neuropsychological Assessment (*NEPSY*) for three school-age children with fetal alcohol syndrome.

The standard scores of all three children on the Problem Behavior Domain of the *SSRS* placed them in the "clinical range." Results of the *NEPSY* revealed that the three children demonstrated an array of processing deficits. These findings are consistent with the variable processing abilities reported by Kodituwakku et al. (1995), Carmichael Olson et al. (1998) and Kerns et al. (1997). Timler and Olswang (2001) have also suggested that processing limitations may interfere with both social performance and complex language performance of children with FAS, especially as environmental demands increase.

V. SOCIAL INTERACTION

A diverse collection of social problems has been reported for children with prenatal alcohol exposure. The evidence has been gathered from three different perspectives: (1) parental report (e.g., Caldwell, 1993; Dorris, 1989; Wright, 1992); (2) case study (e.g., Rathbun, 1993); and (3) controlled clinical investigations (e.g., Carmichael Olson et al., 1998; Thomas et al., 1998; Timler, 2000). All three lines of inquiry have documented the difficulty these children have in establishing and maintaining social relationships. Overall, it appears that many of the social problems exceed what would be expected for IQ level. Moreover, the evidence suggests that these problematic behaviors become more challenging as children grow older and social demands increase.

Hinde (1993) has observed that children with alcohol spectrum disorders have "a hard time figuring out what is going on in social life and how they should behave in different situations" (p. 139). Caldwell (1993) has noted that children with prenatal alcohol exposure also seem to have genuine difficulty anticipating the consequences of their actions, which is compounded by the seeming inability to empathize.

Clinical researchers have also documented an array of social problems in this population. Steinhausen, Willms, and Spohr (1993) investigated 158 participants with FAS and prenatal alcohol exposure who ranged in age from 3 to 18. The Steinhausen research team followed their participants for various intervals, ranging from 3 to 10 years. During the study, caregivers and teachers completed several adaptive behavior measures over the course of the school-age years. Compared to the normative sample, Steinhausen's alcohol-exposed participants were deficient when it came to solving social problems. Moreover, these deficits were consistent over time and observed by both parents and teachers. The limited "social savvy" displayed by this clinical population seriously compromised their interpersonal interactions and social uses of communication and placed them at heightened risk for "secondary disabilities," such as mental health problems, disruptions in school or employment and legal trouble (Streissguth et al., 1996).

Streissguth et al. (1997) have provided evidence from a large cohort that links social problems with heavy prenatal alcohol exposure. The research team interviewed the caregivers of 415 participants with alcohol spectrum disorders who were between the ages of 6 and 51 to determine the nature and prevalence of "secondary disabilities." The Streissguth team defined "secondary disabilities as problems in lifestyle and daily function believed to be a consequence of primary cognitive difficulties." Mental health problems were found in 94% of the sample, whereas 60% of the older participants experienced disrupted school experiences. Closer examination of caregiver interview data for 80 adolescent and adult participants revealed that more than 50% had limited ability to use language to manage socially frustrating experiences. Not surprisingly, all of these participants reported employment difficulties.

Social problems associated with teratogenic levels of prenatal alcohol exposure are not solely the result of decreased cognitive functioning (Streissguth et al., 1996; Thomas et al., 1998). Thomas et al. (1998) compared the social behaviors of 15 children with the complete expression of FAS to 15 children with similar verbal IQ scores (VIQ) and 15 typically developing controls (TDC), all between the ages of 5;7 and 12;11 years. Social behaviors were measured with the *Vineland Adaptive Behavior Scales—Summary Version* (*VABS*) via interviews with caregivers. The research team found significant between-group differences on the *VABS*, with TDC > VIQ > FAS. Differences persisted even when socioeconomic status was controlled. An inspection of the Socialization subtest of the *VABS* revealed that "interpersonal relationships" was the most substantially impaired area of Socialization for the FAS group. Further, there was a significant positive correlation between age and performance for the FAS participants but not for the other two groups. Thomas and colleagues argued that socialization deficits in children with FAS went beyond what could be explained by lower IQ. They suggested that these children were not simply developmentally delayed in their social skills, as would be the case if they continued to lag a few years behind same-age peers. Instead, they reasoned that "children with FAS appear to plateau in social abilities at about the 4- to 6-year level, which suggests arrested development" (p. 532).

Timler (2000) documented the social difficulties of nine children with high levels of prenatal alcohol exposure through the use of parent and teacher reports. She examined social behaviors using two norm-referenced behavioral rating scales of social competence: *Social Skills Rating System* (*SSRS*) (Gresham & Elliot, 1990) and *Taxonomy of Problematic Social Situations for Children* (*TOPS*) (Dodge, McClaskey, & Feldman, 1985). As noted above, the *SSRS* uses rating scales to identify children at risk for social behavior difficulties and poor academic performance. The *TOPS* is a 44-item, five-point rating scale used to identify the presence and severity of children's social difficulties across six distinct situations: (1) peer entry (e.g., child does not attempt to join a group at recess); (2) response to peer provocation (e.g., child responds aggressively to peer teasing); (3) response to failure (e.g., child does not ask for assistance when needed); (4) response to success (e.g., child performs better than a peer at a game); (5) social expectations (e.g., child does not cooperate with peers during group activity); and (6) teacher expectations (e.g., child does not follow classroom directions).

Using these scales, Timler compared the social skills of the nine children with FAS and clinical conditions associated with prenatal alcohol exposure to nine typically developing peers matched for age, gender, and receptive vocabulary. None of the children in Timler's study had been formally diagnosed with a social–emotional or behavioral disorder. Teachers completed the *SSRS* and *TOPS*, and parents rated the occurrence of problem behaviors using the *SSRS*. The data revealed significantly higher scores for the alcohol-exposed group from their parents and teachers on the Problem Behaviors domain of the *SSRS*. Further, compared to the typically developing peers, the participants with high prenatal alcohol exposure had significantly higher scores on four situation subscales of the *TOPS*: peer entry; response to peer provocation; response to failure; and social expectations. These results suggest that peer-related social problems observed in children with prenatal alcohol exposure may reflect a compromised ability to effectively deploy problem-solving strategies rather than an underlying social–emotional/behavioral disorder (Redmond & Rice, 1998).

In an effort to describe these social problems further, Timler (2000) presented 12 *social conflict vignettes* to her participants. Each hypothetical vignette described a conflict with a peer that the children were to resolve. A sample conflict vignette follows.

> "You and some friends are playing soccer. It is a close game and you are excited to see who will win. The soccer ball flies off the field and another friend who is not in the game runs to get it. She/he will not give the ball back to you."

Children were shown each vignette via computer presentation then asked an open-ended statement to elicit strategies for resolving the conflict (i.e., "Tell me all the things you can say or do!"). Following the open-ended statement, they were presented with possible choices of strategies for resolving the conflict (i.e., "Tell me what is the first thing you would say or do." "If you said or did *child's 'first' strategy here*, what will your friends say or do?"). Finally, they were asked what they hoped to accomplish with the strategies (e.g., "Tell me why you would say or do that.").

Results indicated no significant differences in the goals that the nine children selected. However, significant between-group differences were found in the strategies selected to achieve those goals. In the open-ended condition, typically developing children selected more *pro-social* strategies.

Pro-social strategies included accommodating the needs of both parties, suggesting ways to compromise, asking for more information, or making polite requests. The nine children in the alcohol-exposed group selected *anti-social* strategies (hostile/coercive comments, assertive behaviors, adult-seeking and passive remarks) more often than their matched peers. Further, all but one typically developing child produced more pro-social than anti-social strategies; conversely, eight of the nine children with an alcohol spectrum disorder produced more anti-social strategies than pro-social strategies. In the forced-choice condition, again the typically developing children produced significantly more pro-social conflict resolution strategies. In contrast, the alcohol-exposed children produced significantly more hostile-coercive strategies. These results suggest that children with high prenatal alcohol exposure are likely to have considerable difficulty acquiring or using the social abilities necessary to resolve social conflicts, specifically those involved in strategy selection.

VI. Language and Social Communication

To date, the preponderance of evidence regarding language behavior in this clinical population has been gathered using standardized, norm-referenced tests (Abkarian, 1992; Becker, Warr-Leeper, & Leeper, 1990; Church, Eldis, Blakley, & Bawle, 1997; Fried, O'Connell, & Watkinson, 1992; Gentry, Griffith, & Dancer, 1998; Janzen et al., 1995). The overall goal of these studies has been to determine how well children with teratogenic levels of prenatal alcohol exposure comprehend and/or produce the form (i.e., syntax, morphology and phonology) and content (i.e., semantics) of their language. Although the findings from these investigations have revealed a variety of language limitations, no core deficit or identifiable profile has yet emerged.

A few researchers have used nonstandardized, criterion-referenced measures to explore the language performance of children with FAS and related clinical conditions. Rather than concentrating on the structural aspects of language in artificial testing contexts, Hamilton (1981) and Coggins et al. (1998) considered language within social contexts. The findings from these investigations suggest that children with FAS have difficulty using language appropriately as context variables increase. If substantiated, this finding may help investigators to interpret performance variability in the clinical and experimental literature.

In one of the better-controlled investigations, Becker et al. (1990) administered a battery of standardized language tests to six prenatal alcohol exposed Native American Indian (NAI) children and six nonexposed NAI children. The mean age of the alcohol exposed group was 6;5 years (range: 4;8–9;4 years) and the mean age of the nonalcohol exposed group was 5;7 years (3;7–6;7 years). Participants were also matched on a measure of nonverbal intelligence. The investigators administered four standardized language measures: *Test of Auditory Comprehension of Language*, *TOKEN Test*, *Illinois Test of Psycholinguistic Abilities* and the *Clinical Evaluation of Language Fundamentals*. The investigators found several quantitative differences in the semantic and syntactic abilities of the alcohol exposed children when compared to typically developing peers matched for chronological age. The youngsters with high prenatal alcohol exposure did not comprehend as many single words, morphological structures or syntactic forms as the nonalcohol exposed controls. Further, these children generated fewer accurate and complete sentences in their spontaneous productions. However, when the investigators compared the alcohol exposed children with MA matched controls, no significant differences emerged.

Hamilton (1981) used both standardized measures and an analysis of spontaneous language to document developmental patterns of 10 youngsters with the complete FAS diagnosis. The 10 participants, ranging in age from 4;5–6;10 years, were matched with two groups of nonalcohol exposed controls. One control group was comprised of younger peers whose average mean length of utterance (mean length of utterance/morphemes = 3.78) was similar to that of the FAS group (mean length of utterance/ morphemes = 3.80). The second control group was made up of intellectually matched (IQ) same-age peers. IQ was established using either the *Stanford-Binet* or the *Weschsler Preschool and Primary Scale of Intelligence*. The participants completed three standardized language measures: *Detroit Test of Learning Aptitudes*, *Northwestern Syntax Screening Test and Peabody Picture Vocabulary Test*. Hamilton also collected a 100-utterance language sample during a low structured interaction with each participant. Hamilton found that although the participants with FAS performed more poorly than language-matched controls in forming grammatically complete sentences, they outperformed 10 cognitively matched typical control participants on all standardized syntactic and semantic measures.

Arguably, Hamilton's most interesting discovery concerned her participants' spontaneous language during conversational interactions. The one significant difference between children with FAS and their language-matched peers was the number of communicatively *adequate* responses during conversation. Children with high prenatal alcohol exposure produced significantly fewer responses that extended or elaborated their conversational partner's utterances. For example, to the question, "what is on your shoes?" children with FAS were far less likely to respond "dirt" (an adequate response) than they were to say, "I have new shoes (an "inadequate" response) or "I don't want to tell you" (an ambiguous response). This conversational profile was inconsistent with their general cognitive ability. The significant number of inadequate responses suggests that children with FAS were attempting to fulfill their conversational obligation to participate with little apparent regard for whether their utterances were communicatively appropriate. Hamilton's study was the first to document a dissociation between conversational behaviors in children with fetal alcohol exposure and their general cognitive and language abilities.

Coggins et al. (1998) have provided further evidence that older alcohol exposed children may have compromised language, particularly in using language in social contexts. This clinical research team examined the narrative abilities of adolescents with FAS. Narratives are extended units of discourse that occur frequently in a variety of meaningful social contexts. Children who can handle the communicative demands inherent in a narrative are able to access multiple pieces of information with which to capture and convey complex events in words (Berman & Slobin, 1994).

A narrative was gathered from two adolescents with FAS using Mercer Mayer's (1969) *Frog, Where are You?*, an adventure story about a boy and his dog who search for a missing frog. Both adolescents (14;3 years, 16;10 years) had full-scale IQ scores within the average range and were enrolled in regular public school classrooms (though both received resource room assistance). For purposes of comparison, Coggins et al. (1998) also collected, transcribed and scored *Frog* narratives from 12 typically developing students. Six narratives were from students with a mean age of 14;3 years, and six were from older students with a mean age of 16;7 years.

The narratives for all participants were examined for "story cohesion" (i.e., the ability to connect a series of events into logical systems or structures) and "story coherence" (i.e., the ability to clearly express essential story elements). According to Trabasso and Rodkin (1994), a cohesive narrative is built around a plot structure that consists of an initiating event and a series of related episodes. The initiating event in the *Frog* story (a pet frog escapes through an open window) is followed by a series of logically related episodes each consisting of a goal (i.e., desire or intention of characters), attempts (i.e., overt actions to satisfy or obtain goals) and an outcome (i.e., attainment or nonattainment of goals). To be given credit for a story episode, all three components must be encoded. Story coherence is concerned with being informative. The ability to communicate unambiguous information to a listener often means going beyond listing the contents of pictures, beyond commenting on the obvious and beyond the static descriptions of the characters. A coherent narrative requires that a narrator leave no doubt in the listener's mind as to what is intended.

The performance profiles of the adolescents with FAS and their typically developing, chronological-age matched peers were clearly different. Whereas the *Frog* narratives of the typically developing adolescents reflected logical organizational schemes, neither FAS participant generated stories that contained a basic plot structure. Both youngsters lacked an initiating event and failed to use language to link goals, attempts and outcomes into story episodes. As a result, their *Frog* stories were, for all intent and purposes, a truncated set of utterances largely devoid of hierarchical connections.

In sum, literature exploring the language abilities of children with prenatal alcohol exposure has yet to reveal a distinctive profile. However, most of the evidence on which this observation rests has been gathered in contrived contexts using standardized instruments. Interestingly, when language is examined under conditions that resemble unstructured, naturalistic environments, including conversations and narratives, performance is more limited than would be predicted from standardized tests, and dissimilar to chronological age-matched and even mental-age matched, non alcohol-exposed peers. This finding suggests that contextual variables may exert a powerful influence on the language performance of children with FAS and associated clinical conditions. Following this argument, one might expect a child to have more difficulty using language in real world social situations that demand higher levels of inference, social reasoning and information processing. Understanding the complex relationship between these underlying competencies and language performance is critical for the development of efficacious assessment and intervention.

VII. A FRAMEWORK FOR EXAMINING COMMUNICATIVE BEHAVIOR IN SOCIAL INTERACTIONS

A. Communication and Context

The following discussion presents the reader with a conceptual framework for considering social communication competence. We believe that this framework provides a reference for understanding and examining why children with alcohol spectrum disorders have such difficulty using language in interpersonally appropriate ways. In our view, this social communicative framework may also function as a viable structure for future research and clinical services that address children with high prenatal alcohol exposure.

A solid linguistic foundation is necessary for successful and satisfying social interactions (Brinton, Fujiki, Spencer, & Robinson, 1997; Guralnick, 1999). In order to communicate effectively in social situations, children must be able to use their language to handle a variety of sophisticated environmental demands. Researchers have argued that a communicatively competent speaker is one who can retain and process multiple pieces of incoming information in the context of, and embedded in, real time events (Chapman, 1992; Mattson et al., 1999; Sullivan, Zaitchik, & Tager-Flusberg, 1994). Children who have language limitations, in addition to limitations in processing capacity, stand at high risk for social communication deficits.

The literature has revealed a variety of language problems in children with high prenatal alcohol exposure. Researchers have not, however, been able to identify a common performance profile in these children or establish a core set of linguistic deficits. In our view, there are at least two important reasons that the search for a common profile is unlikely to yield a recognizable pattern. First, the teratogenic effects of alcohol typically result in diffuse organic brain involvement rather than a specific type of brain dysfunction. Not only is there a wide variety in the types of damage and places in the brain for damage to occur, but also the degree of damage varies tremendously (Clarren & Astely, 1997). Given this variability, it would be rather surprising to find a similar set of linguistic deficits in such a heterogeneous population. Second, we believe that the organic abnormalities linked to prenatal alcohol exposure may not compromise the basic linguistic abilities children need to perform appropriately in highly structured contexts (e.g., standardized testing). Rather, diffuse brain dysfunction seems to impair one's aptitude to recruit those abilities to meet the often implicit, and challenging demands, of unstructured situations that constitute daily social interactions. This belief is supported by the fact that most children with prenatal alcohol exposure who have been assessed with standardized language measures score broadly within the normal range (Abkarian, 1992; Church & Kaltenbach, 1997; Janzen et al., 1995; Weinberg, 1997). In short, language problems in this clinical population are not typically manifested under highly structured conditions with tasks that create discrete response opportunities.

Language problems in fetal alcohol exposed children become increasingly obvious during unstructured social interactions that are more typical of everyday life. The ability to use language in interpersonally appropriate ways, particularly in social interactive contexts, is frequently compromised. Children often seem perplexed in situations that require an array of attentional, social, linguistic, and nonlinguistic information processing resources (e.g., entering a peer group; resolving a conflict).

In these more complex social contexts, they give little evidence of knowing about the social aspects of language use.

Being a socially competent communicator requires more than simply having the necessary language for social interactions. Socially competent communicators know how and when to use language appropriately in dynamic interactions occurring in real time. A competent communicator is able to integrate, synthesize and organize knowledge and resources across sequences of social exchanges in order to solve the diverse and complex challenges encountered in daily living. Presently, we can only speculate whether children with FAS and associated conditions are aware of the rules governing the use of language in different social contexts. Appreciating the factors that influence children's social communicative competence is an important step in understanding the relationship between language and the problematic social behaviors that these children exhibit.

B. A Conceptual Framework

Figure 3 presents a conceptual model of social communication competence. The model is an attempt to understand basic factors that interact and influence school-age children's communication during social interactions. The model reflects the social information processing paradigm proposed by Crick and Dodge (1994), the social behavior construct advanced by Campbell and Siperstein (1994) and Guralnick's (1999) model of peer-related social competence.

As illustrated in Figure 3, social communicative competence is governed by three interrelated components. The language component includes the necessary syntactic, semantic and pragmatic abilities that school-age children need to be competent social communicators. The social cognitive component focuses on social understanding and is concerned with a child's ability to appreciate what others think, know or believe. The third foundational component is executive function. The primary goals of executive functions are decision-making and strategic planning. We have nested language and social cognitive components within higher-order executive functions because socially competent communicators must integrate, sequence and/or modify their language and social cognitive abilities in accordance with demands of particular situations. The purposeful integration of abilities of more fundamental components results in social communicative behaviors. These communication behaviors are the actions children perform that characterize social communicative competence. A disruption in one or more of the fundamental components is likely to result in less capability, if not impaired ability, to use language appropriately during interpersonal interactions. We also believe that the extent and nature

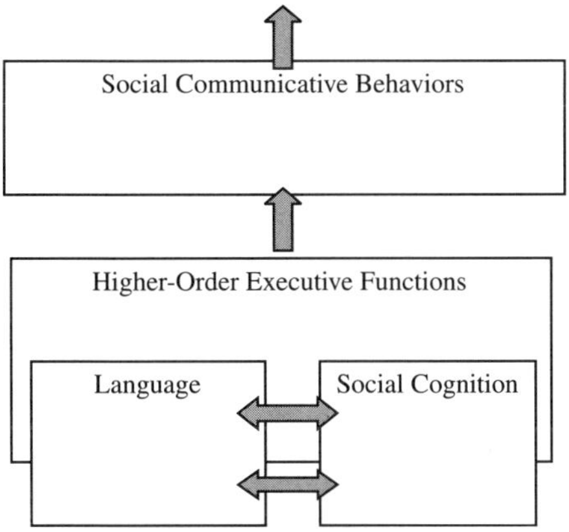

FIG. 3. A model of social communication.

of these disruptions are likely to vary across children, which inevitably results in variable social communicative abilities. Each of the fundamental components is described in greater detail in the following sections.

1. LANGUAGE BEHAVIORS

Social communicative competence is predicated on linguistic competence (Guralnick, 1999). Indeed, language is the primary means by which children succeed in establishing and maintaining social relationships at home, school and with peers. The pivotal role that language plays in interpersonal interactions places children with compromised language not only at a social communicative risk, but also jeopardizes their ability to participate in social environments (Gresham, 1998).

A socially competent communicator must have basic and advanced semantic, syntactic and pragmatic abilities. Semantic skills include having the vocabulary to allow for sophisticated forms of information exchange as needed in social exchanges. Lack of flexibility in word knowledge can create misunderstandings in interpersonal communication and confusion when deciphering linguistic information. For example, appropriately offering help or resolving conflicts necessitates an adequate vocabulary and production of word relations. Very often successful interpersonal relations among school-aged children requires an ability to appreciate synonyms, analogies, idioms and other forms of figurative language (e.g., "Are you going back on your word?" "Don't let the cat out of the bag." "Are you biting off more than you can chew?").

School-age social communication also requires adequate syntax for formulating complex sentences. Facility with comprehension and production of complex constructions, especially embedded clauses, is necessary for elaboration of abstract ideas that occur in social interactions. Syntax used for such social behaviors as negotiating interactions is typically rather sophisticated, including compound and complex sentence types (e.g., "I'd like to help, but I'm late for school." "If the movies are over early, we can go bowling afterwards.").

Finally, school-aged children must have advanced pragmatic knowledge. Arguably, this may be the most significant component of language as it relates to communicative competence in social situations. Pragmatics refers to how children use semantic and syntax abilities in interactions with others. It reflects a child's knowledge of how communication should vary in different contexts, allowing a child to know how to talk and behave in different situations with different people. For example, consider two children trying to decide who gets the first turn on the classroom computer. To resolve this potential peer conflict, one child might use language to accommodate the needs of other the other child (e.g., "I know, let's flip a coin"). These are the abilities that are necessary for determining how to appropriately behave in the classroom as a child interacts with peers and teachers.

2. SOCIAL-COGNITIVE ABILITIES

Children strive to make sense of their worlds. Although they actively seek to interpret the physical events in their world, they also spend much of their time trying to understand the social world in which they live. Because language is learned during dynamic social interactions with other people, children are naturally curious about people around them. They try and make sense of social situations by figuring out why people act in particular ways and what they are likely to do next. Social cognition focuses is concerned with how children conceptualize and think about their social world—the people they observe, the relations between people, and the groups in which they participate.

An important area of social cognitive research is Theory of Mind (TOM). The primary focus of TOM has been on child's knowledge of mental states. The TOM paradigm is concerned with how child learn to appreciate, imagine or represent states of mind in themselves and other people in order to make sense of social interactions, and behave competently in social situations. Because communication is the vehicle for social interaction, children would seem to need a well-defined TOM in order to exchange information, initiate and develop satisfying social relationships, cope with changing environmental demands and appropriately assert their needs, desires and preferences. The TOM literature has revealed that preschool and school-age children have extensive and sophisticated skills for interpreting the behavior of other people in terms of mental states.

Crick and Dodge (1994) have postulated six social cognitive processes that operate while children try and interpret social interactions. The six processes are: (1) encoding of cues (children selectively attending to and encoding particular situational and internal cues); (2) interpretation of cues (making inferences about the perspectives of others in the situation, including inferences regarding the meaning of prior and present exchanges); (3) clarification of goals (selecting a desired outcome relative to the situation at hand); (4) response access or construction (generating verbal and nonverbal strategies to achieve selected goal); (5) response decision (evaluating strategies and selecting the one most likely to achieve desired goal); and (6) behavioral enactment (implementing the chosen strategy). Difficulties in any of these processes can lead to ineffective strategies.

3. EXECUTIVE FUNCTIONS

The over-arching component in our model is executive function. Executive functions are higher-order, decision-making and planning processes invoked in the face of novel challenges (Singer & Bashir, 1999). These processes encompass a range of abilities that over-arch "all contexts and content domains" (Denkla & Reader, 1993, p. 443). As such, executive functions allow children to disengage from the immediate context and reason about interpersonal goals; a fundamental ability in forming and maintaining positive social relationships.

Executive functioning is primarily concerned with the ability to utilize information. In other words, these functions play a role in deciding how children use what they know. Although different disciplines have defined higher-order executive functions in somewhat different terms, there is general agreement regarding the following six control components: (1) inhibiting actions; (2) restraining and delaying responses; (3) attending selectively; (4) setting goals; (5) planning strategically; and (6) maintaining and shifting sets.

The ability to communicate in social situations requires intact executive functioning. According to Tannock and Schachar (1996), executive strategies that are involved in social communication include: (1) recognizing social and information demands in the situation; (2) knowing the appropriate linguistic forms to use to code underlying meaning for the situation at hand; (3) organizing and encoding thoughts through several modalities simultaneously; and (4) making rapid, "on-line" changes according to real time changes in the situation. Dysfunction in any of these strategies, alone or in combination, could compromise a child's social communicative competence.

4. SOCIAL COMMUNICATION BEHAVIORS

Social communication behaviors are specific, observable actions. The decision to place these behaviors near the top of our model reflects Campbell and Siperstein's (1994) social behavior hypothesis. This research team has identified a series of important social behaviors that communicatively competent children use during verbal interactions with peers. Some principle social behaviors include entering peer groups, collaborating with peers, explaining behaviors, resolving conflicts and negotiating interactions. The execution of these behaviors in particular social situations provides the evidence for determining how effectively a child has integrated underlying components processes and abilities. A child who effectively and appropriately uses these communicative behaviors during social interactions, either in isolation or combination, would be judged a competent social communicator (Guralnick, 1999).

5. SUMMARY

The essential focus of our social communication model is its emphasis on the dynamic relationships between language, social cognitive and executive function components. Indeed, the essence of social communication is the successful integration and execution of these underlying components in relation to important environmental variables and demands. Social interactive contexts serve as the basis for interpreting both the effectiveness and appropriateness of children's social communicative behaviors. Communicative differences that exist among children should be reflected during important social interactions, such as entering a peer group or resolving a conflict, where performance and expectations vary as a function of environmental demands. The effectiveness and appropriateness with which children use language to resolve diverse problems of a social nature is a primary basis for determining communicative competence.

C. Implications for Research and Practice

Researchers and clinicians have relied heavily on standardized language instruments to provide an overall appraisal of children's functioning. These global measures, which occur under controlled and contrived conditions, have allowed investigators to compare an individual child's performance to normative data. The obtained results, however, may provide little insight into how children perform during everyday social interactions.

Different social interactions have different demands that require different amounts of effort for communication to be successful. Moreover, as context demands increase, the processing resources a child utilizes may increase proportionally (Evans, 1996). Unfortunately, it is not possible to predict how any given child will deploy his or her resources to meet the demands of a particular task or social interaction. Thus, communication must be sampled under conditions that more accurately reflect the integration, organization and sequencing required of children to solve most interpersonal problems. Only in this way will researchers and clinicians be able to reconcile variability in children's social communication performance (Coggins, Olswang, & Guthre, 1987).

From this perspective, a representative sample of a child's social communication is likely to be gathered in natural contexts. Direct (behavioral) observation is perhaps the most socially valid method of collecting authentic and functional performance because it is embedded within actual communicative contexts (Kovarsky & Damico, 1997; Sillman & Wilkinson, 1994; Westby, Stevens-Dominguez, & Oetter, 1996). Because direct observation allows an examination of language performance in real time, it allows inspection of how environmental variables support or impede social interactions. Although behavioral observation is a useful methodology for discriminating children with social communicative deficits, observing children in natural contexts presents nontrivial challenges with respect to both data collection and data reduction (Olswang et al., 2001). The social communication model we have proposed provides an initial response to these methodological challenges.

As discussed above, problems with specific social communication behaviors may arise because of limitations in one or more underlying components. Figure 4 presents an experimental questionnaire that we have begun to use with school-based, speech-language pathologists to profile the source(s) of problematic social communication in their students (see http://depts.washington.edu/soccomm).

The questionnaire is organized around the three foundational components we believe are necessary for children to use social communicative behaviors appropriately: language, social-cognition and executive functioning. The specific items for each developmental process were gleaned from the clinical and experimental research literature in child development, thus, content validity appears robust. The judgments made by speech-language pathologists are summary, evaluative conclusions based on first-hand observations of a "child of concern" during important school settings. As a general principle, the professionals who complete the questionnaire are clinically competent, have a basic understanding of standardized and nonstandardized testing and adequate overall knowledge of child development. In completing the questionnaire, speech-language pathologists draw on their direct observations during real-time social interactions that occur across different school contexts.

I. Does this child have difficulty with any of the following language abilities?

___ Using a diverse vocabulary

___ Using mental state verbs (e.g., think, know, believe)

___ Using emotion words (e.g., like, hate, confused)

___ Using complex syntactic forms

  ___ Relative clauses

  ___ Causal conjunctions

___ Clear referents for pronouns

___ Stating conversational topics

___ Maintaining conversations

___ Asking the right questions for needed information

___ Answering questions to provide relevant and sufficient information

___ Being polite

II. Does this child have difficulty with any of the following social cognitive abilities?

___ Interpreting social cues

___ Speculating why an event has occurred

___ Knowing what to do next in social situations

___ Appreciating beliefs, ideas and knowledge of others

___ Formulating and pursuing goals involving others

___ Selecting and using effective strategies for:

  ___ Entering a group

  ___ Resolving conflicts

  ___ Maintaining play

___ Using alternative strategies in solving social dilemmas

___ Understanding consequences of decisions

III. Does this child have difficulty with any of the following executive functions?

___ Planning for future activities, tasks or situations

FIG. 4. An experimental questionnaire for examining major components, behaviors and settings contributing to children's communicative competence during social interactions.

___ Inhibiting competing or irrelevant responses

___ Analyzing situations before acting

___ Staying engaged with a task of appropriate length of time

___ Altering approach when confronted with failure

___ Adjusting style of interaction

___ Managing task-related anxiety

___ Use of self-talk to control behavior

___ Managing social interactions

___ Coordinating multiple pieces of information

IV. Does this child have difficulty using communicative behaviors in the following social interactions?

___ Entering peer groups

___ Collaborating

___ Asking permission

___ Waiting for turn

___ Telling the truth

___ Explaining behaviors

___ Negotiating with peers

___ Making and keeping friends

V. In which school settings do these social communicative problems occur?

___ Classroom

    ___ Free time

    ___ Cooperative activities

    ___ Study time

    ___ Silent reading

    ___ Group discussion

    ___ Computer time

___ Recess

___ Lunch

___ Assembly

___ Transition between periods

FIG. 4. (Continued)

Their responses can reveal the source(s) of a child's social communicative impairment (i.e., language, social-cognitive and/or executive function), type of social behavior problem (e.g., entering peer groups, resolving conflicts) and/or how context might be influencing performance (e.g., school situations). We trust that the profile may ultimately become an important nonstandardized assessment tool for those who seek a more functional assessment of a child's social communicative competence.

VIII. CONCLUSION

Over the last three decades, we have learned much about the panoply of problems that characterize children with prenatal alcohol exposure. The revealing results of our colleagues lead us to hypothesize that the difficulty these children exhibit in being competent communicators during social situations is a key deficit in this clinical population. In this paper, we have suggested that the variability in social performance associated with children who have teratogenic alcohol exposure may, in part, be a reflection of underlying difficulties in how language, social-cognitive and/or executive function fuse together to meet the demands of varying social interactions. We have offered this perspective as a framework for studying children who do not adequately communicate in real world (i.e., school) situations.

REFERENCES

Abkarian, G. (1992). Communication effects of prenatal alcohol exposure. *Journal of Communication Disorders*, *25*, 221–240.

Astley, S., & Clarren, S. (2000). Diagnosing the full spectrum of fetal alcohol exposed individuals: introducing the 4-Digit Diagnostic Code. *Alcohol & Alcoholism*, *35*, 400–410.

Astley, S., & Clarren, S. (2001). Measuring the facial phenotype of individuals with prenatal alcohol exposure: correlations with brain dysfunction. *Alcohol & Alcoholism*, *36*, 147–159.

Astley, S., Clarren, S., Stachowiak, J., & Clausen, C. (2001). FAS screening in a foster care population using the FAS DPN computerized facial photographic screening tool: interim results. *Alcoholism: Clinical and Experimental Research*, *25*, 77A.

Astely, S., Magnuson, S., Omnell, L., & Clarren, S. (1999). Fetal alcohol syndrome: changes in craniofacial form with age, cognition and timing of ethanol exposure in the macaque. *Teratology*, *59*, 163–172.

Becker, M., Warr-Leeper, G., & Leeper, H. (1990). Fetal alcohol syndrome: a description of oral motor, articulatory, short term memory, grammatical and semantic abilities. *Journal of Communication Disorders*, *23*, 97–124.

Berman, R., & Slobin, D. (1994). *Relating events in narrative: A cross linguistic development study*. Hillsdale, NJ: Lawrence Erlbaum Asociates, Inc.

Brinton, B., Fujiki, M., Spencer, J., & Robinson, L. (1997). The ability of children with specific language impairment to access and participate in ongoing interaction. *Journal of Speech, Language and Hearing Research*, *40*, 1011–1025.

Caldwell, S. (1993). Nuturing the delicate rose. In J. Kleinfeld, & S. Wescott (Eds.), *Fantastic Antone succeeds! Experiences in educating children with fetal alcohol syndrome* (pp. 97–129). Anchorage, AK: University of Alaska Press.

Campbell, P., & Siperstein, G. (1994). *Improving social competence*. Allyn & Bacon Publishing.

Carmichael Olson, H., Feldman, J. J., Streissguth, A. P., Sampson, P. D., & Bookstein, F. L. (1998). Neuropsychological deficits in adolescents with fetal alcohol syndrome: clinical findings. *Alcoholism: Clinical and Experimental Research, 20*, 1998–2012.

Carmichael Olson, H., Gendler, B., Kraegel, P., Rosengren, D., Clarren, S., & Astley, S. (under review). A targeted approach to FAS prevention: the FAS DPN first bridges program. *Alcoholism: Clinical and Experimental Research.*

Carmichael Olson, H., Morse, B. A., & Huffine, C. (1998). Development and psychopathology: FAS and related conditions. *Seminars in Clinical Neuropsychiatry, 3*, 262–284.

Chapman, R. (1992). *Processes in language acquisition and disorders*. St. Louis, MO: Mosby.

Church, M., Eldis, F., Blakley, B., & Bawle, E. (1997). Hearing, language, speech, vestibular and dentofacial disorders in fetal alcohol syndrome. *Alcoholism: Clinical and Experimental Research, 21*, 227–237.

Church, M., & Kaltenbach, J. (1997). Hearing, speech, language and vestibular disorders in the Fetal Alcohol Syndrome: a literature review. *Alcoholism: Clinical and Experimental Research, 21*, 495–512.

Clarren, S., & Astely, S. (1997). The development of fetal alcohol syndrome diagnostic and prevention network in Washington State. In A. Streissguth, & J. Kanter (Eds.), *The challenge of fetal alcohol syndrome: Overcoming secondary disabilities* (pp. 40–51). Seattle, WA: University of Washington Press.

Clarren, S., Carmichael Olson, H., Clarren, S., & Astley, S. (2000). A child with fetal alcohol syndrome. In M. Guralnick (Ed.), *Handbook of clinical assessment for young children with developmental disabilities* (pp. 307–326). Baltimore, MD: Paul H. Brookes.

Clarren, S., & Smith, D. (1978). Fetal alcohol syndrome. *New England Journal of Medicine, 298*, 1063–1067.

Coggins, T., Friet, T., & Morgan, T. (1998). Analyzing narrative productions in older school-age children and adolescents with fetal alcohol syndrome: an experimental tool for clinical applications. *Clinical Linguistics & Phonetics, 12*, 221–236.

Coggins, T., Olswang, L., & Guthre, J. (1987). Assessing communicative intents in young children: low structured observation or elicitation tasks? *Journal of Speech and Hearing Disorders, 532*, 44–49.

Coles, C. D., Platzman, K. A., Raskind-Hood, C. L., Brown, R. T., Falek, A., & Smith, I. E. (1997). A comparison of children affected by prenatal alcohol exposure and attention deficit hyperactivity disorder. *Alcoholism: Clinical and Experimental Research, 21*, 150–161.

Conry, J. (1990). Neuropsycholoigcal deficits in fetal alcohol syndrome and fetal alcohol effects. *Alcoholism: Clinical and Experimental Research, 14*, 650–655.

Crick, N., & Dodge, K. (1994). A review and reformulation of social information-processing mechanisms in children's social adjustment. *Psychological Bulletin, 11*, 74–101.

Denkla, M., & Reader, M. (1993). Education and psychological interventions. Executive dysfunction and its consequences. In R. Kulan (Ed.), *Handbook of Tourette's syndrome and related tic and behavior disorders* (pp. 431–451). New York: Marcel Dekker.

Dodge, K., McClaskey, C., & Feldman, E. (1985). A situational approach to the assessment of social competence in children. *Journal of Consulting and Clinical Psychology, 53*, 344–353.

Dorris, M. (1989). *The broken cord.* New York, NY: Harper Perennial.

Driscoll, C., Streissguth, A., & Riley, E. (1990). Prenatal alcohol exposure: compariability of effects in humans and animal models. *Neurotoxicology and Teratology*, *12*, 2231–2237.

Evans, J. (1996). Plotting the complexities of language sample analysis: linear and nonlinear dynamic models of assessment. In K. Cole, P. Dale, & D. Thal (Eds.), *Communication and language intervention series: Assessment of communication and language* (Vol. 6, pp. 207–256). Baltimore: Brookes.

Fried, P., O'Connell, C., & Watkinson, B. (1992). 60 and 72-month follow-up of children prenatally exposed to marijuana, cigarettes and alcohol: cognitive and language assessment. *Developmental and Behavioral Pediatrics*, *13*, 383–391.

Gentry, B., Griffith, L., & Dancer, J. (1998). Prenatal alcohol exposure and communication, behavior and nonverbal intelligence of 3 school-age children. *Perceptual and Motor Skills*, *86*, 1089–1090.

Gresham, F. (1998). Social skills training with children: Social learning and applied behavioral analytic approaches. In T. Watson, & F. Gresham (Eds.), *Handbook of Child Behavior Therapy* (pp. 475–497). New York: Plenum Press.

Gresham, F., & Elliot, S. (1990). *Social Skills Rating System*. Circle Pines, MN: American Guidance Service, Inc.

Guralnick, M. (1999). Family and child influences on the peer-related social competence of young children with developmental delays. *Mental Retardation and Developmental Disabilities*, *5*, 21–29.

Hamilton, M. (1981). Linguistic abilities of children with fetal alcohol syndrome. Unpublished doctoral dissertation. Seattle: University of Washington.

Hinde, J. (1993). Early intervention for alcohol-affected children. In J. Kleinfeld, & S. Wescott (Eds.), *Fantastic Antone succeeds! Experiences in education children with Fetal Alcohol Syndrome* (pp. 131–147). Anchorage, AK: University of Alaska Press.

Institute of Medicine, U.S. (1996). Division of Biobehavioral Sciences and Mental Disorders, Committtee to Study Fetal Alcohol Syndrome. In K. Stratton, C. Howe, & F. Battaglia (Eds.), *Fetal alcohol syndrome: Diagnosis, epidemiology, prevention, and treatment*. Washington, DC: National Academy Press.

Jacobson, J., & Jacobson, S. (1997). Prenatal exposure to alcohol: Is there a distinctive neurobehavioral profile. Extramural Scientific Advisory Board Meeting on FAS. May 12–13, 1997.

Janzen, L., Nanson, J., & Block, G. (1995). Neuropsychological evaluation of preschoolers with Fetal Alcohol Syndrome. *Neurotoxicology and Teratology*, *17*, 273–279.

Jones, K., & Smith, D. (1973). Recognition of the fetal alcohol syndrome in early infancy. *Lancet*, *22*, 999–1001.

Kerns, J., Don, A., Mateer, C., & Streissguth, A. (1997). Cognitive deficits in nonretarded adults with fetal alcohol syndrome. *Journal of Learning Disabilities*, *30*, 685–693.

Kleinfeld, J., & Wescott, S. (1993). *Fantastic Antone succeeds! Experiences in educating children with Fetal Alcohol Syndrome*. Anchorage, AK: University of Alaska Press.

Kodituwakku, P., Handmaker, N., Cutler, S., Weathersby, E., & Handmaker, S. (1995). Specific impairments in self-regulation in children exposed to alcohol prenatally. *Alcoholism: Clinical & Experimental Research*, *19*, 1558–1564.

Kopara-Frye, K., Dehaene, S., & Streissguth, A. (1996). Impairments of number processing induced by prenatal alcohol exposure. *Neuropsychologica*, *34*, 87–1196.

Korkman, M., Kirk, U., & Kemp, S. (1998). *A developmental neuropsychological assessment*. New York: The Psychological Corporation.

Kovarsky, D. & Damico, J. (1997). Language and context: some issues of practice. *Language, Speech, and Hearing Services in Schools*, *28*, 308–313.

Mattson, S., Goodman, A., Caine, C., Delis, D., & Riley, E. (1999). Executive functioning in children with heavy prenatal alcohol exposure. *Alcoholism: Clinical and Experimental Research, 23*, 1808–1815.

Mattson, S., & Riley, E. (1998). A review of the neurobehavioral deficits in children with fetal alcohol syndrome or prenatal exposure to alcohol. *Alcoholism: Clinical & Experimental Research, 22*, 279–294.

Mayer, M. (1969). *Frog, where are you?* New York: Dial Book for Young Readers.

Nanson, J. (1990). Behavior in children with fetal alcohol syndrome. In W. Fraser (Ed.), *Key issues in mental retardation research.* London: Blackwell.

National Institute on Alcohol Abuse & Alcoholism (NIAAA) (1997). Ninth special report to the U.S. Congress on Alcohol and Health, NIH Publication, No. 97–4017. Washington, DC: U.S. Department of Health & Human Services.

Olswang, L., Coggins, T., & Timler, G. (2001). Outcome measures for school-age children with social communication problems. *Topics in Language Disorders, 22*, 50–73.

O'Malley, K., & Hagerman, R. (1998). Developing clinical practice guidelines for pharmacological interventions in alcohol-affected children. In K. O'Malley, & R. Hagerman (Eds.), *Intervening with children affected by prenatal alcohol exposure.* Monograph from the Interagency Coordinating Committee on Fetal Alcohol Syndrome Special Focus Session. Chevy Chase, MD: Centers for Disease Control and Prevention.

Plumridge, D., Bennett, R., Dinno, N., & Branson, C. (1993). *The student with a genetic disorder: Educational implications for special education teachers and for physical therapists, occupational therapists and speech pathologists.* Springfield, IL: Charles C. Thomas.

Rathbun, A. (1993). Overcoming the cycle of failure and frustration. In J. Kleinfeld, & S. Wescott (Eds.), *Fantastic Antone succeeds! Experiences in educating children with fetal alcohol syndrome* (pp. 295–313). Anchorage, AK: University of Alaska Press.

Redmond, S., & Rice, M. (1998). The socio-emotional behaviors of children with SLI: social adaptation or social deviance? *Journal of Speech, Language and Hearing, 41*, 688–700.

Redmond, S., & Rice, M. (2002). Stability of behavioral ratings of children with SLI. *Journal of Speech, Language and Hearing Research, 45*, 190–201.

Roebuck, T., Mattson, S., & Riley, E. (1999). Behavioral and psychosocial profiles of alcohol-exposed children. *Alcoholism: Clinical and Experimental Research, 23*, 1070–1076.

Rosett, H., & Weiner, L. (1984). *Alcohol and the Fetus: A Clinical Perspective.* New York: Oxford.

Sampson, P., Kerr, B., Carmichael Olson, H., Streissguth, A., Hunt, E., Barr, H., Bookstein, F., & Thiede, K. (1997). The effects of prenatal alcohol exposure on adolescent cognitive processing: a speed-accuracy tradeoff. *Intelligence, 24*, 329–353.

Sillman, E., & Wilkinson, C. (1994). *Observation is more than looking.* New York: Merrill Publishing.

Singer, B., & Bashir, A. (1999). What are executive functions and self-regulation and what do they have to do with language-learning disorders? *Language, Speech and Hearing Services in Schools, 30*, 265–273.

Spohr, H.-L., Willms, J., & Steinhausen, J.-C. (1993a). Prenatal alcohol exposure and long-term developmental consequences. *Lancet, 341*, 907–910.

Spohr, H.-L., Willms, J., & Steinhausen, J.-C. (1993b). The fetal alcohol syndrome in adolescence. *Acta Paediatrica, 83*, 19–26.

Steinhausen, H.-C., Willms, J., & Spohr, H.-L. (1993). Long-term psychopathological and cognitive outcome of children with fetal alcohol syndrome. *Journal of the American Academy of Child and Adolescent Psychiatry, 32*, 990–994.

Streissguth, A. (1997). *Fetal alcohol syndrome: A guide for families and communities.* Baltimore: Paul H. Brookes Publishing Co.

Streissguth, A., Barr, H., Kogan, J., & Bookstein, F. (1996). Understanding the occurrence of secondary disabilities in clients with fetal alcohol syndrome (FAS) and fetal alcohol effects (FAE): Final report to the Centers for Disease Control and Prevention on Grant No. R04/CCR008515 (Tech. Report No. 96060). Seattle: University of Washington Fetal Alcohol and Drug Unit.

Streissguth, A., Barr, H., Kogan, J., & Bookstein, F. (1997). Primary and secondary disabilities in fetal alcohol syndrome. In A. Streissguth, & J. Kanter (Eds.), *The challenge of fetal alcohol syndrome: overcoming secondary disabilities* (pp. 25–39). Seattle, WA: University of Washington Press.

Sullivan, K., Zaitchik, D., & Tager-Flusberg, H. (1994). Preschoolers can attribute second-order beliefs. *Developmental Psychology*, *30*, 395–402.

Tannock, R., & Schachar, R. (1996). Executive dysfunction as an underlying mechanism of behavior and language problems in attention deficit hyperactivity disorder. In J. Bleitchman, N. Cohen, M. Konstantareas, & R. Tannock (Eds.), *Language, learning, and behavior disorders*. Cambridge, UK: Cambridge University Press.

Thomas, S., Kelly, S., Mattson, S., & Riley, E. (1998). Comparison of social abilities of children with fetal alcohol syndrome to those of children with similar IQ scores and normal controls. *Alcoholism: Clinical and Experimental Research*, *22*, 528–533.

Timler, G. (2000). Investigation of social communication skills during peer conflict tasks in school-age children with alcohol-related disabilities. Unpublished doctoral dissertation. University of Washington, Seattle, WA.

Timler, G., & Olswang, G. (2001). Variable structure/variable performance: Caregiver and teacher perspectives of a school-age child with fetal alcohol syndrome. *Journal of Positive Behavior Interventions*, *3*, 48–56.

Timler, G., Olswang, L., & Coggins, T. (under review). Do I know what I need to do? A treatment package for school-age children with social communication deficits.

Trabasso, T., & Rodkin, P. (1994). Knowledge of goal/plans: a conceptual basis for narrating *Frog, Where Are You?* In D. Berman, & D. Slobin (Eds.), *Relating events in narrative: A cross-linguistic developmental study*. Hillsdale, NJ: Lawrence Erlbaum.

Uecker, A., & Nadel, L. (1996). Spatial locations gone awry: object and spatial memory deficits in children with fetal alcohol syndrome. *Neuropsychologia*, *34*, 209–223.

Weinberg, N. (1997). Cognitive and behavioral deficits associated with prenatal alcohol use. *Journal of the American Academy of Child and Adolescent Psychiatry*, *36*, 1177–1186.

Westby, C., Stevens-Dominguez, M., & Oetter, P. (1996). A performance/competence model of observational assessment. *Language, Speech and Hearing Services in Schools*, *27*, 144–156.

Wright, R. (1992). One step forward: using information about FAE to help my son. *Iceberg*, *1*, 3–4.

Zucker, R., Fitzgerald, H., Refior, S., Puttler, L., Pallas, D., & Ellis, D. (2000). The clinical and social ecology of childhood for children of alcoholics: description of a study and implications for a differentiated social policy. In H. Fitzgerald, B. Lester, & B. Zuckerman (Eds.), *Children of addiction: Research, health, and public policy* (pp. 109–142). New York: Falmer Press.

Memory, Language Comprehension, and Mental Retardation

EDWARD C. MERRILL, REGAN LOOKADOO, and STACY RILEA

DEPARTMENT OF PSYCHOLOGY, UNIVERSITY OF ALABAMA, TUSCALOOSA, ALABAMA

I. INTRODUCTION

There is a long history of research conducted on memory systems and processes of persons with mental retardation. In fact, the relation between memory ability and general intellectual ability was part of many of the earliest intelligence tests (see Estes, 1982). In terms of basic memory systems, researchers have evaluated the performance of persons with mental retardation relative to persons without mental retardation in short-term, immediate, or working memory (e.g., Cohen & Sandberg, 1980; Ellis, 1970), long-term memory (e.g., Prehm & Mayfield, 1970; Sperber, Greenfield, & House, 1973), semantic memory (e.g., Glidden, 1986; Sperber & McCauley, 1984), episodic memory (Stan & Mosley, 1988), tacit memory (Atwell, Conners, & Merrill, 2003), and the possible interactions of some of the various memory systems (e.g., Cody & Borkowski, 1977; Winters, 1986). In terms of memory processes, considerable research attention has been devoted to the study of meta-memory and the use of task-specific memory strategies by persons with and without mental retardation (e.g., Borkowski & Cavanaugh, 1979; Brown & Campione, 1977; Justice, 1986), automatic versus effortful memory retrieval processes (e.g., Ellis, Palmer, & Reeves, 1988; Ellis, Woodley-Zanthow, & Dulaney, 1989), memory scanning (e.g., Merrill, 1990; Phillips & Nettelbeck, 1986), semantic priming (e.g., Sperber, Davies, Merrill, & McCauley, 1982; Sperber, Ragain, & McCauley, 1976), and semantic inhibition (e.g., Cha & Merrill, 1994; Merrill & Taube, 1996).

Memory has always played an important role in the study of language comprehension in cognitive psychology (see Lorch & van den Brock, 1997). In fact, discourse comprehension is often viewed as the cognitive equivalent of constructing a coherent memory representation of the text or discourse during its processing and early models of discourse comprehension relied

0074-7750/2003 $35.00

heavily on many of the same mechanisms and processes developed for the processing of semantic knowledge (see Lorch, 1998). Hence, cognitive research on language comprehension has typically involved investigating the type of information that is included in the memory representation of units of discourse (single sentences or multiple sentence passages) and the systems and processes that facilitate the construction of the memory representation. This is the view of language comprehension that has directed our review.

Language comprehension is a complex cognitive activity and obviously involves the use of multiple memory systems and multiple memory processes. The intent of this review is to examine the role of the mechanisms and processes associated with memory for verbal information on language comprehension differences between persons with and without mental retardation. In our analysis, language comprehension involves no less than three separate memory systems: working memory, semantic memory, and tacit, or procedural, memory. Working memory provides space for the temporary storage of important components of the discourse during comprehension and resources for the retrieval and incorporation of relevant information from semantic memory into the memory representation of the discourse. Semantic memory reflects our knowledge about the world and provides the fundamental context for language comprehension activities. Among the most important functions of semantic memory is to promote coherence during comprehension by filling in details, such as causal relations or implied instruments, that are seldom made explicit during written or oral discourse. Tacit, or procedural, memory usually refers to a storage system of relatively complex knowledge of how to do things (very broadly defined), and is typically not accessible to conscious inspection. Many features of language (e.g., word order rules of grammar) occur with a consistency that may be accessible to a form of learning, called implicit learning, that takes place below the level of conscious awareness (see Reber, 1976, 1989). The knowledge gained through implicit learning is stored in tacit memory. Hence, differences in the use of tacit memories may also be related to language comprehension differences.

Obviously, other memory systems are likely to be involved in various aspects of language comprehension (e.g., episodic memory would assist in distinguishing between sources of language activities), however, the three systems on which we focus in this review have the most direct relation to general language comprehension. Although acknowledging the deficiencies inherent in reviews that treat mechanisms and processes of memory as functionally independent from other mechanisms and processes of memory, we review each system separately in the sections that follow. Within each section, we attempt to describe the basic components of the memory system under consideration, discuss each system's role in language comprehension as revealed by research conducted on skilled language users, evaluate research conducted with persons with mental retardation, and assess how differences between persons with and without mental retardation in language comprehension may be related to the operation of each memory system.

Virtually all of the studies that include persons with mental retardation that we discuss in this review include at least one comparison group. We generally favored studies that matched on the basis of some estimate of Mental Age rather than Chronological Age. In some ways, this choice reflects the assumptions that guide our own research. More specifically, we tend to include chronological age comparison groups when studying what we consider to be basic cognitive processes and abilities and mental age comparison groups when studying what we consider to be cognitive skills (the products of basic processes and abilities). Our rationale is relatively straightforward. Because mental retardation is defined in terms of performance relative to others of the same chronological age, it has made sense to us to catalog pockets of similarity and differences in basic cognitive abilities between persons with and without mental retardation who are similar on chronological age (see for example, Burack, Evans, Klaiman, & Iarocci, 2001 for an alternative perspective on matching). One of the important general results of research using chronological age matches is the observation that there are many similarities in basic abilities between persons with and without mental retardation of the same chronological age (see for example, Atwell et al., 2003; Merrill & Jackson, 1992b; Merrill, McCown, & Kelley, 2001). Hence, we have learned that mental retardation is not characterized by a deficit in all cognitive abilities nor even all situations when ability differences have been observed. In contrast, when evaluating cognitive skills such as language comprehension we tend to favor a comparison of individuals who are matched on mental age. Albeit a relatively gross measure, we have accepted mental age as a construct indicating current ability/performance levels in general cognitive functioning. Therefore, our basic question when investigating cognitive skills focuses on whether or not persons with mental retardation are able to utilize current ability/performance in general cognitive functioning to achieve similar levels of skilled performance as persons without mental retardation of the same mental age. One of the important general results of research using the mental age match is the observation that there are many differences in skilled performance between persons with and without mental retardation of the same mental age (see for example, Courbois, 1996; Merrill & Marr, 1987; Merrill et al., 1987; Spitz & Borys, 1977).

Our review also focuses primarily on research conducted on adolescents with mild mental retardation. The notable exceptions will be studies in which a wide range of ability levels are considered that includes mild retardation as well as more severe levels of mental retardation. This decision was made because we are more confident that the models of memory and language comprehension that we use to guide our research are applicable to adolescents with mild mental retardation than to younger individuals with mental retardation or adolescents with more severe mental retardation. In addition, the procedures designed to measure memory performance and language skill tend to be more reliable for adolescents with mild mental retardation than for persons in the other classifications. As a result, the research that we discuss typically involves persons with mental retardation whose measured IQs fall between 50 and 70 and estimated mental ages fall between 6 and 9 years. Hence, our conclusions are not necessarily appropriate for other persons with mental retardation.

With the exception of a brief discussion of the relation between vocabulary acquisition and phonological processing, we have also focused on language comprehension activities involved in sentence and discourse processing. This choice was made for two reasons. First, it is in the context of understanding larger units of discourse that memory has its greatest direct impact on language comprehension activities. Second, it is in the processing of larger units of discourse that language serves its primary functions of providing the means for communication, reasoning, and problem solving.

II. WORKING MEMORY

Working memory is now the preferred term to identify the cognitive system responsible for the temporary storage and simultaneous manipulation of information. This system is fundamental to the performance of a variety of complex cognitive tasks. One role of working memory in language comprehension is a storage function to provide access to referents necessary for comprehension. Understanding a full sentence requires that we be able to remember words from initial phrases when we reach the end of the sentence. Understanding larger units of discourse of requires access to referents from several sentences back. In addition, working memory provides and coordinates cognitive resources necessary for the integration of information across sentences, the retrieval of relevant information from semantic memory, and the use of strategies and goals to facilitate language comprehension activities.

The most influential model of working memory currently available identifies working memory as a multi-component system consisting of a central executive and two subordinate slave systems: an articulatory–phonological loop and a visuo-spatial sketchpad (Baddeley, 1986; Baddeley & Hitch, 1974). The two slave systems operate as basic short-term storage mechanisms, whereas the central executive acts to coordinate resources necessary for the processing and manipulation of information. Several theorists have described the prime function of the central executive as the coordination of resources throughout the cognitive system, with the memory storage function of working memory being one of a number of basic operations that may make demands on the central executive (e.g., Baddeley, 1986; Schneider & Detweiler, 1987). In fact, the central executive is typically assumed to be responsible for a wide range of functions that traditionally have been assigned to attentional processing, such as the retrieval of information from various long-term memory systems and regulating the flow of information among the components of working memory and between the components of long-term memory and working memory (see e.g., Baddeley, 1986; Engle, Tuholski, Laughlin, & Conway, 1999).

In the next two sections, we review the role of working memory in language comprehension activities of individuals with and without mental retardation focusing on the articulatory-loop and the central executive. In the first section we discuss working memory functions related to language comprehension of individuals without mental retardation. As discussed below, the storage function associated with the articulatory–phonological loop appears to play a limited role in discourse comprehension (with the exception of learning to read), but a more prominent role in vocabulary acquisition. However, the central executive, typically measured in terms of working memory capacity (Daneman & Carpenter, 1980), appears to be involved in many aspects of language comprehension. In the second section we review studies that assess the working memory of individuals with mental retardation and compare working memory performance of individuals with and without mental retardation.

A. Working Memory and Language Comprehension: Individuals Without Mental Retardation

Two of the three components of working memory would logically be expected to correlate highly with general language comprehension: the articulatory–phonological loop and the central executive. We do not rule out a possible relation between language comprehension and the visuo-spatial sketchpad in the form of, for example, the processing of visual context to facilitate online comprehension. Unfortunately, much of the research on the visuo-spatial sketchpad has focused on demonstrating a dissociation between its operation and cognitive activities assumed to be related to the articulatory–phonological loop. Hence, data on this issue, especially data that may be relevant to language comprehension by persons with mental retardation, are not available.

Despite the logical relation between the operation of the articulatory–phonological loop and language comprehension, many studies have reported a relatively weak relation between them in the general population. For example, Waters, Caplan, and Hildebrandt (1987) reported that articulatory suppression (forcing participants to engage in a secondary articulation task and limit the role of the phonological loop in sentence comprehension) interfered with the processing of two proposition sentences but not the processing of one proposition sentence. The authors concluded that the phonological representation stored in working memory served as a backup when particularly demanding sentences would overload on-line comprehension processes but was not necessary when on-line comprehension was relatively easy. Martin and Feher (1990) evaluated the role of the articulatory–phonological loop in the language comprehension of patients with short-term memory impairments. They presented sentences with and without printed forms that remained available for as long as the participants wished. They assumed that having a printed form available would limit the working memory requirements of the task because the sentence was physically available. There was no difference in correct interpretation associated with printed versus unprinted versions of the sentences except for Token Test sentences containing many content words (e.g., "Touch the large blue square and the small red triangle") that were considerably more difficult for their patients to process. For even syntactically complex sentences, having a printed version available did not increase correct interpretation of the sentences, indicating a relatively limited role for the phonological loop in sentence comprehension. Butterworth and colleagues (Butterworth, Campbell, & Howard, 1986; Campbell & Butterworth, 1985) have gone so far as to suggest that the phonological loop may not be a critical component of auditory language comprehension on the basis of results from a college student who exhibited severe phonological memory impairment, but unimpaired language comprehension skills.

A number of researchers have noted that the role of the articulatory–phonological loop in language comprehension may be greater for children than it is for adults. For example, Gathercole and Baddeley (1993) have suggested that one important role of phonological memory is to support comprehension off-line, and that it is logical to expect that young children will be required to do more off-line processing when learning to master complex sentence constructions. Hence, it may not be appropriate to assume that the failure to find a clear relation between phonological working memory and comprehension in skilled language users would necessarily generalize to children, and for our discussion, persons with mental retardation. Unfortunately, we were not able to find systematic research on the role of phonological working memory on language comprehension of children independent of learning to read. Therefore, there is no clear and convincing support for this possibility. More recently, Baddeley, Gathercole, and Papagano (1998) have argued that the use of the phonological loop for retaining sequences of familiar words during comprehension may actually be secondary to its use in the storing of unfamiliar sound patterns during the construction of more permanent memories of new words.

Although it may be that the articulatory–phonological loop is not directly related to the language comprehension abilities of skilled language users, it does appear to play an important role in two other facets of language use: learning to read and vocabulary acquisition. The role of the articulatory–phonological loop in learning to read in the general population has been well established (see Gathercole & Baddeley, 1993). This particular literature and the role of working memory in learning to read by persons with and without mental retardation is reviewed elsewhere in this volume (see Conners) and will not be addressed directly in this review.

Gathercole and Baddeley (1993) present data that indicate a relatively strong relation between phonological memory skills and vocabulary acquisition for children between the ages of 4 and 8 years old. Using nonword repetition as their measure of phonological memory, they found positive correlations between phonological memory and measures of receptive vocabulary that ranged between 0.50 and 0.60 for children at ages 5, 6, and 7. The correlation was only half as large when children were 8 years old. Cross-lagged correlations indicated that the direction of causality actually changed across the age range tested, with phonological memory driving the relationship for the 4- and 5-year-old children and vocabulary skills driving the relationship for the older children. They suggested that the manner in which good phonological memory facilitates the acquisition of new vocabulary is by producing more discriminable and persistent phonological traces that are more likely to be semantically linked with the appropriate referent than would less discriminable and weaker memory traces. This would be most evident with young children.

Despite the lower correlations of phonological memory and vocabulary acquisition exhibited by children over the age of 6 years, research has also indicated that phonological memory may play an important role in the acquisition of new words by adults as well as children. Papagno, Valentine, and Baddeley (1991) presented adults with familiar and unfamiliar words while they were or were not concurrently performing an articulatory suppression task. The suppression task caused greater impairment in memory for the unfamiliar words than for the familiar words. They concluded that phonological memory skills played an important role in the learning of unfamiliar words for which there is no semantic code that can facilitate memory. Papagno and Vallar (1992) reported that phonological similarity impaired memory for word–novel word pairs more than it impaired memory for word–familiar word pairs, and hence, reached a similar conclusion.

The contribution of the phonological–articulatory loop to basic language comprehension skill may be mostly an indirect one; however, it is clear that the central executive has a direct and more general influence on language comprehension (see Carpenter, Miyake, & Just, 1995; Daneman & Merickle, 1996). The central executive controls available resources and can influence how they are distributed to the storage and processing functions of working memory. In fact, in practice it is often equated with working memory capacity. To assess this feature of working memory, Daneman and Carpenter (1980) developed a measure of working memory span that required individuals to use both the storage and processing components of working memory: they had individuals read or listen to a series of unrelated sentences and, after the entire set was presented, recall the last word of each sentence. Working memory capacity was defined as the number of sentences that individuals could process and still recall the last word of each sentence. In an assessment of good and poor readers, Daneman and Carpenter found that working memory span varied reliably across individuals (two to five final words for college students), and observed that working memory span correlated more highly with global measures of language comprehension than did traditional measures of static memory span. The relation between working memory capacity and language comprehension was assumed to reflect the added processing requirements associated with language comprehension activities for the poor language comprehenders. More specifically, the general claim was that language comprehension activities required more of the available resources of the central executive for the poor comprehenders and left fewer resources for storing and retrieving the last word of the sentences.

Over the last 20 years, this approach to assessing working memory capacity has been used by many groups of researchers who have replicated the basic result that working memory span is highly correlated with general language comprehension (e.g., Daneman & Tardif, 1987; Dixon, LeFevre, & Twilley, 1988; Masson & Miller, 1983; Turner & Engle, 1989). A meta-analysis conducted by Daneman and Merickle (1996) also indicated that measures that reflect the combined processing and storage functions of working memory are better predictors of general language comprehension ability than are those that reflect only the storage component. Further, they report that working memory span predicted language comprehension skill even when the measure of working memory span did not involve language processing (as long as some form of symbolic processing was involved).

Working memory capacity can influence language comprehension in a variety of different language processing situations (see Just and Carpenter, 1992). For example, Daneman and Carpenter (1980) report that a strong relation exists between working memory capacity, as measured by reading span, and the distance over which readers can integrate information across text constituents. Low working memory capacity has also been shown to be related to a reduction in the speed and accuracy with which sentences can be processed, with increasing difficulty being manifested as sentences become more complex in structure (King & Just, 1991). In addition, Just and Carpenter (1992) report that higher working memory capacity increases the likelihood that individuals will use nonsyntactic information to avoid being led down the garden path by syntactic ambiguity. There is also evidence that individuals with a higher working memory capacity were more likely to represent more than one interpretation of a syntactic ambiguity during on-line processing until disambiguating information was presented at some later time (MacDonald, Just, & Carpenter, 1992).

The general influence of working memory capacity on language comprehension can be summarized as follows. When increasing demands are placed on working memory capacity during language comprehension activities, language comprehension performance is likely to suffer. Individuals with lower working memory capacity or who must use more of their available capacity for language processing activities will exhibit a greater decline in comprehension performance than will individuals with higher working memory capacity as processing demands associated with language increases.

B. Working Memory and Language Comprehension: Individuals with Mental Retardation

Assessments of the working memory system of persons with mental retardation have generally shown that a basic similarity exists between the structure of working memory for persons with and without mental retardation. For example, researchers have demonstrated the expected dissociation between measures of verbal memory (reflecting the operation of the articulatory–phonological loop) and measures of visuo-spatial memory (reflecting the operation of the visuo-spatial sketch pad) (e.g., Jarrold, Baddeley, & Hewes, 1999; Wang & Bellugi, 1993). What has also been observed in many of these studies is that individuals with Down syndrome exhibit relative deficiencies in verbal memory and strengths in visuo-spatial memory, whereas individuals with Williams syndrome exhibit the opposite pattern (Grant et al., 1997; Wang & Bellugi, 1994). We will return to the relation between these results and language performance below.

Recently, Numminen et al. (2000) conducted a systematic evaluation of working memory structure of persons with mental retardation. They presented individuals with IQs between 35 and 70 with a battery of tests representing measures of phonological processing, visuo-spatial processing, central executive functions, intelligence, language skills, general academic skills, and everyday memory. Factor-analytic procedures isolated two separate components of working memory: one corresponding to the articulatory–phonological loop, and one corresponding to a combined visuo-spatial sketch pad and central executive that they considered a general component of working memory. On the surface, this may seem contrary to the model described by Baddeley. However, as noted by the authors, recent research has shown that the sensitivity of particular tasks in assessing components of working memory may vary with intellectual level (Engle et al., 1999) and with developmental level (Gathercole & Pickering, 2000). Thus, rather than assuming that working memory is structurally different for these different groups, they concluded that it is more reasonable to expect that the structures are similar but that individuals probably responded to the basic tasks differently.

Comparing working memory performance to participants' performance on the various skills tests, Numminen et al. reported that measures of general intelligence (Raven's and Similarities of the WAIS-R) were related to the general component of working memory, but not related to the articulatory–phonological loop. All academic measures (reading, writing, vocabulary, sentence comprehension, mathematics, and everyday memory) were also related to the general component of working memory. Reading, writing, and sentence comprehension were related to the phonological loop; however, other aspects of language skills were not (vocabulary and story recall). This pattern of performance is fundamentally the same as is typically observed for individuals without mental retardation: measures that reflect general intelligence are associated with the central executive while measures that reflect more specific competencies are associated with the slave systems. In this study, Numminen et al. were able to isolate one slave system and found that it was specific to some language skills. The failure to observe significant relationships between the functioning of the phonological loop and vocabulary or story recall was not particularly surprising. First, as mentioned previously, the correlations between current vocabulary level and phonological memory are not particularly strong as developmental level increases and the participants of Numminen et al. appear to have represented a wide range of ability levels. Second, story recall does not appear to rely heavily on phonological working memory.

Research specific to evaluating aspects of the articulatory–phonological loop with persons with mental retardation has been conducted to compare processing and memory differences among different etiologies. In many respects, this research has taken the opposite approach from working memory research in the general literature. That is, rather than evaluating working memory and then trying to predict language performance, researchers have observed differences in language skills among different etiologies of mental retardation and have tried to predict differences in working memory performance. The typical evaluation consists of comparing performance on a digit span or word span task with performance on some version of the Corsi blocks task (Milner, 1971). In the Corsi blocks task, the experimenter points to a block or several blocks in sequence and the participant is required to point to the same blocks in order. The digit and word span tasks are presented aurally and reflect the operation of the articulatory–phonological loop, whereas the Corsi blocks task is presented visually and reflects the operation of the visuo-spatial sketchpad. Individuals with Down syndrome exhibit difficulties with language processing that are greater than would be predicted by measures of general intellectual functioning and also exhibit shorter digit and word spans relative to Corsi block spans than control participants matched on general intellectual functioning (e.g., Jarrold & Baddeley, 1997; Marcell & Cohen, 1992; Vicari, Carlesimo, & Caltagirone, 1995). Individuals with Williams syndrome exhibit stronger language processing skills than would be predicted based on measures of general intellectual functioning and exhibit digit and word spans that are often equivalent to persons without mental retardation matched on chronological age, but exhibit shorter Corsi block spans (e.g., Grant et al., 1997). Hence, a general relation between phonological working memory and language performance by persons with mental retardation has been demonstrated.

The operation of the phonological loop is related to vocabulary acquisition in typically developing children (ages 4 and 5) and the rate at which unfamiliar words are learned by adults (Gathercole & Baddeley, 1993). Unfortunately, relatively few studies assessing the relation between phonological processing and vocabulary have been conducted on persons with mental retardation. Investigations across etiologies have generally established that persons with Williams syndrome and persons with Down syndrome exhibit very different behavior profiles with respect to language development. These differences in language performance also include differences in vocabulary performance: individuals with Williams syndrome exhibit better performance on most measures of vocabulary than do individuals with Down syndrome (e.g., Jarrold et al., 1999; Klein, & Mervis, 1999; Mervis, & Robinson, 2000; Wang & Bellugi, 1994). Hence, we observe that groups of individuals who exhibit relatively greater impairments on measures of phonological memory processes also exhibit relatively greater impairments on measures of vocabulary development. This pattern of performance corresponds with the prediction that phonological processing is positively correlated with vocabulary acquisition across etiologies. However, the results of research that has investigated the relation between vocabulary knowledge and phonological processing within etiologies has been less consistent. In single-participant analysis of a 23-year-old woman with Down syndrome, Vallar and Papagno (1993) describe an individual who exhibited relatively preserved functioning of phonological memory processes and also exhibited an excellent vocabulary and strong foreign language learning skills. These results suggest that preserved phonological processing corresponds with preserved vocabulary development and learning. In contrast, Jarrold & Baddeley (1997) did not find significant correlations between auditory digit span and vocabulary comprehension for groups of children with Down syndrome, indicating a potentially weaker link between phonological working memory and vocabulary acquisition for persons with Down syndrome than reported by Gathercole and Baddeley (1993) for typically developing children.

There are at least a couple of reasons why the relation between vocabulary acquisition and phonological working memory may appear weaker for individuals with Down syndrome than for typically developing children (see Numminen et al., 2000). First, a great deal of special attention is paid to the vocabulary development of children with Down syndrome (Girolametto, Weitzman, & Clements-Baartman, 1998; Kumin, 2001; Kumin, Councill, & Goodman, 1998). It is reasonable to expect that relations that hold during normal development may be attenuated when extraordinary means of instruction are employed. Second, it may be that word and digit span measures are influenced by factors other than phonological processing for persons with mental retardation more than they are for persons without mental retardation. Recently, Connors, Carr, and Willis (1998) evaluated differences in word span for individuals with undifferentiated mental retardation and individuals without mental retardation who were matched for either chronological or mental age. Significant differences in word span were substantially reduced when measures of central executive processing were taken into account.

Laws (1998) recently reported a study comparing phonological memory and language skills for persons with Down syndrome using nonword repetition as her measure of phonological memory. Participants were required to listen to and repeat nonwords read to them by the experimenter that varied from one to five syllables in length. Laws compared the relation between nonword repetition and vocabulary comprehension with the relation between auditory digit span and vocabulary comprehension. Partial correlations were conducted among the measures to remove the effects of age and nonverbal cognitive ability. The correlation between nonword repetition and vocabulary comprehension was substantially larger than the correlation between auditory digit span and vocabulary comprehension (0.44 vs 0.18, respectively). Hence, the relation between phonological memory and vocabulary may depend, in part, on the measure of phonological memory that is used (cf., Comblain, 1999).

A more direct relation between the operation of the central executive and language comprehension has been reported in the literature on persons without mental retardation (Daneman & Carpenter, 1980; Daneman & Merickle, 1996; Gathercole & Baddeley, 1993; Just & Carpenter, 1992). This relation has been observed comparing both individual differences in working memory capacity (Daneman & Carpenter, 1980) and group differences in working memory capacity (Kemper, 1986) to measures of language comprehension. Such differences may be manifested in a variety of ways, but generally reflect the observation that differences in language comprehension increase between groups differing in memory capacity when increasing demands are placed on working memory.

One theoretical perspective that is consistent with the notion that differences in working memory capacity lead to differences in language comprehension skills between persons with and without mental retardation has been developed by Kail (1992). Kail has suggested that one primary difference between persons with and without mental retardation involves the speed of information processing. Further, after a careful review of 45 studies in which persons with mental retardation performed more slowly on speeded tasks than did persons without mental retardation, he concluded that some global mechanism, such as limited processing resources, was responsible for group differences on speeded tasks. Because the allocation of processing resources is a function of the central executive, differences in general processing speed may be considered to reflect differences in working memory capacity.

Merrill and Marr (1987) assessed the relation between increased processing demands and the speed of language processing for adolescents with mild mental retardation and children matched on mental age by presenting sentences and passages at varying rates of speed. Using a compressed speech technique, it was possible to present materials at rates ranging from 100 to 300 words per minute. In one experiment, participants were played individual sentences followed by word probes that were either included or not included in the sentence. Increasing the rate of presentation did not create group differences in the ability to determine whether or not individual words were part of the presented sentences. However, in a second experiment, four-sentence passages were presented at varying rates and comprehension rather than simple storage was assessed. Differences in comprehension were produced by increasing the presentation rate of sentences: persons with mental retardation exhibited relatively poorer language comprehension when the passages were presented at faster speeds. Language comprehension differences between persons with and without mental retardation emerged when working memory resources were extended even though simple phonological storage differences did not emerge under the same conditions.

The ability to suppress contextually irrelevant and inappropriate meanings of words presented in sentences is generally assumed to be related to working memory capacity as well. Many current models of sentence processing suggest that sentences are encoded and understood in a series of steps (Kintsch & Mross, 1985; Till, Mross, & Kintsch, 1988). Initially, word recognition involves the activation of both context-appropriate and context-inappropriate aspects of a word's meaning. It is only over time (less than a second) that comprehension activities focus on context-appropriate meanings, with context-inappropriate meanings being suppressed or allowed to fade as words in the sentence are semantically integrated. In a series of studies, my colleagues and I evaluated the relative abilities of persons with and without mental retardation to restrict meanings of words to context-appropriate features during language comprehension.

Merrill and Bilsky (1990) compared the sentence representations constructed during language processing by persons with and without mental retardation. The participants with mental retardation were adolescents with mild mental retardation and the participants without mental retardation were matched on either mental age or chronological age. During the experiment they were presented with a series of sentences, after which their memory for the sentences was tested using a cued recall paradigm. The cues were either the noun of the original sentence, the verb of the original sentence, or the noun plus verb of the original sentence. The logic underlying the cue manipulation was that the two-word cue would be relatively better to the extent that participants had created a semantically integrated representation of the sentence during processing that focused on context-appropriate meanings of the words (the two-word cue and the sentence representation would only include context-appropriate word meanings, whereas the one-word cues would contain both context-appropriate and context-inappropriate word meanings). If they did not construct integrated representations, then the two-word cue would not be any better than the combined performance to the two one-word cues, because the one-word cues would be providing the same information as the two-word cue (i.e., both would include context-appropriate and context-inappropriate information). The results indicated that the chronological age-matched participants without mental retardation exhibited the greatest two-word cue advantage, whereas the participants with mental retardation exhibited the smallest two-word cue advantage. It was concluded that the participants with mental retardation exhibited a difficultly in language processing that reflected a deficiency in semantically integrating words in a sentence during auditory sentence processing.

Merrill and Jackson (1992a,b) conducted two follow-up investigations that indicate that the semantic processing difficulties exhibited by persons with mental retardation in the Merrill and Bilsky experiment may be due to working memory capacity differences. Merrill and Jackson (1992b) conducted a similar study to Merrill and Bilsky (1990) except that in one condition a pictorial representation of the sentence was included with the auditory presentation of the sentence. Although presenting a picture with the sentence probably does many different things, one likely change in processing is that the working memory capacity requirements associated with sentence processing are considerably less when a picture is presented with the sentence than when a picture is not presented with the sentence. The results indicated that participants with mental retardation exhibited a similar two-word cue advantage as chronological age-matched participants without mental retardation when the working memory capacity requirements of semantic integration were lessened by the picture manipulation.

Merrill and Jackson (1992a) manipulated working memory capacity by presenting sentences in which the individual words were more semantically related (e.g., The hunter shot the rabbit) or less semantically related (e.g., The photographer chased the rabbit). The logic was that a sentence consisting of semantically related words would require fewer working memory resources to construct a semantically integrated representation than would a sentence consisting of semantically unrelated words. Consistent with expectations, individuals with and without mental retardation matched on chronological age performed in a similar manner when processing sentences constructed from semantically related words. However, the participants with mental retardation did not perform as well as the participants without mental retardation when the sentences were constructed from semantically unrelated words. The results of this series of experiments supports the suggestion that differences in sentence processing between persons with and without mental retardation may be closely related to general working memory capacity.

C. Summary

Two components of working memory are directly or indirectly related to general language comprehension: the articulatory–phonological loop and the central executive (typically assessed by reference to working memory capacity). The phonological loop has primary responsibility for vocabulary acquisition and the learning of novel words. The best available evidence indicates that this relation holds for persons with mental retardation as well as persons without mental retardation. The best available evidence also indicates that differences in phonological processing are not directly related to differences in auditory language comprehension between persons with and persons without mental retardation. On the other hand, working memory capacity, which is highly correlated with measures of general intelligence, also appears to be highly correlated with measures of language comprehension. Unfortunately, we cannot tell from the research we have reviewed whether working memory capacity is a better predictor of language comprehension than are our measures of general intelligence or if we are simply measuring the same thing in more than one manner.

We offer one caveat to these specific conclusions. Research on persons who exhibit normal to above normal working memory capacity has not produced evidence of a direct relation between the activities of the articulatory–phonological loop and language comprehension. It may be that differences in phonological processing can be ameliorated if individuals possess at least a normal working memory capacity. The fact that persons with mental retardation are generally characterized by below average working memory capacity may limit their ability to overcome other deficiencies, such as those that may be associated with the phonological loop. It is quite possible that persons with mental retardation will exhibit correlations between memory mechanisms and comprehension that are not exhibited by persons without mental retardation in some instances. Hence, it would be inappropriate to conclude that the operation of the articulatory–phonological loop is not related to language comprehension for persons with mental retardation on the basis of results obtained in research on persons without mental retardation. Numminen et al. (2000) provide a good starting point for evaluating working memory structure and operations associated with mental retardation without worrying about how they compare to persons without mental retardation. This type of research should continue. It would also be interesting to evaluate the role of the articulatory–phonological loop when working memory capacity is experimentally equated (e.g., test at individually determined half and full working memory capacity being utilized for other tasks) across individuals. Correlations that are not observed when working memory capacity is allowed to vary may emerge when it is experimentally equated.

III. SEMANTIC MEMORY

As mentioned earlier, language comprehension has typically been equated with the construction of a coherent semantic representation of discourse (see Lorch & van den Brock, 1997). Lorch (1998) has noted that early models of text comprehension (e.g., Kintsch & van Dijk, 1978) relied heavily on the mechanisms described by models developed for understanding the representation and processing of semantic knowledge (e.g., Anderson & Bower, 1973; Collins & Loftus, 1975; Kintsch, 1974). This emphasis is also evident in current theoretical approaches (e.g., Gerrig & McKoon, 1998; Kintsch, 1988; McKoon, Gerrig, & Greene, 1996). One important change in emphasis associated with the more recent models involves a consideration of the role of how individuals use their background knowledge during language comprehension activities (Lorch, 1998). Hence, for many current theorists, language comprehensions activities are assumed to engage a highly automated memory retrieval process (e.g., Myers & O'Brien, 1998). Current debate centers on the degree to which memory retrieval during language processing is restricted to only those aspects of discourse and background knowledge that are relevant to the interpretation of the text (e.g., Albrecht & O'Brien, 1993; Fletcher & Bloom, 1988; Glenberg & Langston, 1992; O'Brien, Rizzella, Albrecht, & Halleran, 1998) and the degree to which language comprehension requires an evaluative, constructivist component as well as a resonance based, automatic memory retrieval component (e.g., Noordman & Vonk, 1992; Singer, Graesser, & Trabasso, 1994). Regardless of the outcome of these debates, it is clear that semantic memory is generally considered integral to language comprehension.

Semantic memory, as we use it here, refers to a context-free repository of knowledge about concepts, words, and nonword symbols. Semantic memory is generally assumed to be highly organized (Anderson, 1983, 1993; Collins & Loftus, 1975; McClelland, Rumelhart, & Hinton, 1988). Many semantic memory models view semantic memory as a network of interrelated conceptual nodes linked together by labeled pathways that specify particular relations between the nodes (Anderson, 1983, 1993; Collins & Loftus, 1975; Collins & Quillian, 1972). For example, the concept "canary" may be linked to the concept "bird" by a "member of" pathway and to the concept of "yellow" by a "property of" pathway. In these models, several assumptions are made about the basic processes that operate on semantic memory that may impact language comprehension. First, memory retrieval, or accessing the meaning of a concept, involves the automatic activation of the node above its resting state when the word or symbol representing the node is encountered. Second, when an individual node is activated, activation spreads from that node to other conceptual nodes with which it is linked in the network. Further, this activation spreads from these newly activated nodes to others with which they are linked, resulting in the full elaboration of meaning for any given word or symbol that is encountered.

Third, much of what we know are things that we never directly learned, but can easily infer from evaluating interconnections of activated conceptual nodes. For example, most of us did not directly learn that a canary has wings. Rather, we learned that a bird has wings and that a canary is a bird. From these two pieces of information, we "know" that a canary has wings.

In addition to knowledge about basic concepts, people also have knowledge about general objects and events that are often constructed from multiple concepts. These units of knowledge have often been referred to as schemas (e.g., Rumelhart & Ortony, 1977) or scripts (Schank & Abelson, 1977). The script or schema is assumed to reflect typical information about common events rather than a specific episode. Hence, we would have a schema for going to a restaurant but not for going to a restaurant with Carol last Wednesday night. Scripts are assumed to be flexible and can vary in their degree of abstractness. Script knowledge allows us to infer actions that are not explicitly stated in a conversation or text. For example, if you hear that I went to a restaurant with Carol last Wednesday night, ate some enchiladas, and left a big tip, it is likely that you would infer a variety of other actions occurred, as well. It is likely that I sat down, ordered from a menu, enjoyed my food, was pleased with the service, paid my check, and left the restaurant. None of these activities was stated in the description, but they are part of our understanding of the event I described. Scripted knowledge is assumed to facilitate general comprehension of information with which individuals are reasonably familiar.

In the next two sections, we consider the role of semantic memory in discourse comprehension. In the first of these sections, we review the basic findings from research on persons without mental retardation. The intent of this review is to demonstrate the basic influence of semantic memory on discourse processing. Most of the studies that we discuss in this section are relatively older. However, the basic findings have not changed over the years, only the theoretical constructs used to explain them. In the second section, we first review studies that evaluate the basic similarities and differences of semantic memory for persons with and without mental retardation. This is followed by a review of research that compares similarities and differences in how semantic memory influences discourse comprehension processes for persons with and without mental retardation.

A. Semantic Memory and Language Comprehension: Persons without Mental Retardation

It is reasonable to assume that language comprehension is related to semantic knowledge in fundamental ways. In a series of studies, Anderson and colleagues (e.g., Anderson, 1977; Anderson et al., 1976; Anderson & Ortony, 1975) have revealed a number of important ways that semantic knowledge facilitates language comprehension. For example, semantic knowledge provides the basic framework for assimilating text information. In a sense, the semantic framework has slots that can be filled with new information consistent with the framework and facilitates the learning and remembering of the new information. In addition, semantic knowledge directs attention during the comprehension process. Attention is directed to aspects of the verbal material that are deemed important and relevant by the semantic framework. Finally, semantic knowledge facilitates inferential elaboration and reconstruction. Comprehension typically involves making reasonable guesses about information that is not directly given as we listen and read. Semantic knowledge provides the basis for the memory search, editing, and summary processes that make our guesses more likely to be correct than incorrect. Following are several examples of the influence of top–down processing on language comprehension.

Anderson and Ortony (1975) reported that it is common for persons to instantiate specific exemplars consistent with sentence context and general world knowledge when they encounter superordinate labels during discourse processing. For example, they found that when participants were presented sentences such as "The container held the cola" they were likely to remember the container as a "bottle" and when presented sentences such as "The container held the apples" they were likely to remember the container as a "basket." The degree to which these instantiations are made spontaneously is influenced by many factors, including the amount of context available to support the instantiation and the degree to which the specific term is a typical or atypical member of the general category (Rosch, 1975). Nevertheless, it is clear that the ability to perform this operation requires a reasonably well-developed semantic knowledge base, and the specificity of comprehension depends on the ability to perform this operation.

Owens, Bower, and Black (1979) illustrated the importance of activated semantic knowledge providing a semantic framework in basic comprehension activities. They had college students read paragraphs such as the following:

> "Nancy went to see the doctor. She arrived at the office and checked in with the receptionist. She went to see the nurse, who went through the usual procedures. Then Nancy stepped on the scale and the nurse recorded her weight. The doctor entered the room and examined the results. He smiled at Nancy and said, "Well, it seems my expectations have been confirmed." When the examination was finished, Nancy left the office." (p. 186)

Two groups of participants read the story, with the only difference between the two groups being that the one group read a brief thematic statement before they read the story that included the following information:

> "Nancy woke up feeling sick again and she wondered if she really were pregnant. How would she tell the professor she had been seeing? And the money was another problem." (p. 185)

Twenty-four hours later, the participants were asked to recall the story. Participants who had read the thematic statement before they read the passage were able to recall many more facts that were stated in the passage than those who were not provided the theme ahead of time. In addition, they recalled many more facts that were inferred from the passage, but were not directly stated in the passage. The theme, which resulted in an activated base of knowledge for comprehending the passage, allowed for a much richer interpretation of the passage and a more durable memory of what was read (and inferred).

Anderson and Pichert (1978) illustrated how comprehension is influenced by contextual and situational biases. Participants in their study were asked to read a story about the home of a fairly wealthy family from the standpoint of someone considering either the purchase or the burglary of the house. Included in the description of the house were features such as a leaky roof, musty basement, fireplace, coin collection, silverware, and television set. Consistent with expectations, memory about specific features described in the passage was influenced by the participants suggested role: the "burglars" remembered more information about the valuable contents of the house and the "prospective-buyers" remembered more information about the condition of the home. In this case, a selectively activated knowledge base associated with the reader's purpose encouraged a selective encoding and comprehension of information in the passage.

Bower, Black, and Turner (1979) demonstrated that familiarity in the form of activated knowledge may also have a cost if verbatim comprehension and recall is the goal. They presented participants with brief passages such as the following:

> "Bill had a toothache. It seemed forever before he finally arrived at his dentist's office. Bill looked around at the various dental posters on the wall. Finally the dental hygienist examined and X-rayed his teeth. He wondered what the dentist was doing. The dentist said that Bill had a lot of cavities. As soon as he'd made another appointment, he left the dentist's office." (p. 190)

In testing, Bower et al. presented old sentences (The dentist said Bill had a lot of cavities), new related sentences (Bill checked in with the dentist's receptionist), and new unrelated sentences (The receptionist took out the coffee pot and filled it with water). Participants often mistakenly reported that new related sentences were actually a part of the original passage.

Despite the fact that accessing prior knowledge may contribute to less accurate verbatim memories during language comprehension, it is generally accepted that language materials that are consistent with activated prior knowledge are easier to comprehend and remember (e.g., Bransford, 1979; Bransford & Stein, 1984). However, distinctive and unusual events may be exceptions to this generalization (see e.g., Bellezza, 1983; Bellezza, & Bower, 1981; Graesser, 1981). It appears that novel and unexpected objects that find their way into events are typically much better remembered than irrelevant events. Atypical events may, in fact, receive more processing than typical events (Bellezza, 1983; Bellezza, & Bower, 1981) and be better remembered as a result.

More recently, the concept of "mental model" has been applied to the understanding of text comprehension by adults without mental retardation (see Johnson-Laird, 1983). According to Johnson-Laird, mental models are structural analogues of the environment and can encompass many different concepts and schemas and the relations between them. An important feature of mental models is that they are dynamic and are continually updated as comprehension proceeds. Morrow, Greenspan, and Bower (1987) had participants learn the locations of various objects in several rooms of a building. The building was used as the setting for a narrative that was subsequently presented to the participants. During the narrative, a test sentence was presented, such as "Wilber walked from the library into the reception room." Following the test sentence, the participants were presented with probes that consisted of two of the objects whose locations they had previously memorized. Their task was to determine whether or not the two objects were in the same room. They found that decision times were shorter if the objects were located in the current room of the individual depicted in the narrative, suggesting that the participants were constructing and updating dynamic representations of the narrative during comprehension activities (see also Glenberg, Meyer, & Lindem, 1987). Additional research has found that similar updating occurs for temporal information (e.g., Bestgen & Vonk, 1995), features of the primary characters (e.g., Myers, O'Brien, Albrecht, & Mason, 1994), and goals and intentions of the characters (e.g., Dopkins, 1996; Long, Golding, & Graesser, 1992).

B. Semantic Memory and Language Comprehension: Persons with Mental Retardation

Many aspects of semantic memory appear to operate in a similar manner for persons with and without mental retardation of the same chronological age (Cody & Borkowski, 1977; Glidden, 1986; Sperber & McCauley, 1984; Sperber et al., 1976; Winters & Cundari, 1979). In the majority of these studies, semantic memory has been evaluated in terms of the relatively spontaneous activation of related concepts when a picture or word representing a particular concept is presented. For example, Sperber and his colleagues used semantic priming procedures to evaluate the organization of semantic memory of adolescents with and without mental retardation of equal chronological age. For both groups of participants, they observed that the processing of a target picture was faster when it was preceded by a semantically related prime relative than when it was preceded by a semantically unrelated prime. In addition, the magnitude of facilitation observed for the two groups was virtually identical. Sperber et al. (1976) and Sperber and McCauley (1984) suggested that these data indicate that the basic organization and operation of semantic memory was similar for persons with and without mental retardation.

Winters and Cundari (1979) used a release from proactive interference procedure and found that the spontaneous influence of semantic knowledge on short-term memory was similar for persons with and without mental retardation of the same chronological age. In this procedure, participants are presented with a short list of words from a single semantic category to commit to short-term memory. As additional lists of words from the same category are subsequently presented, we generally see an increase in intrusions from previous lists. When a list from a new category is presented, interference from previous lists is eliminated (Wickens, 1970). Persons with and without mental retardation exhibit a similar pattern of performance on these tasks, suggesting that semantic memory exerts a similar influence on the basic encoding processes of both groups of individuals.

Researchers have also demonstrated that the "typicality effects" (Rosch, 1973, 1975) characteristic of adult semantic organization are also characteristic of persons with mental retardation. More specifically, category membership is not an "all or none" feature. For adults without mental retardation, some members are better examples of a category than are others and are given preferential treatment when category information is employed in language comprehension and decision-making. For example, a "robin" is a more typical bird than is an "ostrich." When asked the question "Do birds fly?", most individuals respond "yes" because most birds are like the typical robin that does fly rather than like the atypical ostrich that does not fly. Children and persons with mental retardation exhibit typicality effects that operate in a manner similar to adults without mental retardation. However, there is some evidence indicating that the category exemplars that are considered typical versus atypical may vary with age and intelligence (see Bjorklund & Thompson, 1983; Glidden & Mar, 1978).

One potentially important difference in the processing of basic semantic information by chronological age-matched persons with and without mental retardation was reported by Sperber, Davies, Merrill, and McCauley (1982). They classified categories as "perceptual" or "nonperceptual" on the basis of raters' judgments of the similarity or distinctiveness of the exemplars of the category. For example, categories such as "four-legged mammals" and "land vehicles" were judged to be perceptual categories because many of the exemplars share similar perceptual features whereas categories such as "furniture" and "clothing" were judged to be "nonperceptual" because exemplars share relatively few perceptual features. Participants in their study included adolescents with mental retardation and second-, fifth-, and eleventh-grade participants without mental retardation. In the procedure, participants were presented with a prime (the name of the category or a neutral word) followed by a picture and had to identify the picture. All participants benefited from the category prime when identifying pictures from perceptual categories; however, only the eleventh grade participants benefited from the category prime when identifying pictures from nonperceptual categories. Apparently, all conceptual information is not created equally. We now consider the distinction between perceptual and nonperceptual categories to reflect something analogous to the distinction made by Keil and others (see Keil, 1989; Keil, Smith, Simons, & Levin, 1998) between concept formation based on similarity and concept formation based on rules. Similarity-based concepts appear to operate the same for persons with and without mental retardation, whereas rule-based concepts, which are not typically acquired until children reach a more advanced developmental level, operate differently. Hence, demonstrating equivalence in the use of semantic knowledge in language comprehension for one set of concepts may not necessarily generalize to all other concepts.

There are a few studies that have evaluated the use of semantic information during sentence comprehension activities by persons with and without mental retardation. For example, Bilsky, Walker, and Sakales (1983) evaluated the likelihood that adolescents with mental retardation would instantiate specific instances of general concepts during sentence processing. Participants were presented with experimental sentences of the type "The bug stung her arm" or control sentences of the type "The bug crawled up her arm." The former was intended to constrain comprehension by inferring that a specific exemplar was involved (e.g., the bug was a bee) and the latter was not. Using a cued recall measure, they presented either the specific term or the general term to cue the recall of these sentences. They found that the specific cues (e.g., bee) were more effective as a cue for the experimental sentence than for the control sentence, and the specific term was just as effective in cueing the experimental sentence as the general term. More importantly, they reported that the adolescents with mental retardation benefited from the use of the specific cue just as much as did a group of children without mental retardation with whom they were matched on mental age. Apparently, both groups were able to infer the specific instance during sentence comprehension activities and did so to the same degree. Hence, it appears that semantic memory processes influenced comprehension equally for persons with and without mental retardation in this study.

An extensive search of the literature produced limited results concerning more systematic evaluation of the influence of semantic knowledge on language comprehension processes of persons with mental retardation. However, there is some research that is relevant to the issue. For example, Kim and Lombardino (1991) found that script-based training was more effective than nonscript based training in teaching young children with mental retardation to understand a variety of sentences constructions. The students were four children with mental retardation with measured mental ages ranging between 23 and 30 months and chronological ages between 61 and 78 months. For the script based treatment conditions, the sentence constructions were embedded in the context of popcorn-, pudding-, or milkshake-making. For the nonscript based treatment conditions, the sentence constructions were trained in the context of "playing with some toys." The researchers found that the training of sentence constructions was more effective in the script conditions for three of the four children.

Bilsky, Blachman, Chi, and Chan-Mui (1986) compared the performance of adolescents with mental retardation and mental age-matched children without mental retardation on the ability to generate inferences from story passages. The participants were presented with ambiguous story passages that permitted story-based inferences or computational inferences. Prior to the presentation of the passages, the participants were given instructions that encouraged the processing of the passage as a story, a math problem, or neutral instructions. For all participants, story inferences were processed more accurately under story and neutral set instructions than under math set instructions (Experiment 1). In a second experiment, the desired processing context was further encouraged by embedding target items in story passages or math problems. In this experiment, the accuracy of computational inferences generated by the participants was increased under math set conditions. These results are generally consistent with the notion that different comprehension strategies are employed in contexts that encourage the interpretation of texts as either math problems or stories. Hence, it appears that activation of the appropriate knowledge base is an important contributor to the comprehension processes of both persons with and without mental retardation.

C. Summary

The results of the studies we have described reveal a fundamental similarity in the ways in which semantic knowledge influences language comprehension for persons with and without mental retardation of the same chronological age. However, we suggest considerable caution in accepting this general conclusion for several reasons. First, activation of the appropriate knowledge base does not appear to be done spontaneously by persons with mental retardation as regularly or effectively as it is done by persons without mental retardation of the same mental age. It is good that semantic knowledge provides a similar basis for comprehension for persons with and without mental retardation, but it is only effective when semantic knowledge is accessed. Similar deficiencies in other aspects of the conscious use of semantic information by persons with and without mental retardation of the same mental age have been noted over the years (Cody & Borkowski, 1977; Davies, Sperber, & McCauley, 1981; Glidden & Mar, 1978; Sperber et al., 1976). Second, each of these studies provides data about relatively rudimentary aspects of semantic knowledge on language comprehension. It is likely that there are differences in the details of semantic knowledge that are available to persons with and without mental retardation, and these details may lead to important differences in aspects of comprehension not assessed in the studies described here. Third, the use of semantic knowledge in comprehension requires that knowledge be applied in a flexible manner. For example, in our discussion of a restaurant script earlier, we indicated that a reasonable inference would be that Carol and I sat down at a table and ordered food from a menu. There are restaurants at which an individual is more likely to sit or even stand at a counter and order from a menu over the top of the food counter. A script or story schema must be flexible enough to handle these changes. It is reasonable to question whether scripts used by persons with mental retardation are as flexibly employed as those by persons without mental retardation. Fourth, the activation and use of semantic knowledge during comprehension may commonly involve working memory. To the extent that this is true, we would expect differences in comprehension performance between persons with and without mental retardation even when all differences in semantic memory are controlled. Fifth, the ability of persons with mental retardation to construct and efficiently use mental models to maintain coherence during discourse processing has yet to be evaluated. This avenue of research should prove fruitful. Clearly, there is a lot of research yet to be conducted on semantic memory processes of persons with mental retardation.

IV. TACIT MEMORY

Tacit, or procedural, memory refers to a system of memories that are used to perform skills, but are not directly accessible for conscious inspection; that is, procedural knowledge will allow us to perform many activities efficiently and accurately, but not allow us to explain exactly how we have performed them (Anderson, 1982). Many researchers have suggested that language comprehension and production include important contributions from a tacit memory system (e.g., Chang, Dell, Bock, & Griffin, 2000; Dell, Reed, Adams, & Meyer, 2000; Mathews, 1997; Nagy & Genter, 1990). This conclusion is based on two general observations. First, people typically are able to make judgments about the grammaticality of sentences but are often unaware of the reasons underlying their judgments. Second, at least some of the ability to judge grammaticality is learned. Because some sentence constructions are grammatical in some languages and not other languages, it is reasonable to claim that some aspects of grammar are learned rather than innate (see Lachter, 1994). To the extent that these assumptions are true, then language comprehension can be viewed as a learned skill.

Another line of research that implicates the tacit memory system in language activities has recently been reported by Saffran and her colleagues (Aslin, Saffran, & Newport, 1998; Saffran, Aslin, & Newport, 1996; Saffran, Newport, & Aslin, 1996; Saffran, Newport, Aslin, Tunick, & Barruecco, 1997). For example, Saffran et al. (1996) presented 8-month-old infants with artificial languages consisting of "words" that were made up of three nonsense syllables. These words were presented continuously in random order for a period of 2 min. The infants were then tested for their ability to discriminate these words from part words and nonwords made from the same nonsense syllables. During testing, the infants attended to part words and nonwords for a longer period of time then they attended to the words, indicating an ability to distinguish the words from the nonwords and part words with only limited exposure. Because no other information was available to the infants, Saffran et al. concluded that the infants' learning and discrimination performance was based on statistical information associated with transitional probabilities between successive syllabi (see also Aslin et al., 1998). We consider this tacit learning and memory because it is unlikely that the infants were consciously aware of these transitional probabilities. Hence, some aspects of language processing appear to be accessible to a tacit memory system at a very young age.

It is also the case that efficient use of the tacit memory system is generally considered indispensable in the performance of virtually all skilled behavior (Anderson, 1983; Keil, 1989; Sun, Merrill, & Peterson, 2001; VanLehn, 1991). As skill develops, the performance of the skill becomes more and more automatic, requiring less attention to be performed and interfering less with other ongoing cognitive activities (Anderson, 1982). When a skill reaches this stage, the procedures used to carry out the skill are assumed to reflect the operation of a tacit, not accessible to consciousness, memory system. An early and interesting demonstration of the automatization of skill was reported by Spelke, Hirst, and Neisser (1976). Their participants performed a reading comprehension task while taking dictation. At first, combining the two tasks was extremely difficult. However, after several weeks of practice the participants' reading comprehension returned to pre-experimental levels while performing near perfect dictation. Interestingly, they could not remember any of the words they were transcribing, suggesting that conscious memory was not responsible for performance on the dictation task. To the extent that language comprehension reflects a skilled behavior, it is likely that tacit memory plays an important role in general language comprehension as well. Therefore, it is necessary to evaluate differences in the acquisition of tacit memories and the use of the tacit memory system by persons with and without mental retardation and to consider the contribution of these differences to language comprehension. Because the relations between tacit memory and language comprehension have not been studied directly, we will focus on the development of tacit memories in the next section.

A. Tacit Memory Research on Persons without Mental Retardation

Tacit memory of persons without mental retardation is generally studied in the context of skill acquisition (Anderson, 1982, 1983; Keil, 1989; VanLehn, 1995). One way that tacit memories are acquired is through "proceduralization." For Anderson (1982), the initial stages of skill acquisition are characterized by the acquisition of basic declarative (i.e., explicit) knowledge about the task to be performed. More specifically, people often learn specific rules and steps that enable them to perform the task first, and the task can only be performed with careful attention directed toward each step (the classic example is learning to drive a car). Through extensive practice, performance of the task becomes proceduralized, which is accomplished by converting explicit, declarative knowledge in the form of instructions into production rules. Production rules allow people to perform the task without attending to declarative knowledge about how to perform the task, and in many cases without awareness of any of the details of task performance. Other researchers have described a similar progression from declarative to procedural, or tacit, memory in the areas of general skill acquisition (Fitts & Posner, 1967), concept formation (Keil, 1989), and verbal information reasoning (Sun, 1994).

Several lines of research have developed in recent years that indicate that people may also learn to perform complex skills without learning extensive declarative knowledge first (e.g., Lewicke, Hill, & Czyzewska, 1992; Mathews et al., 1989; Reber, 1989; Reber & Lewis, 1977). This process has been called "implicit learning." For example, in the domain of artificial grammar learning Reber and colleagues have conducted an extensive series of studies on the possibility that relatively complex rules can be acquired without learning declarative knowledge in the domain (Reber & Lewis, 1977; Reber, 1967, 1976, 1989). Participants were asked to commit a series of letter strings to memory, where the letter strings were formed on the basis of a set of probabilistic rules or were formed randomly. They were not told of the rules or informed that rules were used to construct the letter strings. After experience with "rule-based" letter strings, participants were able to commit new rule-based strings to memory more rapidly than they were able to do without prior experience of the strings. In addition, they were able to classify new strings as grammatical or not grammatical at levels significantly above chance. However, they were not able to explicitly state the rules of grammar that allowed them to classify the new letter strings. Although somewhat controversial because it is difficult to demonstrate with certainty that conscious learning does not play a role in laboratory investigations of these tasks, many researchers believe that implicit learning plays an important role in the learning of language, communication, and social skills (e.g., Lachter, 1994; Mathews, 1997).

B. Tacit Memory Research on Persons with Mental Retardation

Studies of proceduralization have not been conducted on persons with mental retardation. However, Merrill, Goodwyn, and Gooding (1996) have examined the role of extensive practice in the development of automatic processing in a relatively simple visual search task by persons with and without mental retardation. Participants with and without mental retardation (matched on chronological age) were given extensive practice searching through sets of two, three, and four pictures for instances of a designated target category (e.g., clothing). Over a period of 4 days, participants received approximately 1200 search trials. Automatic processing was indexed by a reduction in search rates that indicated that search times were not influenced by the number of items in the search set. This measure was used because automatic processing is assumed to allow parallel processing, whereas conscious processing is assumed to operate in serial fashion (see Schneider & Shiffrin, 1977; Shiffrin & Schneider, 1977). When search times are unaffected by set size, the indication is that the items in the set are being searched in parallel. In the experiment, the participants without mental retardation exhibited evidence of automatic processing after about 2 days of practice, whereas the participants with mental retardation did not exhibit evidence of automatic processing until they completed 4 days of practice. Assuming that we can generalize the results of this experiment to the proceduralization of more complex activities, we would conclude that persons with mental retardation require much more extensive practice to develop a functional tacit memory of a complex procedure relative to persons without mental retardation of the same chronological age. No corresponding study comparing persons with and without mental retardation on mental age has been conducted.

Atwell et al. (2003) recently reported the results of an experiment designed to evaluate implicit learning by persons with and without mental retardation. Participants in this experiment were also adolescents with and without mental retardation matched on chronological age. The procedure of the experiment was a modified artificial grammar learning task. In this case, participants were exposed to strings of colored geometric figures that were formed on the basis of a set of rules. Following exposure, the participants were shown a series of previously seen strings or new strings that were formed in accordance with the same set of rules or were formed randomly. They had to determine if the strings were previously presented or not. Atwell et al. reasoned that if participants had learned features of the rules that were used to form the original strings, they would be more likely to confuse new strings formed on the basis of the same rules as old strings than they would new strings that were formed randomly. Both groups of participants exhibited more confusions with the rule-based strings than they did with random strings. In addition, the degree to which the groups exhibited differential interference as a function of type of string was essentially identical. One difference between groups was observed, however. To exhibit the same level of implicit learning as the participants without mental retardation, the participants with mental retardation required about twice as many presentations of the original series of geometric forms.

C. Summary

Based on the admittedly limited research conducted to date, we can tentatively conclude that persons with and without mental retardation exhibit the ability to acquire tacit memories, and that they appear to do so in fundamentally the same ways. However, it is also clear that persons with mental retardation require more experience/practice with the acquisition materials before they exhibit the same degree of tacit knowledge as persons without mental retardation of the same chronological age. Research has not been conducted that examines how persons with and without mental retardation use tacit knowledge during language comprehension. In addition, research has not been conducted that investigates the relative limits of the abilities of persons with and without mental retardation to acquire tacit knowledge and use it in relatively complex skills. To date, research has only demonstrated that persons with mental retardation can acquire tacit memories for relatively simply materials through implicit learning. It may be that the fundamental difference between persons with and without mental retardation in tacit memory reflects a difference in the degree of complexity of information that can be proceduralized with practice or learned implicitly.

V. CONCLUSION

In this chapter, we have outlined several ways that memory is related to the language comprehension activities of persons with mental retardation. We focused on three memory systems: working memory, semantic memory, and tacit memory. Semantic memory probably plays the biggest role in language comprehension activities. It is in the semantic system that word meanings are stored and organized in a manner that supports language comprehension. However, it is working memory that has been given the majority of credit for explaining individual differences in language comprehension. The role of working memory is to provide resources for and coordinate the retrieval and incorporation of relevant information from semantic memory into developing memory representations that reflect on-line comprehension. Tacit memory may play a relatively indirect, but necessary role in language comprehension. Implicit learning, or the process that is involved in the creation of tacit memories, appears to be involved in the learning of lower-level regularities of language. In particular, research has demonstrated that even children as young as 8-months-old can detect regularities associated with word boundaries. This is a fundamental skill for the development of language abilities.

As is typical of research comparing the performance of persons with and without mental retardation, we found that most studies revealed a basic similarity in the structure and operation of the various memory systems. Language materials are processed and used in fundamentally the same ways by persons with and without mental retardation. However, the level of language comprehension achieved by persons with mental retardation is considerably less than that achieved by persons without mental retardation. In many instances, comprehension falls below expectations based on measures of general mental age.

Working memory plays a prominent role in on-line language comprehension activities and appears to be closely tied to differences in language comprehension between persons with and without mental retardation. Working memory is also the component of memory assumed to be most closely associated with language comprehension difficulties of persons without mental retardation. More specifically, it is working memory capacity that underlies individual differences in language comprehension. However, in light of the research conducted on persons with Down syndrome and Williams syndrome that we have reviewed, this conclusion may be too general. One important outcome of etiology specific research such as this is the observation that differences in the operation of the articulatory–phonological loop may be responsible for some differences in language comprehension, at least for persons with mental retardation. A reassessment of the role of phonological processing in language comprehension processes of persons with mental retardation resulting from different causes may benefit from procedures that do not allow working memory capacity to vary.

We are cautiously optimistic about the similarities in the use of semantic memory during language comprehension by persons with and without mental retardation. Semantic memory appears to serve very similar functions and operate in much the same way during language comprehension activities for persons with and without mental retardation. Our note of caution reflects the fact that persons with mental retardation do not appear to access semantic memory to facilitate language comprehension activities as readily as persons without mental retardation access semantic memory. This may be due to several factors, with working memory capacity involved here as well. Working memory is used in the retrieval of information from semantic memory. If working memory capacity is insufficient to process language on-line and access semantic memory at the same time, language comprehension is likely to suffer. Another possibility is that persons without mental retardation have a greater expectation that language activities should result in comprehension than do persons with mental retardation. Hence, they actively access semantic memory to facilitate comprehension when they do not understand whereas as persons with mental retardation do not.

Based on our general search of the literature, we have concluded that research considering semantic memory and semantic memory processes and the role of semantic memory in the language comprehension activities of persons with mental retardation has slowed considerably in recent years. Perhaps this has been the result of discovering fundamental similarities, rather than important differences in the structure and organization of semantic memory for persons with, relative to persons without, mental retardation. However, there are many aspects of how semantic memory is used in general cognitive skills, including language comprehension, by persons with mental retardation that require some research attention. Specific areas that will benefit from further investigation include the following. We would like to see research that evaluates differences between persons with and without mental retardation in the amount of contextual support necessary to spontaneously activate and retrieve relevant background knowledge from semantic memory during language comprehension. We would like to see additional research on whether persons with mental retardation are able to use semantic knowledge in as flexible a manner as necessary for language comprehension activities. In conjunction with the previous suggestion, we believe that research on language comprehension processes by persons with mental retardation would benefit from a consideration of the concept of mental models. To the extent that comprehension of discourse involves a continual updating of information presented in the narrative, mental models provide the features for considering how the updating mechanism operates.

We are intrigued by the possibility that tacit memory may play an important role in language comprehension activities and may be related to differences in the language comprehension of persons with and without mental retardation. It appears that persons with mental retardation do not benefit as much from extensive practice/experience with stimuli as do persons without mental retardation of the same chronological age. Saffran and colleagues (Saffran et al., 1996) have demonstrated that typically developing children as young as 8-months-old benefit from exposure to regularities that occur in language-like materials. Corresponding research on infants at risk for mental retardation and infants diagnosed with syndromes associated with mental retardation would be very informative. If persons with mental retardation are not as sensitive to covariations in the environment as are persons without mental retardation, then we would expect that natural language learning would be much more difficult for the persons with mental retardation. Therefore, research concerning the acquisition and use of tacit memory by persons with mental retardation may prove to be a fruitful area of investigation.

ACKNOWLEDGMENTS

Preparation of this chapter was supported by NICHD Grant # HD 30263 awarded to the first author.

REFERENCES

Albrecht, J. E., & O'Brien, E. J. (1993). Updating a mental model: maintaining both local and global coherence. *Journal of Experimental Psychology: Learning, Memory, and Cognition, 19*, 1061–1070.

Anderson, J. R. (1977). Memory for information about individuals. *Memory & Cognition, 5*, 430–442.

Anderson, J. R. (1982). Acquisition of cognitive skill. *Psychological Review, 89*, 369–406.

Anderson, J. R. (1983). *The architecture of cognition*. Hillsdale, NJ: Lawrence Erlbaum Associates, Inc.

Anderson, J. R. (1993). *Human mind*. Hillsdale, NJ: Lawrence Erlbaum Associates, Inc.

Anderson, J. R., & Bower, G. H. (1973). *Human associative memory*. Washington, D.C.: Winston & Sons.

Anderson, R. C., & Ortony, A. (1975). On putting apples into bottles: a problem of polysemy. *Cognitive Psychology, 7*, 167–180.

Anderson, R. C., & Pichert, J. (1978). Recall of previously unrecallable information following a shift in perspective. *Journal of Verbal Learning and Verbal Behavior, 17*, 1–12.

Anderson, R. C., Pichert, J. W., Goetz, E. T., Schallert, D. L., Stevens, K. V., & Trollip, S. R. (1976). Instantiation of general terms. *Journal of Verbal Learning and Verbal Behavior, 15*, 667–679.

Aslin, R. N., Saffran, J. R., & Newport, E. L. (1998). Computation of conditional probability statistics by 8-month-old infants. *Psychological Science, 9*, 312–324.

Atwell, J. A., Conners, F. A., & Merrill, E. C. (2003). Implicit and explicit learning in young adults with mental retardation. *American Journal on Mental Retardation, 108*, 56–68.

Baddeley, A. D. (1986). *Working memory*. Oxford: Oxford University Press.

Baddeley, A. D., Gathercole, S., & Papagano, C. (1998). The phonological loop as a language learning device. *Psychological Review, 105*, 158–173.

Baddeley, A. D., & Hitch, G. J. (1974). Working memory. In G. Bower (Ed.), *The psychology of learning and motivation* (Vol. 8, pp. 47–90). New York: Academic Press.

Bellezza, F. S. (1983). Recalling script-based text: the role of selective processing and schematic cues. *Bulletin of the Psychonomic Society, 21*, 267–270.

Bellezza, F. S., & Bower, G. H. (1981). Remembering script-based texts. *Peotics, 11*, 1–23.

Bestgen, Y., & Vonk, W. (1995). The role of temporal segmentation markers in discourse processing. *Discourse Processes, 19*, 385–406.

Bilsky, L. H., Blachman, S., Chi, C., & Chan-Mui, A. (1986). Comprehension strategies in math problems and story contexts. *Cognition and Instruction, 3*, 109–126.

Bilsky, L. H., Walker, N., & Sakales, S. R. (1983). Comprehension and recall and sentences by mentally retarded and nonretarded individuals. *American Journal of Mental Deficiency, 87*, 558–565.

Bjorklund, D. F., & Thompson, B. E. (1983). Category typicality effects in children's memory performance: qualitative and quantitative differences in the processing of information. *Journal of Experimental Child Psychology, 35*, 329–344.

Borkowski, J., & Cavanaugh, J. (1979). Maintenance and generalization of skills and strategies by the retarded. In N. R. Ellis (Ed.), *Handbook of mental deficiency: Psychological theory and research* (2nd ed., pp. 569–617). Hillsdale, NJ: Erlbaum.

Bower, G. H., Black, J. B., & Turner, T. J. (1979). Scripts for memory in text. *Cognitive Psychology, 11*, 177–220.

Bransford, J. D. (1979). *Human cognition: Learning, understanding, and remembering*. Belmont, CA: Wadsworth.

Bransford, J. D., & Stein, B. S. (1984). *The ideal problem solver*. New York: W.H. Freeman & Co.

Brown, A. L., & Campione, J. (1977). Training strategic study time apportionment in educable retarded children. *Intelligence*, *1*, 94–107.

Burack, J. A., Evans, D. W., Klaiman, C., & Iarocci, G. (2001). The mysterious myth of attention deficits and other defect stories: contemporary issues in the developmental approach to mental retardation. In L. M. Glidden (Ed.), *International review of research in mental retardation* (Vol. 24, pp. 299–317). New York: Academic Press.

Butterworth, B., Campbell, R., & Howard, D. (1986). The uses of short-term memory: a case study. *Quarterly Journal of Experimental Psychology*, *38A*, 705–737.

Campbell, R., & Butterworth, B. (1985). Phonological dyslexia and dysgraphia in highly literate subjects: a developmental case with associated deficits of phonemic processing and awareness. *Quarterly Journal of Experimental Psychology*, *37A*, 435–476.

Carpenter, P., Miyake, A., & Just, M. A. (1995). Language comprehension: sentence and discourse processing. *Annual Review of Psychology*, *46*, 91–100.

Cha, K.-H., & Merrill, E. C. (1994). Facilitations and inhibition in visual selective attention processes of persons with and without mental retardation. *American Journal on Mental Retardation*, *98*, 594–600.

Chang, F., Dell, G. S., Bock, K., & Griffin, Z. M. (2000). Structural priming as implicit learning: a comparison of models of sentence production. *Journal of Psycholinguistic Research*, *29*, 217–229.

Cody, W. J., & Borkowski, J. G. (1977). Proactive interference and its release in short-term memory of mildly retarded adolescents. *American Journal of Mental Deficiency*, *82*, 305–308.

Cohen, R. L., & Sandberg, T. (1980). Intelligence and short-term memory: a clandestine relationship. *Intelligence*, *4*, 319–331.

Collins, A. M., & Loftus, E. F. (1975). A spreading-activation theory of semantic processing. *Psychological Review*, *82*, 407–428.

Collins, A. M., & Quillian, M. R. (1972). How to make a language user. In E. Tulving, & W. Donaldson (Eds.), *Organization of memory* (pp. 309–351). New York: Academic Press.

Comblain, A. (1999). The relevance of a nonword repetition task to assess phonological short-term memory in individuals with Down syndrome. *Down syndrome: Research and Practice*, *6*, 76–84.

Connors, F. A., Carr, M. D., & Willis, S. (1998). Is the phonological loop responsible for intelligence-related differences in forward digit span? *American Journal on Mental Retardation*, *103*(1), 1–11.

Courbois, Y. (1996). Evidence for visual imagery deficits in persons with mental retardation. *American Journal on Mental Retardation*, *101*, 130–148.

Daneman, M., & Carpenter, P. A. (1980). Individual differences in working memory and reading. *Journal of Verbal Learning and Verbal Behavior*, *19*, 450–466.

Daneman, M., & Merickle, P. M. (1996). Working memory and language comprehension: a meta-analysis. *Psychonomic Bulletin & Review*, *3*, 422–433.

Daneman, M., & Tardif, T. (1987). Working memory and reading skill re-examined. In M. Coltheart (Ed.), *Attention and performance XII* (pp. 491–508). Hillsdale, NJ: Erlbaum.

Davies, D., Sperber, R. D., & McCauley, C. (1981). Intelligence-related differences in semantic processing speed. *Journal of Experimental Child Psychology*, *31*, 387–402.

Dell, G. S., Reed, K. D., Adams, D. R., & Meyer, A. S. (2000). Speech errors, phonotactic constraints, and implicit learning: a study of the role of experience in language production. *Journal of Experimental Psychology: Learning, Memory, and Cognition*, *26*, 1355–1367.

Dixon, P., LeFevre, J., & Twilley, L. C. (1988). Word knowledge and working memory as predictors of reading skill. *Journal of Educational Psychology*, *80*, 465–472.

Dopkins, S. (1996). Representation of superordinate goal inferences in memory. *Discourse Processes*, *21*, 85–104.

Ellis, N. R. (1970). Memory processes in retardates and normals. In N. R. Ellis (Ed.), *International review of research in mental retardation* (Vol. 4, pp. 1–32). New York: Academic Press.

Ellis, N. R., Palmer, R. L., & Reeves, C. L. (1988). Developmental and intellectual differences in frequency processing. *Developmental Psychology*, *24*, 38–45.

Ellis, N. R., Woodley-Zanthow, P., & Dulaney, C. L. (1989). Memory for spatial location in children, adults, and mentally retarded persons. *American Journal on Mental Retardation*, *93*, 521–526.

Engle, R. W., Tuholski, S. W., Laughlin, J. E., & Conway, A. R. A. (1999). Working, memory, short-term memory and general fluid intelligence: a latent variable approach. *Journal of Experimental Psychology: General*, *128*, 309–331.

Estes, W. K. (1982). Learning, memory, and intelligence. In R. J. Sternberg (Ed.), *Handbook of human intelligence* (pp. 170–224). New York: Cambridge University Press.

Fitts, P., & Posner, M. (1967). *Human performance*. Monterey, CA: Brooks/Cole.

Fletcher, C. R., & Bloom, C. P. (1988). Causal reasoning in the comprehension of simple text. *Journal of Memory and Language*, *27*, 235–244.

Gathercole, S. E., & Baddeley, A. D. (1993). *Working memory and language*. Hillsdale, NJ: Erlbaum.

Gathercole, S. E., & Pickering, S. J. (2000). Assessment of working memory in six- and seven-year-old children. *Journal of Educational Psychology*, *92*, 377–390.

Gerrig, R. J., & McKoon, G. (1998). The readiness is all: the functionality of memory-based text processing. *Discourse Processes*, *26*, 67–86.

Girolametto, L., Weitzman, E., & Clements-Baartman, J. (1998). Vocabulary intervention for children with Down syndrome: parent training using focused stimulation. *Infant Toddler Intervention*, *8*, 109–125.

Glenberg, A. M., & Langston, W. E. (1992). Comprehension of illustrated text: pictures help to build mental models. *Journal of Memory and Language*, *31*, 129–151.

Glenberg, A. M., Meyer, M., & Lindem, K. (1987). Mental models contribute to foregrounding during text comprehension. *Journal of Memory and Language*, *26*, 69–83.

Glidden, L. M. (1986). Semantic processing, semantic memory, and recall. In N. R. Ellis, & N. W. Bray (Eds.), *International review of research in mental retardation* (Vol. 13, pp. 247–278). New York: Academic Press.

Glidden, L. M., & Mar, H. H. (1978). Availability and accessibility of information in the semantic memory of retarded and nonretarded adolescents. *Journal of Experimental Child Psychology*, *25*, 33–50.

Graesser, A. C. (1981). *Prose comprehension beyond the word*. New York: Springer-Verlag.

Grant, J., Karmiloff-Smith, A., Gathercole, S. E., Paterson, S., Howlin, P., Davies, M., & Udwin, O. (1997). Phonological short-term memory and its relationship to language in Williams syndrome. *Cognitive Neuropsychiatry*, *2*, 81–99.

Jarrold, C., & Baddeley, A. D. (1997). Short-term memory for verbal and visuospatial information in Down's syndrome. *Cognitive Neuropsychiatry*, *2*(2), 101–122.

Jarrold, C., Baddeley, A. D., & Hewes, A. K. (1999). Genetically dissociated components of working memory: evidence from Down's and William's syndrome. *Neuropsychologia*, *37*(6), 637–651.

Johnson-Laird, P. N. (1983). *Mental models: Towards a cognitive science of language, inference, and consciousness*. Cambridge, MA: Harvard University Press.

Just, M. A., & Carpenter, P. A. (1992). A capacity theory of comprehension: individual differences in working memory. *Psychological Review*, *99*, 122–149.

Justice, E. M. (1986). Metamemory: an aspect of metacognition in the mentally retarded. In N. R. Ellis, & N. W. Bray (Eds.), *International review of research in mental retardation* (Vol. 13, pp. 79–108). New York: Academic Press.

Kail, R. (1992). General slowing of information-processing by persons with mental retardation. *American Journal on Mental Retardation*, *97*(3), 333–341.

Keil, F. C. (1989). *Concepts, kinds, and cognitive development*. Cambridge, MA: MIT Press.

Keil, F. C., Smith, W. C., Simons, D. J., & Levin, D. T. (1998). Two dogmas of conceptual empiricism: Implications for hybrid models of the structure of knowledge. *Cognition*, *65*, 103–135.

Kemper, S. (1986). Imitation of complex syntactic constructions by elderly adults. *Applied Psycholinquistics*, *7*(3), 277–287.

Kim, Y. T., & Lombardino, L. J. (1991). The efficacy of script contexts in language comprehension intervention with children who have mental retardation. *Journal of Speech and Hearing Research*, *34*, 845–857.

King, J., & Just, M. A. (1991). Individual differences in syntactic processing: the role of working memory. *Journal of Memory and Language*, *30*, 580–602.

Kintsch, W. (1974). *The representation of meaning in memory*. Hillsdale, NJ: Erlbaum.

Kintsch, W. (1988). The role of knowledge in text comprehension: a construction-integration model. *Psychological Review*, *95*, 163–192.

Kintsch, W., & Mross, E. F. (1985). Context effects in word identification. *Journal of Memory and Language*, *24*(3), 336–349.

Kintsch, W., & van Dijk, T. A. (1978). Toward a model of text comprehension and production. *Psychological Review*, *85*, 363–394.

Klein, B. P., & Mervis, C. B. (1999). Contrasting patterns of cognitive abilities of 9 and 10-year olds with Williams syndrome or Down syndrome. *Developmental Neuropsychology*, *16*(2), 177–196.

Kumin, L. (2001). *Classroom language skills for children with Down syndrome: A guide for parents and teachers*. Bethesda, MD: Woodbine House.

Kumin, L., Councill, C., & Goodman, M. (1998). Expressive vocabulary development in children with Down syndrome. *Down Syndrome Quarterly*, *3*(1), 1–7.

Lachter, J. (1994). Consciousness in natural language and motor learning. *Behavioral and Brain Sciences*, *17*, 409–410.

Laws, G. (1998). The use of nonword repetition as a test of phonological memory in children with Down syndrome. *Journal of Child Psychology and Psychiatry and Allied Disciplines*, *39*(8), 1119–1130.

Lewicke, P., Hill, T., & Czyzewska, M. (1992). Nonconscious acquisition of information. *American Psychologist*, *47*, 796–801.

Long, D. L., Golding, J. M., & Graesser, A. C. (1992). A test of the on-line status of goal-related inferences. *Journal of Memory and Language*, *31*, 634–647.

Lorch, R. F., Jr. (1998). Memory-based text processing. *Discourse Processes*, *26*, 213–221.

Lorch, R. F., Jr., & van den Brock, P. (1997). Understanding reading comprehension: Current and future directions of cognitive science. *Contemporary Educational Psychology*, *22*, 213–246.

MacDonald, M. C., Just, M., & Carpenter, P. A. (1992). Working memory constraints on the processing of syntactic ambiguity. *Cognitive Psychology*, *24*(1), 56–98.

Marcell, M. M., & Cohen, S. (1992). Hearing abilities of Down syndrome and other intellectually impaired adolescents. *Research in Developmental Disabilites*, *13*, 533–551.

Martin, R. C., & Feher, E. (1990). The consequences of reduced memory span for the comprehension of semantic versus syntactic information. *Brain and Language*, *38*, 1–20.

Masson, M. E. J., & Miller, J. A. (1983). Working memory and individual differences in comprehension and memory of text. *Journal of Educational Psychology*, *75*, 314–318.

Mathews, R. C. (1997). Is research painting a biased picture of implicit learning? The dangers of methodological purity in scientific debate. *Psychonomic Bulletin and Review*, *4*, 38–42.

Mathews, R., Buss, R., Stanley, W., Blanchard-Fields, F., Cho, J., & Druhan, B. (1989). Role of implicit and explicit processes in learning from examples: A synergistic effect. *Journal of Experimental Psychology: Learning, Memory, and Cognition*, *15*, 1083–1100.

McClelland, J. L., Rumelhart, D. E., & Hinton, G. E. (1988). The appeal of parallel distributed processing. In A. M. Collins, & E. E. Smith (Eds.), *Readings in cognitive science: A perspective from psychology and artificial intelligence* (pp. 52–72). San Mateo, CA: Morgan Kaufmann, Inc.

McKoon, G., Gerrig, R. J., & Greene, S. B. (1996). Pronoun resolution without pronouns: Some consequences of memory-based processing. *Journal of Experimental Psychology: Learning, Memory, and Cognition*, *22*, 919–932.

Merrill, E. C. (1990). Cognitive resource allocation and mental retardation. In N. W. Bray (Ed.), *International review of research in mental retardation* (Vol. 16, pp. 51–88). New York: Academic Press.

Merrill, E. C., & Bilsky, L. H. (1990). Individual differences in the representation of sentences in memory. *American Journal on Mental Retardation*, *95*, 68–76.

Merrill, E. C., Goodwyn, E. H., & Gooding, H. L. (1996). Mental retardation and the development of automatic processing. *American Journal on Mental Retardation*, *101*, 49–62.

Merrill, E. C., & Jackson, T. S. (1992a). Sentence processing by adolescents with and without mental retardation. *American Journal on Mental Retardation*, *97*, 492–500.

Merrill, E. C., & Jackson, T. S. (1992b). Degree of associative relatedness and sentence processing by persons with and without mental retardation. *American Journal on Mental Retardation*, *97*, 173–185.

Merrill, E. C., & Marr, H. H. (1987). Differences between mentally retarded and nonretarded persons' efficiency of auditory sentence processing. *American Journal of Mental Deficiency*, *91*, 406–414.

Merrill, E. C., McCown, S. M., & Kelley, S. (2001). Similarities in negative priming between persons with and without mental retardation. *American Journal on Mental Retardation*, *106*, 113–122.

Merrill, E. C., Sperber, R. D., McCauley, C., Littlefield, J., Rider, E. A., & Shapiro, D. (1987). Picture encoding speed and mental retardation. *Intelligence*, *11*, 169–191.

Merrill, E. C., & Taube, M. (1996). Negative priming and mental retardation: The processing of distractor information. *American Journal on Mental Retardation*, *101*, 63–71.

Mervis, C. B., & Robinson, B. F. (2000). Expressive vocabulary ability of toddlers with Williams syndrome or Down syndrome: A comparison. *Developmental Neuropsychology*, *17*(1), 111–126.

Milner, B. (1971). Interhemispheric differences in the localization of psychological processes in man. *Cortex*, *27*, 272–277.

Morrow, D. G., Greenspan, S. L., & Bower, G. H. (1987). Accessibility and situation models in narrative comprehension. *Journal of Memory and Language*, *26*, 165–187.

Myers, J. L., & O'Brien, E. J. (1998). Accessing the discourse representation during reading. *Discourse Processes*, *26*, 131–157.

Myers, J. L., O'Brien, E. J., Albrecht, J. E., & Mason, R. A. (1994). Maintaining global coherence. *Journal of Experimental Psychology: Learning, Memory, and Cognition*, *20*, 876–886.

Nagy, W., & Genter, D. (1990). Semantic constraints on lexical categories. *Language and Cognitive Processes*, *5*, 169–201.

Noordman, L. G. M., & Vonk, W. (1992). Readers' knowledge and the control of inferences in reading. *Language and Cognitive Processes*, *7*, 373–391.

Numminen, H., Service, E., Ahonen, T., Korhonen, T., Tolvanen, A., Patja, K., & Ruoppila, I. (2000). *Journal of Intellectual Disability Research*, *44*, 579–590.

O'Brien, E. J., Rizzella, M. L., Albrecht, J. E., & Halleran, J. G. (1998). Updating a situation model: A memory-based processing view. *Journal of Experimental Psychology: Learning, Memory, and Cognition*, *24*, 1200–1210.

Owens, J., Bower, G. H., & Black, J. B. (1979). The "soap opera" effect in story recall. *Memory and Cognition*, *7*, 185–191.

Papagno, C., Valentine, T., & Baddeley, A. D. (1991). Phonological short-term memory and foreign-language vocabulary learning. *Journal of Memory and Language*, *30*, 331–347.

Papagno, C., & Vallar, G. (1992). Phonological short-term memory and the learning of novel words: The effects of phonological similarity and item length. *Quarterly Journal of Experimental Psychology*, *44A*, 47–67.

Phillips, C. J., & Nettelbeck, T. (1986). Mild mental retardation and memory scanning. In N. R. Ellis, & N. W. Bray (Eds.), *International review of research in mental retardation* (Vol. 13, pp. 143–179). New York: Academic Press.

Prehm, M. J., & Mayfield, S. (1970). Paired-associate learning and retention in retarded and nonretarded children. *American Journal of Mental Deficiency*, *74*, 622–625.

Reber, A. (1967). Implicit learning of artificial grammars. *Journal of Verbal Learning and Verbal Behavior*, *6*, 855–867.

Reber, A. (1976). Implicit learning of synthetic languages: The role of instructional set. *Journal of Experimental Psychology: Human Learning and Memory*, *2*, 88–94.

Reber, A. (1989). Implicit learning and tacit knowledge. *Journal of Experimental Psychology: General*, *118*, 219–235.

Reber, A., & Lewis, S. (1977). Implicit learning: An analysis of the form and structure of a body of tacit knowledge. *Cognition*, *5*, 333–361.

Rosch, E. (1973). Natural categories. *Cognitive Psychology*, *4*, 328–350.

Rosch, E. (1975). Cognitive representations of semantic categories. *Journal of Experimental Psychology: General*, *104*, 192–233.

Rumelhart, D. E., & Ortony, A. (1977). The representation of knowledge in memory. In R. Anderson, R. Spiro, & W. Montague (Eds.), *Schooling and the acquisition of knowledge* (pp. 99–135). Hillsdale, NJ: Erlbaum.

Saffran, J. R., Aslin, R. N., & Newport, E. L. (1996). Statistical learning by 8-month-olds. *Science*, *274*, 1926–1928.

Saffran, J. R., Newport, E. L., & Aslin, R. N. (1996). Word segmentation: The role of distributional cues. *Journal of Memory and Language*, *35*, 606–621.

Saffran, J. R., Newport, E. L., Aslin, R. N., Tunick, R. A., & Barruecco, S. (1997). Incidental language learning: Listening (and learning) out of the corner of your ear. *Psychological Science*, *8*, 101–105.

Schank, R. C., & Abelson, R. P. (1977). *Scripts, plans, goals, and understanding: an inquiry into human knowledge structures*. Potomac, MD: Lawrence Erlbaum.

Schneider, W., & Detweiler, M. (1987). A connectionist/control architecture for working memory. In G. H. Bower (Ed.), *The psychology of learning and motivation: Advances in research and theory* (Vol. 21, pp. 53–119). New York: Academic Press.

Schneider, W., & Shiffrin, R. M. (1977). Controlled and automatic human information processing: I. Detection, search, and attention. *Psychological Review*, *84*, 1–66.

Shiffrin, R. M., & Schneider, W. (1977). Controlled and automatic human information processing: II. Perceptual learning, automatic attending, and a general theory. *Psychological Review*, *84*, 127–190.

Singer, M., Graesser, A. C., & Trabasso, T. (1994). Minimal or global inference during reading. *Journal of Memory and Language*, *33*, 421–441.

Spelke, E., Hirst, W., & Neisser, U. (1976). Skills of divided attention. *Cognition*, *4*, 215–230.

Sperber, R. D., Davies, D., Merrill, E. C., & McCauley, C. (1982). Cross-category differences in the processing of subordinate–superordinate relationships. *Child Development*, *53*, 1249–1253.

Sperber, R. D., Greenfield, D. B., & House, B. J. (1973). A nonmonotonic effect of distribution of trials on retardate learning and memory. *Journal of Experimental Psychology*, *99*, 186–198.

Sperber, R. D., & McCauley, C. (1984). Semantic processing efficiency in the mentally retarded. In P. Brooks, R. D. Sperber, & C. McCauley (Eds.), *Learning and cognition in the mentally retarded* (pp. 141–163). Hillsdale, NJ: Erlbaum.

Sperber, R. D., Ragain, R., & McCauley, C. (1976). Reassessment of category knowledge in retarded individuals. *American Journal of Mental Deficiency*, *81*, 227–234.

Spitz, H. H., & Borys, S. V. (1977). Performance of retarded and nonretarded children on one- and two-bit logical problems. *Journal of Experimental Child Psychology*, *23*, 415–429.

Stan, E. A., & Mosley, J. L. (1988). Semantic encoding by mentally retarded and nonretarded individuals. *Journal of Mental Deficiency Research*, *32*, 371–382.

Sun, R. (1994). *Integrating rules and connectionism for robust commonsense reasoning*. New York: John Wiley & Sons.

Sun, R., Merrill, E., & Peterson, T. (2001). From implicit skills to explicit knowledge: a bottom-up model of skill learning. *Cognitive Science*, *25*, 203–244.

Till, R. E., Mross, E., & Kintsch, W. (1988). Time course of priming for associate and inference words in a discourse context. *Memory and Cognition*, *16*(4), 282–298.

Turner, M. L., & Engle, R. W. (1989). Is working memory capacity task dependent? *Journal of Memory and Language*, *28*, 127–154.

Vallar, G., & Papagno, C. (1993). Preserved vocabulary acquisition in Down's syndrome: the role of phonological short-term memory. *Cortex*, *29*(3), 467–483.

VanLehn, K. (1991). Rule acquisition events in the discovery of problem solving strategies. *Cognitive Science*, *15*, 1–47.

VanLehn, K. (1995). Cognitive skill acquisition. In J. Spence, J. Darly, & D. Foss (Eds.), *Annual review of psychology* (Vol. 47, pp. 513–519). Palo Alto, CA: Annual Reviews Inc.

Vicari, S., Carlesimo, A., & Caltagirone, C. (1995). Short-term memory in persons with intellectual disabilities and Down's syndrome. *Journal of Intellectual Disability Research*, *39*(6), 532–537.

Wang, P. P., & Bellugi, U. (1993). Williams syndrome, Down syndrome, and cognitive neuroscience. *American Journal of Diseases of Children*, *147*, 1246–1251.

Wang, P. P., & Bellugi, U. (1994). Evidence from two genetic syndromes for a dissociation between verbal and visuo-spatial short-term memory. *Journal of Clinical and Experimental Neuropsychology*, *2*, 317–322.

Waters, G. S., Caplan, D., & Hildebrandt, N. (1987). Working memory and written sentence comprehension. In M. Coltheart (Ed.), *Attention and performance XII* (pp. 531–555). Hillsdale, NJ: Erlbaum.

Winters, J. J. (1986). Proactive inhibition in retarded persons: some clues to short-term memory processing. In N. R. Ellis, & N. W. Bray (Eds.), *International review of research in mental retardation* (Vol. 13, pp. 279–300). New York: Academic Press.

Winters, J. J., & Cundari, L. (1979). Accumulation of and release from proactive inhibition in short-term memory by retarded and nonretarded persons. *American Journal of Mental Deficiency*, *83*, 595–600.

Wickens, D. D. (1970). Encoding categories of words: an empirical approach to meaning. *Psychological Review*, *77*, 1–15.

Reading Skills and Cognitive Abilities of Individuals with Mental Retardation

FRANCES A. CONNERS

DEPARTMENT OF PSYCHOLOGY, UNIVERSITY OF ALABAMA,
TUSCALOOSA, ALABAMA

I. INTRODUCTION

More than ever before, reading plays an important role in daily life. It facilitates independent functioning in one's environment, increases opportunities in the work force, allows opportunities for learning new skills, and provides pleasure as a leisure activity. Educators and researchers have regarded reading as valuable for individuals with mental retardation (MR), as attested by nearly a century of teaching and research activities related to reading skills. The present chapter is a synthesis of the research on this topic.

Reading is the process of extracting meaning from print. It involves recognizing or naming individual words and understanding the meaning conveyed when those words are assembled into sentences and paragraphs. Needless to say, reading is a complex skill requiring the coordination of many cognitive abilities. It is a language skill, yet, unlike many language skills, it usually does not develop naturally as a consequence of maturing brain mechanisms and exposure to language (print in this case). Rather, it almost always must be taught explicitly once the brain mechanisms and the corresponding underlying abilities are ready. Although both cognitive abilities and exposure to instruction are crucial to successful reading acquisition, the present chapter focuses on cognitive abilities and not on instructional techniques. There is a fairly large literature on effectiveness of various instructional techniques to teach reading to individuals with MR, but this literature has been reviewed recently (Browder & Lalli, 1991; Conners, 1992; Katims, 2000; Singh & Singh, 1986) and is beyond the scope of the present chapter. The present chapter addresses the following questions: (1) How well can individuals with MR read? (2) What specific difficulties do they have with reading? (3) Why are some individuals with

0074-7750/2003 $35.00

MR better at reading than others? After a discussion of major contemporary theories of typical reading development, each of these questions will be addressed with a discussion of relevant literature. The chapter ends with conclusions and directions for future research.

To address the three major questions of this chapter, the relevant literature was gathered according to a set of constraints meant to yield a well-defined body of research. The first constraint was that at least one sample in the study would adhere closely to recent American Association on Mental Retardation definitions of mental retardation (i.e., IQ below 70–75 with limitations in multiple areas of adaptive functioning, and manifested by age 18), regardless of the label used to refer to that group. Studies that included a few individuals whose IQs were above 75 were included in the review as long as the mean IQ of the sample was less than 75. Studies with mixed disability groups (e.g., some participants with learning disability, some with mental retardation, others with specific language impairment) were excluded from the review if there was no distinction made between results for participants with MR and those with other disabilities. Also, studies were included only if they had a measure of reading and were published in English. These constraints yielded approximately 80 primary studies, almost all of which involved individuals with mild intellectual limitations (IQ 55–75) of unspecified or unknown/mixed etiology. The results of these studies ultimately provided the conclusions of this chapter.

II. TYPICAL READING DEVELOPMENT

In the past 25 years, researchers have learned quite a lot about the typical development of reading skills (see, Snow, Burns, & Griffin, 1998). It is important to understand what is known about typical reading development before evaluating the difficulties children with MR experience as they learn to read. Gough and Tunmer (1985) suggested that reading ability is the product of word identification ability and language comprehension ability. In the present section, four major theories of reading are described, each of which has a body of empirical research supporting it. Consistent with Gough and Tunmer's framework, two of these theories focus on development of early word identification skills—Ehri's (1999) phase theory and Harm and Siedenberg's (1999) network theory—and two focus on comprehension skills—Gernsbacher's (1997) structure-building framework and Kintsch's (1998) construction-integration theory. The discussion of each theory includes comments on specific cognitive abilities that seem crucial within the context of the theory. These abilities will be important ones to consider when evaluating the reading potential of children with MR. All four theories are compatible and can be integrated into a single conceptualization of the reading acquisition process, as summarized at the end of this section.

A. Early Phases of Reading Development

There is good agreement that children pass through predictable phases on the way to becoming readers (see Ehri, 1999; Frith, 1985; Gough, Juel, & Roper-Schneider, 1983; Marsh, Freidman, Welch, & Desberg, 1981). Ehri's framework is a good example of one that has been documented empirically and updated on a regular basis (e.g., Ehri, 1991, 1994). In Ehri's framework, phases are flexible, not rigid, and fluid, not discrete. This means that a child may show behaviors associated with an advanced phase before showing all the behaviors associated with an earlier phase.

In Ehri's framework, the first phase of reading is the *pre-alphabetic phase*, at which time children learn to identify a small set of words by memory. During this phase, children make little if any use of letter-sound correspondences in their word identification. Rather, they use visual cues and associate them with words they know. For example, they may know that the stop sign means "stop" because of its shape and color cues, not because they know the letters and letter sounds. They may even identify the word "stop" printed on a page because of the way it looks, still without knowing letters and sounds. Thus, word identification may be linked to visual discrimination and associative learning in this phase. Typically developing children who would be in the pre-alphabetic phase would be preschoolers and kindergarteners who have not had reading instruction (age 3–5). Ehri's second phase is the *partial alphabetic phase*, during which children can use one or more letters and their letter sounds to help guess what a word is. It is usually the first or first and last letters of a word that children use to guess a word, particularly if they happen to know the sound of those letters. In this phase, children have limited knowledge of letter-sound correspondences but this knowledge develops rapidly to prepare for the alphabetic phase, which follows. Phonological awareness also comes into play because for the first time, children are using speech segments (i.e., letter sounds) in reading. Also critical is the use of context cues to guess words. Most typically developing children would be in this phase at 4–6 years of age (kindergarten-first grade).

The third phase is the *full alphabetic phase*, in which children can read new words by sounding out letter by letter, or assembling the pronunciation, and then accessing the word in memory. Children in this phase know letter-sound correspondences well, and have begun to learn more sophisticated correspondences between grapheme clusters and phoneme clusters. With this sophistication, reading by analogy becomes possible. This phase of reading must depend heavily on phonological awareness (an understanding of the breakdown and build-up of speech segments in words), working memory, and access of phonological codes from long-term memory. Children might be in the full alphabetic phase at age 5–7 (around first grade). The fourth and final phase in Ehri's framework is the *consolidated alphabetic phase*. In this phase, children make good use of consolidated orthographic units and corresponding phonological units. For example, they know the pronunciation of *–tion* when it occurs at the end of a word. They still assemble the pronunciation, but now use larger units, allowing word identification to be more efficient. They are successful on a wider variety of words, including exception words as well as regular words. Critical to this phase is knowledge of the regularities of English orthography and mapping of these orthographic units to phonological units. Working memory is still important, but its role shifts from managing word identification (which becomes more automatic) to managing comprehension processes. Children in this phase would typically be 6–8 years old (first to third grade).

B. Network Approach to Early Reading Development

Most reading researchers would agree that what goes on in early reading development entails developing correspondences, both small and large, and learning to apply them systematically and efficiently. Thus, Harm and Seidenberg (1999) proposed a network model of reading development, in which phonological units and orthographic units become interconnected with language and text experience (see related models by Plaut, McClelland, Seidenberg, & Patterson, 1996; Seidenberg & McClelland, 1989; Van Orden, Pennington, & Stone, 1990).

This model suggests that in the early years of life, before reading begins, phonological knowledge develops. Phonological knowledge is knowledge of the individual sounds of one's language and how they tend to go together. As young children hear their native language, they learn the patterns of covariances among phonological features and incorporate them into a cognitive network. Connections between phonological feature units become strengthened or weakened and take on positive or negative values. Two phonological features that often co-occur would have a strong positive connection with each other; two that never co-occur would have a strong negative connection with each other. With more exposure to language, weights on connections are adjusted, and the network becomes a more precise representation of the language. By the time children are ready to learn to read, they already have an extensive phonological network in place. Critical abilities at this phase seem to be discrimination, categorization, and association among speech sounds and speech sound patterns.

When children begin to learn letters, their orthographic knowledge develops. Orthographic knowledge is knowledge of the ways in which letters tend to appear together in patterns in one's printed language. As in the phonological network, the weights on connections among the orthographic units (letters) become stronger or weaker with experience and may take on positive or negative values. The integrity of the orthographic network could be assessed by asking children which looks more like a real word *knip* or *znip*? If the children know that *k* and *n* sometimes occur together in this order at the beginning of words—but *z* and *n* do not—they will give *knip* as their answer. It seems that discrimination, categorization, and association of visual patterns would be important abilities for the development of an orthographic network.

According to Harm and Siedenberg (1999), as an orthographic network develops, it is mapped onto the already existing phonological network and reading development proceeds. The ability to read is the ability to map orthographic units to phonological units (presumably there is also a semantic network that connects to the orthographic and phonological networks, but this has not yet been included in Harm and Seidenberg's model). As children experience print and associated pronunciations, the connections between orthographic units and phonological units become weighted and with further exposure and feedback, the weights become revised. Early on, children make mistakes in reading because the weights are not yet optimally refined. Eventually, when presented with text, patterns of orthographic units quickly activate corresponding patterns of phonological units, and the text is automatically decoded. When this happens, reading is more accurate and faster. Establishing and refining connections between orthographic and phonological units seems to involve the ability to make cross-modal associations and to profit from feedback.

C. Reading Comprehension: Structure-Building

With more practice associating orthographic and phonologic units, word reading becomes more automatic and children can process longer sentences with more complex semantic and syntactic content. Thus, with greater automaticity of word identification, comprehension processes become more and more important in determining a child's reading proficiency. A dominant framework for understanding text comprehension is Gernsbacher's structure building framework (Gernsbacher, 1990, 1991, 1995, 1997).

Gernsbacher's framework applies generally to discourse comprehension, which includes listening comprehension, reading comprehension, and comprehension of picture sequences. The framework suggests that the goal of comprehension is to build coherent mental representations, or structures. The building blocks are memory nodes or units of stored information. The first process involved in structure-building is *laying a foundation*, or establishing the initial facts of the discourse. Incoming information activates a set of interconnected memory nodes to lay this foundation. It seems that, in order to lay an appropriate foundation, comprehenders need to have a semantic network or knowledge base already in place. Also, they must know the meanings of words in the discourse and have the syntactic processing skills to comprehend the broad meaning of phrases and sentences.

The second process in structure-building is *mapping*, and this occurs when subsequent incoming information is related to the information in the foundation. The new information activates memory nodes, which connect to the foundation. As long as the incoming information continues to relate to the foundation, it continues to be mapped onto it, and the initial mental structure continues to build. When the topic changes and incoming information is not closely related to the foundation, a *shift* occurs, and a new foundation is laid for a new substructure. By the end of a story, readers may have developed a main mental structure and several connected substructures that represent their understanding of the story. In addition to the abilities needed for laying a foundation, mapping seems to require the maintenance of activation of memory nodes in the foundation, which may be considered working memory. Also, semantic association between discourse units, including the ability to make accurate references and inferences, seems necessary. Finally, to shift appropriately to a new substructure, it would be necessary to evaluate the degree of association between incoming information and the information represented in the foundation.

Laying a foundation, mapping, and shifting are accomplished by way of the mechanisms of *enhancement* and *suppression*. Enhancement is a mechanism by which the activation of memory nodes is increased by the activation of related nodes. This is a way that coherence is supported and topic focus is maintained. Suppression is a mechanism by which the activation of memory nodes is dampened by the lack of activation of related nodes. This is a way that information that is less relevant to the current topic can be suppressed.

D. Reading Comprehension: Construction-Integration

Another well-known model of comprehension is Kintsch's Construction-Integration Model (Kintsch, 1988, 1998; Kintsch & vanDijk, 1978). Similar to Gernsbacher's, this model applies to reading comprehension as well as comprehension of discourse presented in spoken or other formats.

The *construction* part of the model pertains to the immediate construction of meaning from discourse units such as sentences. Incoming information is converted into mental representations called propositions, which represent meaning but do not retain the surface form of the message (i.e., the exact words in the exact order). The formation of propositions requires the activation of concept nodes that exist in memory. The initial propositions form a working text representation. The *integration* part of the model refers to the way in which new information adds to the working text representation. From the first few sentences of the text read, one or two propositions are formed and are activated in working memory. Then, the next few sentences are read and new propositions are formed and linked to the propositions in working memory. Activation levels are adjusted by the degree of relatedness among the propositions, and the one or two propositions with the highest activation level remain in working memory; these are called *central* propositions. The central propositions and the other propositions become integrated in the text model that is developing in long-term memory (or long-term *working* memory, in Kintsch's terms), but only the central propositions remain active in working memory. The process continues until a complex memory structure that represents the meaning of the text exists in long-term memory. Integration is guided by a macro-structure (e.g., schema or script), which provides a general organization for newly integrated propositions and allows for making inferences and filling in missing details. In this model there is an emphasis on working memory, knowledge base, and semantic association.

E. Summary

These models of beginning reading and comprehension suggest that, for typically developing children, reading development begins with general language development. This not only includes vocabulary, semantic associations, and syntactic knowledge, but also the establishment of a phonological feature network. Children begin to read when they first associate print with words they already know. They learn letters and their sounds, and learn to decode words using letter–sound associations. From their experience with print, children develop an orthographic network, which is connected to their phonological network and refined with practice and feedback. Children begin to use larger orthographic units to read, and their reading becomes more precise and automatic. With automaticity, children move on to more complex text, and comprehension processes become more important. Using their related knowledge base or macrostructure for context and guidance, children construct propositions from text, relate them to one another, and build text representations that are organized and coherent.

III. READING ACHIEVEMENT AND MENTAL RETARDATION: THE EMERGING LAG

The development of reading skill involves the coordination of many language and cognitive abilities. For most typically developing children, it takes many years of instruction and practice to learn to read well. How well do children with MR learn to read? The present section focuses on whether the reading achievement of individuals with MR matches, surpasses, or lags behind the level that would be expected given their general cognitive ability. Comparisons between actual and expected reading level can be made in a variety of ways. For example, an age-equivalent score on a reading test can be compared with an estimate of mental age (MA), or a standard score on a reading test can be compared with an estimate of IQ. If the reading age-equivalent score is lower than the MA (or the standard score is lower than the IQ), then there is evidence that reading lags behind the expected level (i.e., reading is a *specific* difficulty). If the reading score is higher, then reading can be said to surpass the expected level. Most common in the literature, however, is the MA-match design, in which individuals with MR are compared with younger typically developing children who have the same MA. If the children with MR perform more poorly than the typically developing children, then their reading can be said to lag behind expectations. If they perform better, then their reading can be said to surpass expectations.

The MA-match design has been criticized on several counts (see Cole, 1998), and so warrants a bit of discussion. It assumes that a single age-equivalent score can summarize a person's cognitive functioning level, when individuals have relative strengths and weaknesses. More importantly, because the design compares an *older* group with MR with a *younger* typically developing group, it introduces group differences due to experience and practice. Nevertheless, MA can be thought of as the average level of various cognitive functions, and can be a quite useful benchmark for comparing specific cognitive skills and abilities and for pooling results from several studies. In the studies reviewed in this section, MA was most often derived from a version of the Stanford-Binet Test of Intelligence. Less often, it was estimated from IQ and chronological age (CA) using the formula $MA = CA \times IQ/100$.

Most evidence suggests that, at low MAs, reading in persons with mental retardation keeps pace with expectations, but at higher MAs reading lags behind. In an early study, Merrill (1924) measured several reading skills in children with and without MR at MAs from 7 to 11. At MA7, children with MR performed better on three comprehensive reading measures than children without MR (though inferential statistical tests were not reported). At MA8, the results were mixed, and, beginning at MA9, the children with MR did worse than those without MR on these tests. The difference between the groups became even greater from MA9 to MA11. Merrill's results suggest that a "reading lag" begins at an MA of 8 or 9, and increases thereafter.

Sheperd (1967) compared cognitive abilities of stronger and weaker readers with MR, as defined by their reading level in relation to MA. He reported that, when he was assembling his sample, he could identify children with MR who were reading above their MA level as long as the MA was below 8 years, 5 month (8-5). Above an MA of 8-5, almost all the children were reading below their MA level. He suggested that first- and second-grade reading material is within the grasp of children with MR with commensurate MA; however, further advancement in reading is difficult, even as MA continues to advance (see also Semmel, Gottleib, & Robinson, 1979). This would suggest that it is the automatization of word identification and shift to comprehension activities which typically occur around MA8-5 that are especially difficult for children with MR (see also Jenkinson, 1989).

Consistent with this pattern are the results of a literature review by Dunn (1954). Dunn reviewed 14 studies from 1918 to 1953 in which actual reading level was compared to the expected reading level in children with MR. The studies used several different ways of comparing actual to expected reading level, but according to Dunn's analysis, 11 of the studies showed that children with MR generally had reading skills below their expected level, whereas 3 studies showed that they had reading skills at or above their expected level. Of the 3 that did not show a reading lag, two had MA range midpoints of 8.5 and 7, and the third had a mean IQ of 75, which suggests a mixed MR/borderline group. Of the 11 that showed a reading lag, most had median MA of about 9. Results from other studies also fit the "emerging lag" pattern. For example, Bos and Tierney's (1980) and Levitt's (1970, 1972) participants with and without MR, at MAs of 8.5 and 7.5, respectively, were equivalent in reading as well as in MA. Yet, Nagle's (1993) participants with MR, at MA12, were reading below the level expected from MA as estimated from IQ and CA.

Recent standardized test data also support the emerging lag pattern. Gronna and her colleagues (Gronna, Jenkins, & Chin-Chance, 1998a,b) reported Total Reading scores from the Stanford Achievement Test 8 for

1060 students with mild MR and 214,443 students without disabilities in the state of Hawaii in grades 3–10 (those with moderate-severe MR were not routinely tested). Overall, children with mild MR scored only about 1.5 standard deviations below children without disabilities on reading, which is better than would be expected based on IQ differences (the IQ cutoff for MR is about 2 standard deviations below the general population mean). However, cross-sequential data suggested a slower rate of improvement of reading skills among students with MR than among students without disabilities from grade 3 to 10. For both groups, the greatest improvement was from grade 3 to 6 and the least was from grade 8 to 10. Children with MR, however, improved slightly more than nondisabled children from grade 3 to 6, the same amount from grades 6 to 8 and somewhat less from grade 8 to 10.

Studies of specific genetic syndromes also follow the emerging lag pattern. Among low-MA individuals with fragile X, Down, and Williams syndromes, there appears to be no reading lag when reading age equivalent is compared with MA or when reading standard score is compared with IQ (Dykens, Hodapp, & Leckman, 1987; Hodapp et al., 1992; Laing, Hulme, Grant, & Karmiloff-Smith, 2001; Pagon, Bennett, LaVeck, Stewart, & Johnson, 1987). However, among higher MA individuals with Prader-Willi syndrome and mixed etiology MR, there does seem to be a reading lag, with reading age lower than estimated MA (Dykens, Hodapp, Walsh, & Nash, 1992) and reading standard scores lower than IQ (Conners, Rosenquist, Atwell, & Klinger, 2000; Roof et al., 2000; but see Roof et al., 2000 for an exception regarding the uniparental disomy subtype).

The emerging lag pattern is discouraging. It suggests that students with MR can only get so far in their reading progress, perhaps not far enough to acquire new knowledge by reading or to enjoy reading as a leisure activity. However, Gronna and her colleagues showed that, despite a slow-down in progress, students with MR continued to gain reading skills through 10th grade—the highest grade examined in the study. Also, three different studies showed that a small minority of students with MR (3–5% who attempted it) were able to pass the reading portion of the high school graduation standards test in their state (Crews, 1988; Serow & O'Brien, 1983; Thompson, Thurlow, Spicuzza, & Parson, 1999). To some degree, the emerging lag pattern could be due to lack of emphasis in reading instruction for children with MR, particularly after students have acquired the skills for single-word reading (see Cegelka & Cegelka, 1970; Jenkinson, 1989). Studies that examine instructional practices targeting students with MR at increasing MAs would be necessary to address this possibility.

IV. SPECIFIC READING SKILLS AND MENTAL RETARDATION

Regardless of MA and whether a reading lag has emerged, reading is a skill that is difficult for children with MR to master. Why? Are there certain aspects of reading that are particularly problematic? Or is each step along the way equally difficult? Does the evidence support Sheperd's (1967) hypothesis that the reading skills that develop at grade 3 and beyond (i.e. automaticity and comprehension processes) are the most difficult? The present section includes a discussion of studies in which groups of individuals with MR are compared with groups of typically developing individuals on one or more specific reading skills. In most studies, the MA-match design was used. The research on reading skills is discussed roughly in order of typical developmental emergence, beginning with sight-word learning, and ending with aspects of reading comprehension. The evidence suggests that, indeed, there are specific difficulties with reading comprehension skills beyond the second-grade level. However, the evidence also suggests that there are specific difficulties earlier on in phonological decoding (i.e., reading by sounding out) as well as in some specific aspects of reading comprehension.

A. Sight-word Learning

When young children first see a stop sign and say, "stop!" they have "read" their first word and are in the pre-alphabetic phase of reading development according to Ehri (1999). At this early phase, reading is associative and there is little if any use of letter–sound correspondences. As children learn more words by association, they are learning sight-words. Under explicit instruction, children with and without MR of equivalent MA are largely similar in their ability to learn sight-words. Gickling, Hargis, and Alexander (1981) found that at MA5, children with MR learned just as many sight-words under the same instruction as children without MR. Also, the two groups were affected similarly by the imagery value of the words, learning more high-imagery words than low-imagery words. Cawley and Parmar (1995) taught children English labels for Czech words. Although this was not exactly the same as teaching real (English) reading words, it was very similar to associative sight-word teaching, of the sort done by Gickling et al. Cawley and Parmar gave children with and without MR, MA10, the same amount of instruction, and found no group difference in number of Czech words learned.

In contrast to these results, however, Laing et al. (2001) found that children and adults with Williams syndrome learned contrived sight words (e.g., LTR) more slowly than typically developing children matched for single-word reading and receptive vocabulary age (about 7). Interestingly, this may have been related to the cognitive profile associated with Williams syndrome. This profile includes relatively good language abilities and relatively poor visuo-spatial abilities. The contrived sight words were either high or low in phonetic similarity (LTR vs LKR for the spoken word *ladder*), and either high or low in imagery value. Although participants with Williams syndrome showed as strong an advantage for high over low phonetic similarity items as typically developing participants, they showed a weaker advantage for high over low imagery items. Thus, their less efficient sight-word learning may have been related to failure to use visuo-spatial/ semantic information. The results of this study compared with the results of the other sight-word studies suggest a specific difficulty in sight-word learning associated with Williams syndrome but not with MR in general. Further research is needed, however, to explore this hypothesis.

B. Letter Knowledge

Early in the development of their reading skills, children learn to identify letters, associate letters with sounds, and use letters as sound cues in single-word reading. Thus, the orthographic network (Harm & Seidenberg, 1999) begins to develop and connections form between orthographic units and phonologic units as children enter the partial-alphabetic phase. There is little evidence to suggest that children with MR have specific problems learning letter names and sounds. In three studies that measured letter knowledge, two clearly indicated similarities between MA-matched participants with and without MR. Cawley and Parmar (1995) found that at MA9, there was no difference between children with and without MR in knowledge of letter names or letter sounds, though both groups performed near ceiling. Also, Blake, Aaron, and Westbrook (1969) found similarities between groups with and without MR (MA8 and MA10) on knowledge of both consonant sounds and vowel sounds. In the one study that indicated poorer performance by individuals with MR, results were mixed. Jenkinson (1992) administered the Woodcock Reading Mastery Tests (WMRT) along with specific experimental tasks in two experiments (see phonological decoding section for details on the two experiments). Although the participant recruitment techniques and resulting samples appeared to be very similar in the two experiments, at MA7, participants with MR performed more poorly on the Letter Identification subtest than participants without MR in one experiment but equivalently in the other. It is difficult to explain why the results for letter identification differed across experiments.

In any case, there is little strong evidence for a specific difficulty with letter knowledge among individuals with MR.

C. Word Identification

Once formal reading instruction has begun, word identification (single-word reading ability) is commonly used as an index of reading proficiency. Word identification is achieved by way of phonological decoding (sounding out) and orthographic decoding (heavily depending on spelling patterns to recognize words). These skills develop when a child has refined the weights on connections between orthographic and phonological units and among orthographic units. They typify the full alphabetic phase and the subsequent consolidated alphabetic phase. When word identification is taken at face value, results are mixed—some studies have shown below-expected performance of children with MR, whereas others have not. For example, in Jenkinson's (1992) two-experiment study, children with MR (MA7) did more poorly on the WMRT Word Identification Test than children without MR in one experiment but not the other. As previously noted, the samples and recruitment were similar for the two experiments. Blake et al. (1969) found no differences between groups with and without MR in rapid word recognition at MA8 and MA10, but Dunn (1954), reported that at MA9, participants with MR did more poorly than participants without MR on a word identification test, a speeded test of word and phrase recognition, and a multiple-choice word/nonword discrimination test. Cawley and Parmar (1995) found no differences between children with and without MR on word identification at MA10. In children and young adults with Down syndrome, three studies showed that, at MA4 to MA8, the level of word identification was higher than the level that would be expected based on MA (Cupples & Iacono, 2000; Fowler, Doherty, & Boynton, 1995; Kay-Raining Bird, Cleave, & McConnell, 2000), whether MA was general or based on receptive vocabulary. In contrast, in adolescents with Williams syndrome (verbal MA about 7), two measures of word identification-age equivalent were several months lower than measures of verbal MA (Laing et al., 2001). None of the studies of Down or Williams syndromes, however, reported statistical tests comparing word identification with MA.

The inconsistency in results for word identification could be due to in part to differences in word lists used in different studies—the difficulty level as well as the proportion of regular vs exception words may have made a difference. Regular words (e.g., staff) can be read successfully by phonological decoding, whereas exception words (e.g., laugh) require orthographic decoding more heavily. Children with MR may have specific difficulty with phonological decoding, as will be argued in the following section, and may be at more of a disadvantage if the word list is made up mostly of regular words. This interpretation could be tested in future research. In contrast to the general inconsistency in the results for word identification, however, the three studies of Down syndrome were consistent in showing that word identification was strong relative to MA among individuals with this syndrome. Future research should explore the possibility of a relative strength in word identification in Down syndrome.

D. Phonological Decoding

Phonological decoding refers to reading by sounding out, and can also be called word attack. It is often measured by having children read pronounceable nonwords such as *glig*. Because *glig* is not a real word, children cannot read it by prior knowledge of the word; rather, they have to use letter–sound correspondences to sound it out. Children with MR can learn to read phonologically, to the point that they can use sounding out skills to read words that they have never seen before (Neville & Vandever, 1973; Vandever & Neville, 1976). There is some evidence that, at MA7, children with MR are capable of learning just as much as children without MR from synthetic (i.e., sounding out) instruction, at least when a contrived alphabet is used (Neville & Vandever, 1973, but see Vandever & Neville, 1976).

However, the reality seems to be that, even at low MAs, phonological decoding skills of individuals with MR lag behind the level expected based on MA. For example, in both of her experiments, Jenkinson (1992) found that the MR group performed more poorly on the WMRT Word Attack subtest than the MA-matched group without MR. In addition, she found that individuals with MR had a less mature pattern of reliance on letter cues than individuals without MR. In Experiment 1, participants reported whether an isolated letter was present in a nonword, real word, or letter string. For real words but not nonwords, participants with MR were quicker to confirm presence of the target letter when it was the first letter of the word compared to subsequent letters; however, participants without MR were quicker when the target letter was either the first or last letter of the word. Experiment 2 was an analysis of errors in oral reading of single words. It showed that, whereas participants with MR made errors that preserved the first letter sound, participants without MR made errors that preserved both the first and last letter sounds. According to Ehri (1999), use of first-letter cues typically emerges before use of last-letter cues in the development of reading skills. Thus, Jenkinson's results suggest that at MA7, students with MR have made less progress toward alphabetic reading than students without MR.

Consistent with Jenkinson's nonword reading results, Cawley and Parmar (1995) found that at MA9, children with MR did worse than children without MR on a test that primarily involved reading phonetically regular nonwords. Interestingly, the groups were similar on all parts of a test that included mostly phonic skills (i.e., skills of relating speech sounds to letters and groups of letters; see also Blake et al., 1969). Apparently, participants with MR could name the sounds of the letters as well as participants without MR, but could not put the sounds together as well to pronounce the nonwords.

Consistent with Jenkinson's findings on oral reading errors, three studies reported that children with MR (MA 7–9) made more errors indicative of weak phonological decoding skills than children without MR. In a study of oral reading errors in single-word reading, Mason (1978) compared children with MR with second graders in a previous study (Mason, 1977), who had the same percent correct on the list of 96 one-syllable words (probably about MA8). Children with MR were more affected by word frequency than children without MR, making more errors on infrequent words relative to frequent words. Also, they were less affected by vowel regularity and complexity than children without MR, making about the same number errors regardless of these factors. These results suggest that, whereas children without MR depend heavily on phonological decoding, children with MR depend more on sight-word reading (see Mason, 1976 for similar results). Mason suggested that this is because children with MR have great difficulty with phonological decoding.

In oral reading of passages, both Levitt (1972) and Dunn (1954) found differences between children with and without MR on errors related to phonological decoding. Levitt's (1972) groups (about MA7) were matched on single-word reading level and read the same passage. Both groups made the same number of oral reading errors, but children with MR gave more "multiple-cue response" errors, which involved combinations of graphemic, phonemic, and contextual cues (e.g., reading *put* for *play*, would be a graphemic–phonemic response error). They also gave more "simple or inferior response" errors which resulted in real-word substitutions, and more morphological errors in which they added or changed a morpheme. Children without MR gave more "no response" errors, and "search for closure response" errors, such as repetitions, self-corrections and regressions. Thus, children with MR struggled most with word identification, especially phonological decoding, whereas children without MR focused on comprehension. Dunn's (1954) participants (MA9) were matched on Stanford-Binet MA. They read paragraphs and single words on their own reading level and error rates were corrected for total number of words read. Participants with MR showed a less mature pattern of phonological decoding—they stalled and asked for help more often, made more errors on vowel sounds (*blend* for *blind*), and omitted sounds more often (*sack* for *stack*). Participants without MR made more repetitions and additions of words.

The bulk of evidence on phonological decoding suggests that it is a specific area of difficulty for individuals with MR, even when the building blocks (i.e., phonics skills) are in place. However, there is some evidence that this may not be true for individuals with Williams and Down syndromes, at least at low MAs. As already noted, Laing et al. (2001) showed that participants with Williams syndrome made just as much use of phonetic cues in sight-word learning as typically developing children matched on receptive vocabulary age (about 7) and word identification. Also, three studies showed that, at MA4 to MA8, the level of nonword reading of individuals with Down syndrome was consistent with or higher than what would be expected based on receptive vocabulary age (Cupples & Iacono, 2000; Fowler et al., 1995; Kay-Raining Bird et al., 2000; see also Evans, 1994, for a similar pattern). For example, Cupples and Iacono's (2000) children with Down syndrome, averaging 8.4 years old, had a mean receptive vocabulary age of 3.9 and a mean word attack age equivalent score of 6.6. Though statistical comparisons were not made between these variables in any of these studies, the consistency across studies is notable. More research is warranted on phonological decoding in Williams, Down, and other syndromes associated with MR.

E. Orthographic Decoding

Eventually, children use more complex orthographic units in their reading, rather than sounding out letter-by-letter. Only one study included a measure that in some way tapped orthographic decoding. Blake et al.'s (1969) spelling patterns test measured children's ability to use Consonant–Vowel–Consonant spelling patterns to help them identify vowel sounds in nonwords, or in other words, to decode by analogy. Decoding by analogy goes beyond letter-by-letter sounding out because it makes use of larger graphemic and phonological units. Blake et al. found that, at both MA8 and MA10, children with MR performed more poorly than children without MR on spelling patterns. Rate of improvement was slower by over 7 months for students with MR than for students without MR at MA8, though equivalent at MA10. Although these results may suggest a specific difficulty with orthographic decoding, the spelling patterns measure also involves phonological decoding. With only the results of one study to go on, it is difficult to decide whether orthographic decoding is a specific area of difficulty in MR. More research is needed.

F. General Reading Comprehension

As children become more skilled in word identification, demands on reading comprehension processes tends to increase. This point in reading development probably corresponds with the point beyond the second grade instructional level that Sheperd (1967) identified as being very difficult for children with MR to master. After all, at this point, semantic and syntactic processes come into play in interpreting incoming information and relating it to background knowledge. Background knowledge, in turn, is used to generate quality inferences essential for comprehension. Central ideas must be identified and details must be related to them such that a mental model is developed that represents the story or text. Given all of the higher-level cognitive demands involved in reading comprehension, it would not be surprising if children with MR had difficulties in it as soon as it could be measured. Yet, Merrill's (1924) comparison of children with and without MR on general reading comprehension measures suggested that the greatest difficulties emerge at MA10. At MA7 through MA9, participants with MR did not differ significantly from participants without MR on three measures of reading comprehension from the Stanford Achievement Test—paragraph meaning, sentence meaning, and word meaning. At MA10, there was still no difference in word meaning, though the group with MR performed more poorly on the other two measures. At MA11, the group with MR performed more poorly on all three comprehension measures. Thus, the pattern for reading comprehension paralleled the overall reading pattern identified in the Merrill study, except that group differences began at MA10 rather than at MA9. Consistent with this pattern, Wood, Buckhalt, and Tomlin (1988) found that at MA10 children with MR performed more poorly than typically developing children on a general reading comprehension measure. Much of the literature on specific aspects of reading comprehension (i.e., story importance, inference generation, etc.) is consistent with Merrill's results—through MA10 children with MR meet the expected level for most skills. However, certain aspects of inference generation, context utilization, and comprehension monitoring lag behind the expected level even before MA 10.

G. Story Importance

Needless to say, the ability to distinguish more important from less important information helps story comprehension and recall. This ability may be fostered by laying a good foundation and keen enhancement and suppression mechanisms (Gernsbacher, 1997), or by accurately maintaining the most highly activated propositions in working memory (Kintsch, 1998).

Children with MR appear to be as sensitive as typically developing children to what facts are important in stories. Luftig and Greeson (1983) had participants listen to a story while they read along, judge the importance of the story's ideas, and recall the story. After correction for response bias, participants with MR were as accurate as MA-matched and CA-matched participants without MR at classifying story idea units as high, medium or low in importance. Although participants with MR *recalled* fewer idea units than participants without MR, their recall of ideas was equally sensitive to importance—all groups recalled more high importance idea units than low or medium importance idea units (see also Luftig & Johnson, 1982).

H. Inference Generation

The ability to make appropriate inferences when information is not stated explicitly in text allows for the development of a coherent text model. Kintsch (1998) would say that assisting in inference-generation is one purpose for a macrostructure, which could be a script or schema, or an otherwise organized body of knowledge. Children with MR appear to be equally good at generating inferences as MA-matched typically developing children if the reading material is narrative or mixed, but not as good if the reading material is exclusively expository.

Blake et al. (1969) questioned children on: (a) cause–effect relationships from sentences, (b) main ideas from paragraphs, and (c) main ideas from stories, which were either directly stated or only implied. At MA8, children with MR did as well as children without MR on all types of directly stated and implied questions. They improved more slowly over 7 months of basal reading instruction on 2 of 3 types of both implied and directly stated questions. At MA10, children with MR did worse than children without MR on 2 of 3 types of both implied and directly stated questions. Over 7 months, they improved more slowly on only one of the types of implied questions. From this pattern, it appears that the groups with MR did not have any specific difficulty with implied information relative to directly stated information.

Bos and Tierney (1980) also found similarities between children with and without MR on inference generation, though the degree of similarity between groups depended on the type of text read. Bos and Tierney asked children with and without MR matched on reading comprehension and similar in MA (MA8) to read narrative and expository texts, free-recall the text content, and then answer questions about information that was implied in the texts. The two groups were equivalent on recognition of words used in the passages and on background knowledge related to the passages.

Children with MR generated the same number of inferences in free recall as children without MR. For a narrative text, which is likely to have associated with it an accessible script, or common sequence of events in a story, the two groups generated the same quality of inferences (number of plausible vs implausible inferences). However, for an expository text, which is less likely to have a universal script associated with it (e.g., topics such as beavers or planets), children with MR generated fewer plausible inferences and slightly more implausible inferences than children without MR. Results from the probe questions yielded the same pattern. Bos and Tierney (1980) suggested that the children with MR had a more difficult time *applying* related background knowledge to help generate plausible inferences and ultimately understand the expository text material.

I. Use of Contextual Cues

Another important reading comprehension skill is use of contextual cues. The first few words of a sentence provide a semantic and syntactic context for words that follow, and as such are helpful in the identification of those words. For example, the context, "Who is knocking at the...?" suggests a small set of possible words that might come next. If the word that follows begin with *d*, it should be easy to identify the word *door*. To the extent that the context helps a child identify the next word or guess what the next word should be, the child is using semantic and syntactic comprehension processes. Research has shown that children with MR who can read short passages are able to take advantage of context cues (Levitt, 1970), even those that are beyond the within-sentence context (Ramanauskas, 1972). Their ability to use context, however, depends on both the predictability of the context and the frequency of the word to be guessed (Allington, 1980). Of course, the ability to use context in reading also depends on being able to read the context accurately.

Of the studies on use of contextual cues that adequately matched or controlled reading level across groups, results are mixed (see Streib, 1976, for background and a review of early research). Taken together, however, they suggest that children with MR perform at the level expected for their MA when they have the benefit of the extensive context of a paragraph, but perform especially poorly when they only have a few words to use as context. Levitt (1970) compared children with and without MR matched on word identification level (about MA7). Children read a set of words in isolation and embedded in text. Both groups read the same number of words correctly and showed the same advantage of context. Also, Crossland (1981) used a cloze task in which children (MA11) read passages with blanks inserted in place of several words and wrote in the words that should go in the blanks. Although the groups were not matched on reading ability, each child read a paragraph at his or her own reading level. Children with MR did better than children without MR at supplying the exact word, though children without MR came up with more grammatically correct synonyms. When exact words and synonyms were combined, the groups were equivalent on cloze performance.

In contrast to these two studies, Goodstein (1970) and Semmel, Barritt, and Bennett (1970) found that children with MR supplied fewer adequate words than children without MR. In these studies, children (MA9 and MA8, respectively) followed along while the experimenter read four-word sentences with one word missing. Thus, they had fewer contextual cues to use than the children who read passages in the Levitt (1970) and Crossland (1981) studies. In spite of supplying fewer adequate words, however, children with MR were equally affected by sentence syntax, position of missing word, form class, and response format. This suggested they were using semantic and syntactic processes similarly, though less efficiently.

J. Comprehension Monitoring

The final aspect of reading comprehension represented in the MR literature is comprehension monitoring. Comprehension monitoring is a process of checking one's own understanding of text and can be indicated by certain reading behaviors. For example, in Levitt's (1972) oral reading error analysis mentioned previously, children with and without MR (about MA7), made the same number of reading errors, yet those with MR made fewer "search for closure" responses than those without MR. These included errors indicative of comprehension-monitoring—self-corrections, repetitions, regressions (going back to the beginning of the sentence). Dunn (1954) also found that participants with MR (MA9) made more repetitions and additions of words in oral reading. Thus, both studies suggest that children with MR lag behind MA expectations in comprehension monitoring.

K. Summary

The research comparing MA-matched children with and without MR on reading skills suggests two main areas of specific difficulty—phonological decoding and comprehension. Phonological decoding problems arise early and persist. Comprehension problems arise in specific forms almost as early as phonological decoding problems. These include inference generation from expository text, use of contextual cues when context is minimal, and comprehension monitoring. General comprehension problems, less well defined, arise later on. Possibly, the early specific difficulties with phonological decoding, inference generation, use of context, and comprehension monitoring develop into a general reading comprehension lag by MA10.

V. INDIVIDUAL DIFFERENCES IN READING AMONG INDIVIDUALS WITH MENTAL RETARDATION

It is clear that individuals with MR have a difficult time learning to read due to their low general cognitive ability. Reading ability correlates moderately with intelligence in the general population (Stanovich, 1985). However, some individuals with MR have an easier time with reading than others. Why? The present section contains a discussion of research on individual differences in reading and related cognitive abilities in participants with MR. Studies were included in this section if they included at least one cognitive ability measure that was statistically compared to reading in a sample of individuals with MR. In several studies, researchers identified stronger and weaker readers and compared these groups on cognitive ability measures. In others, researchers correlated cognitive ability measures with reading measures. The literature suggests that working memory, phonological awareness, visual and orthographic discrimination, associative learning, and semantic/syntactic processing distinguish stronger from weaker readers with MR.

A. Working Memory

Working memory is the part of the memory system in which information is kept active and/or processed actively, and as such, encompasses the earlier concept of short-term memory. It is the center of conscious and effortful processing, so it is important to many cognitive activities, including reading. It is capacity- and time-limited, and if overly limited, problems can occur in many areas of cognition. Indeed, extreme limitations in working memory have been associated with MR (see Hale & Borkowski, 1991; Pulsifer, 1996). Although there are many specific models of working memory (see Gathercole, 1996; Miyake & Shah, 1999), a common feature is a distinction between auditory and visual aspects of working memory. In reading development, working memory is likely to be especially important in the pre-alphabetic phase in which children are sounding out words (Ehri's phase model), and later in comprehension processes such as relating new information to the existing text model (Gernsbacher's model and Kintsch's model).

Working memory may be the single most reliable predictor of reading ability among individuals with MR. Both auditory and visual working memory correlate with reading ability in this population, but auditory working memory is the more consistent correlate of the two. For example, Blackman and Burger (1972) factor analyzed 19 reading readiness variables from tasks completed by children with MR (verbal MA5), along with single-word reading. Then they used the 19 variables to predict single-word reading. Only three variables both loaded on the reading factor and contributed independently to the prediction of word reading ability, one of which was auditory memory for letters. In addition, auditory memory for sentences and visual memory loaded on the reading factor, though they did not contribute independently to the prediction of word reading. Both Sheperd (1967) and Cawley and Parmar (1995) compared stronger and weaker readers with MR (MA8 and about 10, respectively), and either equated groups for MA or controlled MA in analyses. From extensive batteries of tasks, only three discriminated between stronger and weaker readers in each study. In Sheperd's study digit recall distinguished between groups, though a visual memory task did not. In Cawley and Parmar's study, short-term memory for sequences (both auditory and visual) distinguished between groups, though a visual retention task did not.

In nearly every other study that included an auditory working memory measure, it was related importantly to reading. This was true for studies of nonspecific MR (Blackman, Bilsky, Burger, & Mar, 1976; Conners, Atwell, Rosenquist, & Sligh, 2001; Numminen et al., 2000; Parmenter, 1986, 1988; Ramanauskas & Burrow, 1973; Stayton & Fuller, 1974; but see Das & Cummins, 1978; John & Rattan, 1991 for mixed results), as well as for studies of Down syndrome (Fowler et al., 1995; Kay-Raining Bird et al., 2000; Laws, 1998; Laws, MacDonald, & Buckley, 1996). In the only study on Williams syndrome, however, only one of three auditory working memory measures correlated with word identification once age and general ability were statistically controlled (Laing et al., 2001).

Among studies that included a visual working memory measure, some found it to be unrelated to reading (Song & Song, 1969; Sheperd, 1967) some found it to be related (Conners & Detterman, 1987; Fowler et al., 1995, for Down syndrome; Stayton & Fuller, 1974) and some reported mixed results (John & Rattan, 1991; Mandes, Massimino, & Mantis, 1991; Parmenter, 1986). The differences across studies in visual working memory may have to do with the requirement for a drawing response (Stayton & Fuller, 1974), whether the visual stimuli were letters/words vs pictures/designs, the type of reading measure used (single-word reading, reading comprehension, or comprehensive) or the phase of reading of the participants. Very possibly, visual working memory is more important at the earliest phases of reading involving sight-word reading (Ehri's pre-alphabetic stage) than in later phases. Auditory memory, in contrast, appears to be related to reading regardless of the reading measure or phase of reading of the participants.

B. Phonological Awareness

Phonological awareness is measured by tasks that require analyzing words into their phonological parts (e.g., counting syllables or phonemes, comparing first sounds in words, deleting sounds from words) or putting speech sounds together into syllables or words (e.g., sound blending). Phonological awareness is related to reading ability among typically developing children both as a precursor to and a consequence of reading acquisition (Perfetti, Beck, Bell, & Hughes, 1987; Wagner & Torgesen, 1987; Wagner, Torgesen, & Rashotte, 1994). It is one of the major bases for Ehri's partial-alphabetic, full alphabetic, and consolidated alphabetic phases of reading development, and also corresponds closely to Harm and Seidenberg's phonological network. The evidence suggests that better phonological awareness in individuals with MR corresponds with better reading ability, at least when the phonological awareness measure is simple.

Among the simple phonological awareness measures are alliteration, syllable segmentation, phoneme segmentation, phoneme blending, and rhyming. All of these measures except rhyming appear to be related to reading ability in individuals with MR. Alliteration, which requires detecting, matching, or reproducing beginning sounds of words, distinguished between stronger and weaker readers with MR of undifferentiated etiology (Cawley, 1966) as well as with Down syndrome (Cardoso-Martins & Frith, 2001), even when IQ, age, and letter knowledge were covaried out. It also correlated at a marginally significant level with word identification in children with Down syndrome (Cupples & Iacono, 2000). Phoneme blending distinguished between Sheperd's (1967) stronger and weaker readers, loaded with word identification in Blackman and Burger's (1972) factor analysis, and correlated at a marginally significant level with word identification at two different points in time among Cupples and Iacono's (2000) children with Down syndrome. Syllable segmentation distinguished between stronger and weaker readers with MR (Cawley, 1966; Cawley & Parmar, 1995). Phoneme segmentation correlated significantly with word identification among children with Down syndrome and added significantly to the prediction of word identification 9 months later after age, receptive vocabulary and digit span were controlled (Cupples & Iacono, 2000). Only one study did not generally show meaningful relations between simple phonological awareness measures and reading ability (Kay-Raining Bird et al., 2000). The correlations reported from this study of children with Down syndrome spanned 4.5 years, however, and were based on a sample size of 12. Still, in this study, phoneme segmentation correlated marginally significantly with word identification with age and MA partialed out.

Rhyming is the one simple form of phonological awareness that seems clearly *unrelated* to reading among individuals with MR. Of four studies that included a rhyming measure, one reported mixed results and three reported no relationship to reading. Cawley (1966) reported that stronger readers were better at rhyming words than weaker readers, though not at rhyming sounds. Other studies found no significant correlations between rhyming and word identification in children with Down syndrome (Cupples & Iacono, 2000; Kay-Raining Bird et al., 2000) or Williams syndrome (Laing et al., 2001), at least when age and general ability were partialed out. One reason that rhyming might have been unrelated to reading is that it is a very rudimentary form of phonological awareness, and as such, might not have discriminated among readers very well.

Results for the more complex measures of phonological awareness are not as strong as results for the simple measures. The complex measures require both segmentation and blending and perhaps manipulation of speech sounds. For example, a phoneme deletion task requires taking one sound away from a word and saying what is left (e.g., *snip* without the /n/ is *sip*). A spoonerism task requires switching the first sounds of two words, as in *Yew Nork*. Fowler et al. (1995) found that a version of the Auditory Analysis Test (AAT) of syllable/phoneme deletion correlated significantly with word identification among adults with Down syndrome, after correction for general ability. No other study produced a significant relationship, though there were some trends in the expected direction. Kay-Raining Bird et al. (2000) used the AAT with children with Down syndrome, Laing et al. (2001) used a phoneme deletion/spoonerisms composite with adolescents with Williams syndrome, and Conners et al. (2001) used the Lindamood Auditory Conceptualization Test with children with mixed etiology MR. The complexity in this set of phonological awareness tasks may have introduced additional variance in the measures that was unrelated to reading ability, resulting in weaker relationships (e.g., variance related to task comprehension, attentional capacity, etc.).

C. Visual and Orthographic Discrimination

For the present discussion, visual discrimination refers to distinguishing one visual pattern from another. Orthographic discrimination refers to distinguishing common vs uncommon letter patterns. Visual discrimination would be important in pre-alphabetic reading, which occurs before letter–sound correspondences are known. However, reading at any level requires discrimination and identification of visual stimuli (i.e., letters). Orthographic discrimination requires knowledge of how letters tend to combine in one's language, similar to Harm and Seidenberg's orthographic network. Being able to identify common letter clusters allows for faster word identification as well as reading by analogy. The research suggests that stronger readers with MR are better at visual and orthographic discrimination than are weaker readers with MR, especially in the early phases of reading involving pre-alphabetic sight-word reading.

Blackman and Burger (1972) found that, among their 19 reading readiness variables, a visual discrimination measure loaded on the reading factor and correlated moderately with reading among first graders with MR, though it did not contribute independently to the prediction of single-word reading. Consistent with this finding, Conners and Detterman (1987) found that adolescents with moderate MR who were faster at discriminating among six visual matrices were better at learning sight-words, and Conners (1990) found that this was particularly true when the discrimination difficulty in the sight-word learning task was high. Similarly, Evans and Bilsky (1972) found that under some instructional presentations, stronger readers were better at learning visual discriminations than weaker readers. Sheperd (1967), however, found that visual discrimination did not distinguish stronger from weaker decoders. His reading measure was comprehensive, whereas those in the other studies were single-word reading. As suggested for visual working memory, it may be that visual discrimination ability is more important in the sight-word phase of reading than in subsequent phases.

Orthographic discrimination was measured by Blackman and Burger's (1972) visual wordness task. This task was one of the three of 19 that both loaded on the reading factor and contributed independently to the prediction of single-word reading ability. This task measured children's ability to discriminate permissible nonwords made of English letters from those made from Greek, Russian, or Sanskrit letters, and thus tapped their general knowledge of English orthography. Although this task was not used in other studies, its importance to reading in the Blackman and Burger study is very clear, and future research should investigate orthographic discrimination as an index of individual differences in reading in MR.

D. Associative Learning

Associative learning is strongly suggested as important to reading in network models such as Harm and Seidenberg's. These models suggest that reading acquisition is accomplished by forming associations among phonological features and orthographic units (i.e., auditory–visual associations; see Windfuhr & Snowling, 2001, for emipirical evidence). Comprehension models such as Gernsbacher's and Kintsch's also highlight the importance of semantic associations in building coherent text models. Thus, both cross-modal and uni-modal associations are of interest. Results suggest that both types of associative learning correlate with reading, at least if word identification is the criterion.

Studies using cross-modal associative learning tasks have clearly shown that individuals with MR who are better at learning associations are also better at word identification. Blackman and Burger (1972) found that auditory–visual integration and associative learning were highly important to individual differences in reading ability in children with MR. Their auditory–visual integration task required children to choose which of three visual dot patterns corresponded to a series of long and short sounds or taps. It contributed independently to the prediction of single-word reading, though it did not load on the reading factor. An associative learning task called "learning sample" required children to learn spoken words that corresponded to printed words. Number of trials to criterion on this task both contributed independently to the prediction of single-word reading and loaded on the reading factor. In other studies, Stayton and Fuller (1974) showed that learning nonsense syllable names for line drawings correlated significantly with reading among individuals with MR, even when MA and CA were partialed out. Mair (1962) showed that three cross-modal associative learning measures correlated strongly with word identification, whereas MA did not. The measures all involved learning associations between speech sounds (e.g., *eem*) and letter-like shapes. Finally, Laing et al. (2001) reported that performance on their cue-target associative learning task (e.g., LKR = *ladder*) correlated significantly with word identification in adolescents with Williams syndrome, after controlling age and general ability.

Studies using uni-modal associative learning tasks also have demonstrated a link between associative learning and single-word reading in individuals with MR. Blackman et al. (1976) found that a traditional paired-associates learning task both loaded on their reading factor and was one of the best predictors of reading. In this task, participants listened to 15 word pairs and then listened to the first word of each pair and tried to recall its partner word. Feedback was given on each trial, and trials continued until an accuracy criterion was reached. Conners and Detterman (1987) found that learning spatial locations of visual matrix stimuli was related to sight-word learning. In contrast, Mair (1962) found only nonsignificant trends toward correlations between reading and uni-modal associative learning.

Learning associations between two sets of letter-like shapes correlated marginally significantly with reading, but learning associations between two sets of sounds (e.g., ep-sar) did not.

There was a single study in which neither cross-modal nor uni-modal associative learning was related to reading. In this study, Cawley and Parmar (1995) had children make associations between visual stimuli (geometric figures and wordlike stimuli) and pictures of common objects or between visual stimuli and auditory stimuli (presumably words or nonwords). They also had children learn English labels for printed Czech words. There were no differences between stronger and weaker readers with MR on any of these tasks. Ceiling effects, however, might have masked any true differences between groups. Or, it is possible that associative learning relates to single-word reading moreso than to broad reading achievement, which was used to define reader groups in this study. Thus, the best conclusion from the associative learning studies might be that associative learning (particularly cross-modal) is important at least to word identification in individuals with MR; its importance to a broader range of reading abilities needs further documentation.

E. Semantic and Syntactic Processing

Once children have advanced to reading sentences, syntactic and semantic processing become more important, and they begin to use more top-down processing in their reading. Semantic and syntactic context can prime word recognition thereby making it faster and more accurate (Levitt, 1970). In turn, more resources are made available for developing a mental text representation. Semantic associations are particularly important in Kintsch's integration process and Gernsbacher's mapping process, both of which are critical to the development of a mental text representation. Most of the research supports the notion that semantic and syntactic processing abilities are important in distinguishing stronger and weaker readers with MR, though the results are sensitive to measurement parameters.

Measures that primarily reflect semantic processing generally have been related to reading among individuals with MR. These include the Semantic Knowledge subtest of the Bankson Language Screening Test (Parmenter, 1986, 1988), the Vocabulary and Information subtests of the Wechsler Intelligence Scale for Children (though not the Similarities subtest; Ramanauskas & Burrow, 1973), and receptive vocabulary (Blackman & Burger, 1972; Bochner, Outhred, & Pieterse, 2001, Fowler et al., 1995; Laing et al., 2001). Also, Cronin et al. (1986) found that, in a word association task, the tendency to make a more mature, paradigmatic response (e.g., cold–hot) as opposed to a syntagmatic response (cold–outside) correlated with general reading skill, once differences in MA were controlled. These studies included measures of word identification and reading comprehension, and participants with Down syndrome, Williams syndrome, and undifferentiated MR.

Slightly different from the rest of these studies, however, Blackman et al. (1976) found that only three of five semantic classification tasks were related to word identification, though they all loaded together on a "classificatory" factor. Naming (generating category exemplars) and Abstraction (saying how three items are alike) contributed independently to the prediction of word identification, and Sorting (sorting pictures into conceptual categories) loaded on the reading factor. However, Class Inclusion (saying if there are more hammers or tools) and Semantic Oddity (choosing the one that is not in the category) were not related to word identification. The three semantic classification tasks that were related to reading involved generating rather than choosing a response, as did the word identification task. Possibly, variance related to response format was important in this study.

For measures that involve both semantic and syntactic processing, or primarily syntactic processing, results are somewhat mixed. In two studies, stronger readers were better than weaker readers at using contextual cues to guess the next word while reading or listening to phrases and sentences (Cawley & Parmar, 1995; Sheperd, 1967). In two other studies, stronger readers were better than weaker readers on measures involving the Test of Auditory Comprehension of Language, both with Down syndrome (Fowler et al., 1995) and with mixed-etiology MR (Conners et al., 2001). However, Conners et al. reported that the group difference disappeared when age was held constant, and Fowler et al. did not covary age in their analysis. Parmenter (1986) found that knowledge of syntactic rules correlated with various measures of reading, but Sheperd (1967) found no reader group difference in understanding of grammatical structure. Essentially, the measures that tapped syntactic processing more implicitly (cloze measures) were more successful at distinguishing between stronger and weaker readers. The more explicit measures might have been too difficult for at least the younger participants with MR in the studies by Conners et al. and Sheperd. Syntactic processing may be related to reading in individuals with MR when appropriate measures are used.

F. Unrelated Abilities

A few other abilities were measured by more than one study and found not to relate to reading among individuals with MR. These include auditory discrimination (Blackman & Burger, 1972; Mair, 1962; Sheperd, 1967;

Simpson, Haynes, & Haynes, 1984), intermediate/long-term memory (Bilsky & Evans, 1970; Conners & Detterman, 1987; Evans, 1970), visual categorization/classification (Blackman et al., 1976; Blackman & Burger, 1972), use of clustering in recall (Blackman et al., 1976; Evans, 1970; but see Bilsky & Evans, 1970 for an exception), visuo-motor skill (Cellura & Butterfield, 1966; Sheperd, 1967; Song & Song, 1969; but see Blackman & Burger 1972); and full-scale IQ (Blackman et al., 1976; Conners, 1990; Conners et al., 2001; Grossman & Clark, 1984; Naglieri, 1980; Slate, 1995; but see Nagle, 1993 for a weak but significant correlation; Slate, 1995 for a range-correction; and Laing et al., 2001 for an exception with Williams syndrome).

G. Summary

It is fairly certain that working memory, especially auditory working memory, is important to individual differences in reading among children and adults with MR. This is the strongest finding in the literature reviewed. Phonological awareness and semantic/syntactic processing are also important, but relationships depend on which specific measures are used. In general, the simpler measures relate to reading more reliably. Visual discrimination and associative learning are related to sight-word reading ability, though not necessarily to more advanced reading ability. Orthographic discrimination appears to be important to reading, but more research is needed in this area.

VI. CONCLUSION

The research suggests an emerging lag in reading development in children with MR. Early reading skills (i.e., sight-word learning, letter knowledge, and letter–sound correspondences) develop at a pace consistent with MA, but by MA8 or 9, reading becomes a specific area of difficulty, lagging behind MA-based expectations. The emerging lag appears to be due to difficulty in phonological decoding as early as MA7. Most children with MR struggle greatly with sounding out. This difficulty no doubt makes word identification more effortful and slows progress toward automatization. At a point when cognitive resources would normally begin to shift from word identification to comprehension, they are still needed for word identification. The restriction on resources no doubt hampers reading comprehension. But also, the failure to apply background knowledge, to use brief context, and to monitor comprehension result in serious problems in overall reading comprehension that are obvious by MA10. In spite of these generalizations, some children with MR are more successful at learning to read than others. Those who are more successful in sight-word learning and word identification have better visual working memory, visual discrimination, and associative learning abilities. Those who are more successful overall (i.e., in both word identification and reading comprehension) have better auditory working memory, phonological awareness, and semantic processing abilities. More research is needed on orthographic processing, including the relative difficulty of orthographic decoding for children with MR and the degree to which orthographic discrimination is related to individual differences in reading ability. More research is also needed on word identification, phonological awareness, and semantic/syntactic processing to better understand some of the mixed results on these topics.

One of the strongest findings in this literature is that children with MR have tremendous difficulty with phonological decoding (see also Jenkinson, 1989). They learn sight-words, letter names and even letter–sound correspondences relatively easily, but they seem to get stuck on the sounding out. In our own research we have seen children with MR correctly say each sound in the right order, but fail to finally pronounce the word correctly (Conners, Rosenquist, Sligh, Atwell, & Kiser, 2000). Why? One possibility is that when it comes time to sound out a word, children do not *apply* the letter–sound knowledge they have. This argument is similar to the one advanced by Bos and Tierney (1980) in relation to inference generation on expository texts—children with MR had the background knowledge, but apparently did not *apply* it to the reading comprehension task. In other words, it may be that children with MR do not *transfer* their knowledge to the reading task. Transfer of knowledge is documented as very difficult for individuals with MR (e.g., Day & Hall, 1988; Minsky, Spitz, & Bessellieu, 1985). However, Neville and Vandever (1973; Vandever & Neville, 1976) found good transfer by children with MR in the context of sounding out instruction (see also Conners et al., 2000).

Another likely explanation for the phonological decoding difficulty is poor working memory. Certainly, to sound out a word requires accessing sounds in order and holding them in working memory while accessing subsequent sounds. Working memory may be so limited in children with MR, that by the time they get to the third letter sound in a word, they begin to lose the first letter sound, making phonological decoding nearly impossible. As noted earlier in this chapter, researchers have long viewed working memory as an area of extreme difficulty in individuals with MR. Further, working memory—in particular *auditory* working memory—emerged in the present review as the cognitive ability most reliably related to reading ability in children with MR. Finally, in a reading-level matched design, Kabrich and McCutchen (1996) found that children with MR had a smaller advantage for phonologically dissimilar over phonologically similar words in a word list recall task, compared to children without MR. This appeared to reflect a problem in working memory, probably related to rehearsal of phonological codes, and this problem may have been a cause for the poor reading ability of the children with MR.

There are several other possible explanations for the phonological decoding difficulty associated with MR. Perhaps phonological awareness is so poor in children with MR that, though they may get the sounds of the letters, they don't have the awareness that those sounds make up a word—the sounds seem separate, and the idea of blending them together is difficult to grasp. The evidence indicates that children with MR who have better phonological awareness—including sound blending—are better at reading. However, other evidence suggests that phonological awareness is not closely related to intelligence (Conners, Carr, Wang, & Wyatt, 1998; Siegel, 1993), whereas working memory is related (e.g., Fry & Hale, 1996; Miller & Vernon, 1996). In other words, individuals with MR are not necessarily poor in phonological awareness, though they usually are poor in working memory. Another possibility is that poor vocabulary limits the number of words children with MR have access to when they read. They may have the sequence of sounds worked out, but have trouble matching that sequence with a word they know. Research suggests that unfamiliar words are harder to access and pronounce (Connine, Mullennix, Shernoff, & Yelen, 1990; Walker, Barrow, & Rastatter, 2002) as well as to decode (McKague, Pratt, & Johnston, 2001). Researchers need to understand the underlying reasons for the phonological decoding difficulty in individuals with MR so that the most sensible instructional techniques can be developed.

The second major finding to emerge from this review is that the stronger readers with MR are those with the better working memory skills. Visual working memory seems related to reading primarily at MAs associated with the sight-word phase of reading, whereas auditory working memory seems related to reading regardless of MA and regardless of the reading measure. An assumption is that working memory enables development of reading skills, as suggested in the discussion above. This is probably true for children with MR, but there is evidence that, at least for children with Down syndrome, reading ability enables improvement in working memory (Laws, Buckley, Bird, MacDonald, & Broadley, 1995). The fact is that both reading and memory are developing through the school years, and their strong association should be incorporated into instructional techniques. Future longitudinal studies featuring visual and auditory working memory skills and various reading skills should help in this endeavor. This research should involve children with MR of nonspecific etiology, as well as children with fragile X and Down syndromes, who are known to have specific difficulty with working memory.

Several studies reviewed in this chapter featured participants with specific genetic syndromes of MR, most notably Down syndrome and Williams syndrome. In general, results from these studies fit with the results from studies with participants with nonspecific etiology of MR. However, there was some evidence that individuals with Down syndrome functioned higher in word identification and perhaps also in phonological decoding than would be predicted based on their MA or verbal MA. Statistical comparisons were not reported and it is premature to make a conclusion about a relative strength in word identification or phonological decoding in Down syndrome (see Buckley, 1995; Buckley, Bird, & Byrne, 1996a,b for discussions). However, this is certainly an important area for future research. Similarly, there was evidence that participants with Williams syndrome were particularly poor at a mock sight-word learning task in which they showed little use of imagery. This raises the possibility that children with Williams syndrome may have a unique difficulty with sight-word learning due to their poor visuo-spatial ability. This is another important avenue for future research. Insofar as relative cognitive strengths and weaknesses exist in *many* syndromes of MR, there also may exist relative strengths and weaknesses in reading skills that deserve investigation.

A final suggestion for future research is to allow mainstream reading theory to guide investigations of reading difficulty in individuals with MR. Harm and Seidenberg (1999) suggested ways in which the development of the phonological–orthographic network could be faulty, resulting in reading problems. These include problems in the formation, revision, and maintenance of connections among phonological units, lack of experience, degraded input, and inefficient use of hidden/cleanup units. These ideas are supported by simulations, but are still in the early stage of development. They were proposed as ways of explaining phonological and surface dyslexia. Nevertheless, they may be relevant to reading difficulties experienced by individuals with MR. Gernsbacher (1997) has also suggested points of breakdown in the structure-building process that could result in poor comprehension. She suggested that a failure in the suppression mechanism may be the reason for comprehension difficulties of some individuals. Gernsbacher, Varner, and Faust (1990) found that poorer comprehenders showed evidence of shifting when they should have been mapping. They suggested that, when faced with irrelevant information that cannot be mapped onto the existing foundation, poor comprehenders may fail to suppress that information. Instead, they may use it to lay a foundation for a new substructure. The result would be too many poorly connected substructures, and lack of coherence in the mental representation. Kintsch has conducted modeling research that suggests that reduced memory capacity can lead to fewer activated central propositions at a given time, and ultimately, poor comprehension. To date, these ideas have not been applied to the reading difficulties of individuals with MR.

Historically, attitudes about individuals with MR have volleyed back and forth between positive and negative. Attitudes have influenced expectations and quality of services. Judging from the comments made in recent years by numerous authors, attitudes are currently positive and expectations for reading achievement have increased. More children with MR than ever before are being educated in mainstream classrooms, and whenever possible, they are held to the same standards as typically developing children. Yet, the reading problem has not been solved. In fact, the volume of basic research on reading in individuals with MR has slowed to a trickle in the last 15 years, just at a time when it could benefit from advances in the mainstream reading literature as well as the dyslexia literature. We need to know more about what makes reading so difficult for children with MR, and then find out how to facilitate reading. There is much work to do, but a great deal to gain.

ACKNOWLEDGMENTS

Preparation supported in part by NIH Grant HD 37445 from the National Institute of Child Health and Human Development, jointly with the National Down Syndrome Society.

REFERENCES

Allington, R. L. (1980). Word frequency and contextual richness effects on word identification of educable mentally retarded children. *Education and Training of the Mentally Retarded, 15*, 118–121.

Bilsky, L., & Evans, R. A. (1970). Use of associative clustering technique in the study of reading disability: effects of list organization. *American Journal of Mental Deficiency, 74*, 771–776.

Blackman, L. S., Bilsky, L. H., Burger, A. L., & Mar, H. (1976). Cognitive processes and academic achievement in EMR adolescents. *American Journal of Mental Deficiency, 81*, 125–134.

Blackman, L. S., & Burger, A. L. (1972). Psychological factors related to early reading behavior of EMR and nonretarded children. *American Journal of Mental Deficiency, 77*, 212–229.

Blake, K. A., Aaron, I. E., & Westbrook, H. R. (1969). Learning of basal reading skills by mentally handicapped and non-mentally handicapped children. *Journal of Research and Development in Education, 2*(2), 2–123.

Bochner, S., Outhred, L., & Pieterse, M. (2001). A study of functional literacy skills in young adults with Down syndrome. *International Journal of Disability, Development, and Education, 48*, 67–90.

Bos, C. S., & Tierney, R. J. (1980). Inferential reading abilities of mildly mentally retarded and nonretarded students. *American Journal of Mental Deficiency, 89*, 75–82.

Browder, D. M., & Lalli, J. S. (1991). Review of research on sight-word instruction. *Research in Developmental Disabilities, 12*, 203–228.

Buckley, S. (1995). Teaching children with Down syndrome to read and write. In L. Nadel, & D. Rosenthal (Eds.), *Down syndrome: Living and learning in the community* (pp. 158–169). New York: Wiley-Liss, Inc.

Buckley, S., Bird, G., & Byrne, A. (1996a). The practical and theoretical significance of teaching literacy skills to children with Down syndrome. In J. A. Rondal, J. Perera, L. Nadel, & A. Comblain (Eds.), *Down's syndrome: Psychological, psychobiological, and socio-educational perspectives* (pp. 119–128). London: Whurr Publishers.

Buckley, S., Bird, G., & Byrne, A. (1996b). Reading acquisition by young children. In B. Stratford, & P. Gunn (Eds.), *New approaches to Down syndrome* (pp. 268–279). London: Cassell.

Cardoso-Martins, C., & Frith, U. (2001). Can individuals with Down syndrome acquire alphabetic literacy skills in the absence of phoneme awareness? *Reading and Writing, 14*, 361–375.

Cawley, J. F. (1966). Reading performance among the mentally handicapped: a problem in assessment. *Training School Bulletin, 63*(1), 11–16.

Cawley, J. F., & Parmar, R. S. (1995). Comparisons in reading and reading-related tasks among students with average intellectual ability and students with mild mental retardation. *Education and Training in Mental Retardation and Developmental Disabilities, 30*, 118–129.

Cegelka, P. A., & Cegelka, W. J. (1970). A review of research: reading and the educable mentally handicapped. *Exceptional Children, 37*, 187–200.

Cellura, A. R., & Butterfield, E. C. (1966). Intelligence, the Bender-Gestalt test, and reading achievement. *American Journal of Mental Deficiency, 71*, 60–63.

Cole, P. (1998). Developmental versus difference approaches to mental retardation: a theoretical extension to the present debate. *American Journal on Mental Retardation, 102*, 379–391.

Conners, F. A. (1990). Aptitude by treatment interactions in computer-assisted word learning by mentally retarded students. *American Journal on Mental Retardation, 94*, 387–397.

Conners, F. A. (1992). Reading instruction for students with moderate mental retardation: a review and analysis of research. *American Journal on Mental Retardation, 96*, 577–597.

Conners, F. A., Atwell, J. A., Rosenquist, C. J., & Sligh, A. C. (2001). Abilities underlying decoding differences in children with intellectual disability. *Journal of Intellectual Disability Research, 45*, 292–299.

Conners, F. A., Carr, M. D., Wang, A., & Wyatt, B. S. (1998). Phonological processing: a modular ability? In S. A. Soraci, & W. McIlvane (Eds.), *Perspectives on fundamental processes in intellectual functioning* (Vol. 1, pp. 265–286). Norwood, NJ: Ablex.

Conners, F. A., & Detterman, D. K. (1987). Information processing correlates of computer-assisted word learning by mentally retarded students. *American Journal of Mental Deficiency, 91*, 606–612.

Conners, F. A., Rosenquist, C. J., Atwell, J. A., & Klinger, L. G. (2000). Cognitive strengths and weaknesses associated with Prader-Willi syndrome. *Education and Training in Mental Retardation and Developmental Disabilities, 35*, 441–448.

Conners, F. A., Rosenquist, C. J., Sligh, A. C., & Atwell, J. A., & Kiser, T. (2000, August), *Acquisition of phonological reading skills in children with mental retardation.* Presented at the International Association for the Scientific Study of Intellectual Disabilities (IASSID) World Congress, Seattle.

Connine, C. M., Mullennix, J., Shernoff, E., & Yelen, J. (1990). Word familiarity and frequency in visual and auditory word recognition. *Journal of Experimental Psychology: Learning, Memory, and Cognition, 16*, 1084–1096.

Crews, W. B. (1988). Performance of students classified as educable mentally handicapped on Florida's State Student Assessment Test, Part II. *Education and Training in Mental Retardation, 23*, 186–191.

Cronin, V., Pratt, M., Abraham, J., Howell, D., Bishop, S., & Manning, A. (1986). Word association and the acquisition of reading. *Journal of Psycholinguistic Research, 15*, 1–11.

Crossland, C. L. (1981). A comparison of retarded and non-retarded on the ability to use context in reading. *Journal for Special Educators, 17*, 234–241.

Cupples, L., & Iacono, T. (2000). Phonological awareness and oral reading skill in children with Down syndrome. *Journal of Speech, Language, and Hearing Research, 43*, 595–608.

Das, J. P., & Cummins, J. (1978). Academic performance and cognitive processes in EMR children. *American Journal of Mental Deficiency, 83*, 197–199.

Day, J. D., & Hall, L. K. (1988). Intelligence-related differences in learning and transfer and enhancement of transfer among mentally retarded persons. *American Journal on Mental Retardation, 93*, 125–137.

Dunn, L. M. (1954). A comparison of the reading processes of mentally retarded and normal boys of the same mental age. *Monographs of the Society for Research in Child Development, 19*, 7–99.

Dykens, E. M., Hodapp, R. M., & Leckman, J. F. (1987). Strengths and weaknesses in the intellectual functioning of males with fragile X syndrome. *American Journal of Mental Deficiency, 92*, 234–236.

Dykens, E. M., Hodapp, R. M., Walsh, K., & Nash, L. J. (1992). Profiles, correlates, and trajectories of intelligence in Prader-Willi syndrome. *Journal of the American Adademy of Child and Adolescent Psychiatry, 31*, 1125–1130.

Ehri, L. C. (1991). Development of the ability to read words. In R. Barr, M. Kamil, P. Mosenthal, & P. Pearson (Eds.), *Handbook of reading research* (Vol. 2, pp. 383–417). New York: Longman.

Ehri, L. C. (1994). Development of the ability to read words: Update. In R. Ruddell, M. Ruddell, & H. Singer (Eds.), *Theoretical models and processes of reading* (4th ed., pp. 237–269). Newark, DE: International Reading Association.

Ehri, L. C. (1999). Phases of development in learning to read words. In J. Oakhill, & R. Beard (Eds.), *Reading development and the teaching of reading: A psychological perspective* (pp. 79–108). Oxford: Blackwell Science Ltd.

Evans, R. A. (1970). Use of associative clustering technique in the study of reading disability: effects of presentation mode. *American Journal of Mental Deficiency, 74*, 765–770.

Evans, R. (1994). Phonological awareness in children with Down's syndrome. *Down Syndrome Research and Practice, 2*, 102–105.

Evans, R. A., & Bilsky, L. (1972). Discrimination training on the identification of reversible letters by EMR adolescents. *American Journal of Mental Deficiency, 77*, 169–174.

Fowler, A. E., Doherty, B. J., & Boynton, L. (1995). The basis of reading skill in young adults with Down syndrome. In L. Nadel, & D. Rosenthal (Eds.), *Down syndrome: Living and learning in the community* (pp. 182–196). New York: Wiley-Liss, Inc.

Frith, U. (1985). Beneath the surface of developmental dyslexia. In K. E. Patterson, J. C. Marshall, & M. Coltheart (Eds.), *Surface dyslexia: Neuropsychological and cognitive studies of phonological reading* (pp. 301–330). London: Erlbaum.

Fry, A. F., & Hale, S. (1996). Processing speed, working memory, and fluid intelligence: evidence for a developmental cascade. *Psychological Science, 7*, 237–241.

Gathercole, S. E. (1996). *Models of short-term memory*. Hove, UK: Psychology Press.

Gernsbacher, M. A. (1990). *Language comprehension as structure building*. Hillsdale, NJ: Erlbaum.
Gernsbacher, M. A. (1991). Cognitive processes and mechanisms in language comprehension: the structure building framework. In G. H. Bower (Ed.), *The psychology of learning and motivation* (pp. 217–263). New York: Academic Press.
Gernsbacher, M. A. (1995). The structure building framework: what it is, what it might also be, and why. In B. K. Bitton, & A. C. Graesser (Eds.), *Models of text understanding* (pp. 289–311). Hillsdale, NJ: Erlbaum.
Gernsbacher, M. A. (1997). Two decades of structure building. *Discourse Processes*, *23*, 265–304.
Gernsbacher, M. A., Varner, K. R., & Faust, M. (1990). Investigating differences in general comprehension skill. *Journal of Experimental Psychology: Learning, Memory, and Cognition*, *16*, 430–445.
Gickling, E. E., Hargis, C. H., & Alexander, D. R. (1981). The function of imagery in sight-word recognition among retarded and nonretarded children. *Education and Training of the Mentally Retarded*, *16*, 259–262.
Goodstein, H. A. (1970). Performance of mentally handicapped and average-IQ children on two modified cloze tasks for oral language. *American Journal of Mental Deficiency*, *75*, 290–297.
Gough, P., Juel, C., & Roper-Schneider, D. (1983). Code and cipher: a two-stage conception of initial reading acquisition. In J. A. Niles, & L. A. Harris (Eds.), *Searches for meaning in reading/language processing and instruction* (*32nd Yearbook of the National Reading Conference*) (pp. 207–211). Rochester, NY: National Reading Conference.
Gough, P. B., & Tunmer, W. E. (1985). Decoding, reading, and reading disability. *RASE: Remedial and Special Education*, *7*, 6–10.
Gronna, S. H., Jenkins, A. A., & Chin-Chance, S. A. (1998a). The performance of students with disabilities in a norm-referenced, statewide standardized testing program. *Journal of Learning Disabilities*, *31*, 482–493.
Gronna, S. H., Jenkins, A. A., & Chin-Chance, S. A. (1998b). Who are we assessing? Determining state-wide participation rates for students with disabilities. *Exceptional Children*, *64*, 407–418.
Grossman, F. M., & Clark, J. H. (1984). Concurrent validity of WISC-R factor scores for educable mentally handicapped children. *Perceptual and Motor Skills*, *58*, 227–230.
Hale, C. A., & Borkowski, J. G. (1991). Attention, memory, and cognition. In R. W. Reese, & L. Lipsett (Eds.), *Handbook of mental retardation* (pp. 505–528). New York: Pergamon.
Harm, M. W., & Seidenberg, M. S. (1999). Phonology, reading acquisition, and dyslexia: insights from connectionist models. *Psychological Review*, *106*, 491–528.
Hodapp, R. M., Leckman, J. F., Dykens, E. M., Sparrow, S. S., Zelinsky, D. G., & Ort, S. I. (1992). K-ABC profiles in children with fragile X syndrome, Down syndrome, and nonspecific mental retardation. *American Journal on Mental Retardation*, *97*, 39–46.
Jenkinson, J. C. (1989). Word recognition and the nature of reading difficulty in children with an intellectual disability: a review. *International Journal of Disability, Development, and Education*, *36*, 39–56.
Jenkinson, J. C. (1992). The use of letter position cues in the visual processing of words by children with an intellectual disability and nondisabled children. *International Journal of Disability, Development, and Education*, *39*, 61–76.
John, K. R., & Rattan, G. (1991). A comparison of short-term memory tests as predictors of reading achievement for learning-disabled and educable mentally retarded students. *Journal of School Psychology*, *29*, 309–318.
Kabrich, M., & McCutchen, D. (1996). Phonemic support in comprehension: comparisons between children with and without mild mental retardation. *American Journal on Mental Retardation*, *100*, 510–527.

Katims, D. S. (2000). Literacy instruction for people with mental retardation: historical highlights and contemporary analysis. *Education and Training in Mental Retardation and Developmental Disabilities*, *35*, 3–15.

Kay-Raining Bird, E., Cleave, P. L., & McConnell, L. (2000). Reading and phonological awareness in children with Down syndrome: a longitudinal study. *American Journal of Speech–Language Pathology*, *9*, 319–330.

Kintsch, W. (1988). The use of knowledge in discourse processing: a construction-integration model. *Psychological Review*, *95*, 163–182.

Kintsch, W. (1998). *Comprehension: A paradigm for cognition*. Cambridge, UK: Cambridge University Press.

Kintsch, W., & vanDijk, T. A. (1978). Towards a model of text comprehension and production. *Psychological Review*, *85*, 363–394.

Laing, E., Hulme, C., Grant, J., & Karmiloff-Smith, A. (2001). Learning to read in Williams syndrome: looking beneath the surface of atypical reading development. *Journal of Child Psychology and Psychiatry*, *42*, 729–739.

Laws, G. (1998). The use of nonword repetition as a test of phonological memory in children with Down syndrome. *Journal of Child Psychology and Psychiatry*, *39*, 1119–1130.

Laws, G., Buckley, S., Bird, G., MacDonald, J., & Broadley, I. (1995). The influence of reading instruction on language and memory development in children with Down's syndrome. *Down Syndrome Research and Practice*, *3*, 59–64.

Laws, G., MacDonald, J., & Buckley, S. (1996). The effects of a short training in the use of a rehearsal strategy on memory for words and pictures in children with Down syndrome. *Down Syndrome Research and Practice*, *4*, 70–78.

Levitt, E. (1970). The effect of context on the reading of mentally retarded and normal children at the first grade level. *Journal of Special Education*, *4*, 425–429.

Levitt, E. (1972). Higher-order and lower-order reading responses of mentally retarded and nonretarded children at the first-grade level. *American Journal of Mental Deficiency*, *77*, 13–20.

Luftig, R. L., & Greeson, R. L. (1983). Effects of structural importance and idea saliency on discourse recall of mentally retarded and nonretarded pupils. *American Journal of Mental Deficiency*, *87*, 414–421.

Luftig, R. L., & Johnson, R. E. (1982). Identification and recall of structurally important units in prose by mentally retarded learners. *American Journal of Mental Deficiency*, *86*, 495–502.

Mair, K. J. (1962). Coding and literacy in severely subnormal children. *Journal of Mental Deficiency Research*, *7*, 46–52.

Mandes, E., Massimino, C., & Mantis, C. (1991). A comparison of borderline and mild mental retardates assessed on the Memory for Designs and the WAIS-R. *Journal of Clinical Psychology*, *47*, 562–567.

Marsh, G., Freidman, M., Welch, V., & Desberg, P. (1981). A cognitive-developmental theory of reading acquisition. In T. G. Waller, & G. MacKinnon (Eds.), *Reading research: Advances in theory and practice* (Vol. 3, pp. 199–221). New York: Academic Press.

Mason, J. M. (1976). Testing pronunciation skill competence of both normal and retarded readers. *Mental Retardation*, *14*, 36–40.

Mason, J. M. (1977). Questioning the notion of independent processing stages in reading. *Journal of Educational Psychology*, *69*, 288–297.

Mason, J. M. (1978). Role of strategy in reading by mentally retarded persons. *American Journal of Mental Deficiency*, *82*, 467–473.

McKague, M., Pratt, C., & Johnston, M. B. (2001). The effect of oral vocabulary on reading visually novel words: a comparison of the dual-route-cascaded and triangle frameworks. *Cognition*, *80*, 231–262.

Merrill, M. A. (1924). On the relation of intelligence to achievement in the case of mentally retarded children. *Comparative Psychology Monographs* (Vol. 11, Serial No. 10). Baltimore: Williams and Wilkins Company.

Miller, L. T., & Vernon, P. A. (1996). Intelligence, reaction time, and working memory in 4- to 6-year-old children. *Intelligence, 22*, 155–190.

Minsky, S. K., Spitz, H. H., & Bessellieu, C. L. (1985). Maintenance and transfer of training by mentally retarded young adults on the Tower of Hanoi problem. *American Journal of Mental Deficiency, 90*, 190–197.

Miyake, A., & Shah, P. (1999). *Models of working memory: Mechanisms of active maintenance and executive control.* Cambridge, UK: Cambridge University Press.

Nagle, R. J. (1993). The relationship between the WAIS-R and academic achievement among EMR adolescents. *Psychology in the Schools, 30*, 37–39.

Naglieri, J. A. (1980). McCarthy and WISC-R correlations with WRAT achievement scores. *Perceptual and Motor Skills, 51*, 392–394.

Neville, D., & Vandever, T. R. (1973). Decoding as a result of synthetic and analytic presentation for retarded and nonretarded children. *American Journal of Mental Deficiency, 77*, 533–537.

Numminen, H., Service, E., Ahonen, T., Korhonen, T., Tolvanen, A., Patja, K., & Ruoppila, I. (2000). Working memory structure and intellectual disability. *Journal of Intellectual Disability Research, 44*, 579–590.

Pagon, R. A., Bennett, F. C., LaVeck, B., Stewart, K. B., & Johnson, J. (1987). Williams syndrome: features in late childhood and adolescence. *Pediatrics, 80*, 85–91.

Parmenter, T. R. (1986). The relationship between selected information processing variables and reading skills in a sample of mildly retarded adolescents. In J. M. Berg (Ed.), *Science and service in mental retardation* (pp. 205–215). New York: Methuen.

Parmenter, T. R. (1988). An investigation of the strategic behaviour of mildly intellectually handicapped adolescents in acquiring reading skills. In A. J. Watson (Ed.), *Intelligence: Controversy and change* (pp. 135–151). Hawthorn, Victoria, Australia: Australian Council for Educational Research Limited.

Perfetti, C. A., Beck, I., Bell, L. C., & Hughes, C. (1987). Phonemic knowledge and learning to read are reciprocal: a longitudinal study of first grade children. *Merrill-Palmer Quarterly, 33*, 283–319.

Plaut, D. C., McClelland, J. L., Seidenberg, M. S., & Patterson, K. E. (1996). Understanding normal and impaired word reading: computational principles in quasi-regular domains. *Psychological Review, 103*, 56–115.

Pulsifer, M. B. (1996). The neuropsychology of mental retardation. *Journal of the International Neuropsychological Society, 2*, 159–176.

Ramanauskas, S. (1972). Contextual constraints beyond a sentence on cloze of mentally retarded children. *American Journal of Mental Deficiency, 77*, 338–345.

Ramanauskas, S., & Burrow, W. H. (1973). WISC Profiles: above average and MR good and poor readers. *Mental Retardation, 11*(2), 12–14.

Roof, E., Stone, W., MacLean, W., Feurer, I. D., Thompson, T., & Butler, M. G. (2000). Intellectual characteristics of Prader-Willi syndrome: comparison of genetic subtypes. *Journal of Intellectual Disability Research, 44*, 25–30.

Seidenberg, M. S., & McClelland, J. L. (1989). A distributed, developmental model of word recognition and naming. *Psychological Review, 97*, 447–452.

Semmel, M. I., Barritt, L. S., & Bennett, S. W. (1970). Performance of EMR and nonretarded children on a modified cloze task. *American Journal of Mental Deficiency, 74*, 681–691.

Semmel, M. I., Gottleib, J., & Robinson, N. M. (1979). Mainstreaming: perspectives on educating handicapped children in the public school. In D. C. Berliner (Ed.), *Review of research in education* (Vol. 7, pp. 223–279). Itsaca, IL: Peacock.

Serow, R. C., & O'Brien, K. (1983). Performance of handicapped students in a competency testing program. *Journal of Special Education*, *17*(2), 149–155.

Sheperd, D. G. (1967). Selected factors in the reading ability of EMR boys. *American Journal of Mental Deficiency*, *71*, 563–570.

Siegel, L. S. (1993). Phonological processing deficits as the basis of a reading disability. *Developmental Review*, *13*, 246–257.

Simpson, R. G., Haynes, M. D., & Haynes, W. O. (1984). The relationship between performance on the Wepman Auditory Discrimination Test and reading achievement among adolescents. *Educational and Psychological Measurement*, *44*, 353–358.

Singh, N. N., & Singh, J. (1986). Reading acquisition and remediation in the mentally retarded. *International Review of Research in Mental Retardation* (Vol. 14, pp. 165–199). New York: Ablex.

Slate, J. R. (1995). Two investigations of the validity of the WISC-III. *Psychological Reports*, *76*, 299–306.

Snow, C. E., Burns, M. S., & Griffin, P. (1998). *Preventing reading difficulties in young children*. Washington, DC: National Academy Press.

Song, A. Y., & Song, R. H. (1969). Visual memory and reading ability of mental retardates. *American Journal of Mental Deficiency*, *73*, 942–945.

Stanovich, K. E. (1985). Cognitive determinants of reading in mentally retarded individuals. In N. R. Ellis, & N. W. Bray (Eds.), *International review of research in mental retardation* (Vol. 13, pp. 181–214). New York: Ablex.

Stayton, S., & Fuller, R. (1974). Reading level of retardates related to visual and auditory memory, and to paired-associate learning. *Training School Bulletin*, *70*(4), 202–207.

Streib, R. (1976). Context utilization in reading by educable mentally retarded children. *Reading Research Quarterly*, *12*, 32–54.

Thompson, S., Thurlow, M., Spicuzza, R., & Parson, L. (1999). Participation and performance of students receiving special education services on Minnesota's Basic Standards Tests: Reading and Math, 1996 through 1998 (Minnesota Report No. 18). Minneapolis, MN: University of Minnesota, National Center on Educational Outcomes.

Vandever, T. R., & Neville, D. D. (1976). Transfer as a result of synthetic and analytic reading instruction. *American Journal of Mental Deficiency*, *80*, 498–503.

Van Orden, G. C., Pennington, B. F., & Stone, G. O. (1990). Word identification in reading and the promise of subsymbolic psycholinguistics. *Psychological Review*, *97*, 488–522.

Wagner, R. K., & Torgesen, J. K. (1987). The nature of phonological processing and its causal role in the acquisition of reading skills. *Psychological Bulletin*, *101*, 192–212.

Wagner, R. K., Torgesen, J. K., & Rashotte, C. A. (1994). Development of reading-related phonological processing abilities: new evidence of bi-directional causality from a latent variable longitudinal study. *Developmental Psychology*, *30*, 73–87.

Walker, M. M., Barrow, I., & Rastatter, M. P. (2002). The effect of dimension and vocabulary age on rapid picture naming in children. *Journal of Communication Disorders*, *35*, 1–10.

Windfuhr, K. L., & Snowling, M. J. (2001). The relationship between paired associate learning and phonological skills in normally developing readers. *Journal of Experimental Child Psychology*, *80*, 160–173.

Wood, T. A., Buckhalt, J. A., & Tomlin, J. G. (1988). A comparison of listening and reading performance with children in three educational placements. *Journal of Learning Disabilities*, *21*, 493–496.

Language Interventions for Children with Mental Retardation

NANCY C. BRADY and STEVEN F. WARREN

SCHIEFELBUSCH INSTITUTE FOR LIFE SPAN STUDIES
UNIVERSITY OF KANSAS, KANSAS

I. INTRODUCTION

The topic of language intervention for children with mental retardation is necessarily broad and reflects the variability in degree of language impairment associated with mental retardation. Moreover, interventions designed to improve a specific aspect of language in children with mental retardation are obviously going to differ greatly from interventions aimed at fostering the beginnings of a communication system. Yet the underlying goal for all children with mental retardation participating in language intervention is to improve their quality of life by improving their language and communication.

Within this chapter, we have selectively reviewed research on language intervention for children with mental retardation. We have focused on research completed within the last 10 years because earlier literature has been thoroughly reviewed elsewhere (e.g., Goldstein & Hockenberger, 1991). We have also focused on studies reporting results from interventions aimed at teaching early communication forms, such as prelinguistic communication responses. We have excluded most of the research on augmentative and alternative communication because a separate chapter within this volume is devoted to this topic.

Our discussion of recent research on communication intervention for children with mental retardation pertains to four related questions. These questions reflect new knowledge of communication and mental retardation gained from recent research on these topics, as well as changes in attitudes about appropriate interventions for children with mental retardation. We will introduce these questions briefly in this introductory section, then address each question more fully in subsequent sections of this chapter.

INTERNATIONAL REVIEW OF RESEARCH IN
MENTAL RETARDATION, Vol. 27

0074-7750/2003 $35.00

The first question is: *How should intervention be adapted to the child's specific diagnosis?* Can knowing a child's diagnosis help determine an appropriate course of communication intervention? Increasingly, both descriptive and experimental studies of communication in children with mental retardation have focused on participants with a known diagnosis, such as Down syndrome or autism. Some studies have compared performances by groups of participants with different etiologies (e.g., children with Down syndrome vs children with fragile X syndrome). As the communication characteristics associated with specific etiologies become better understood, intervention approaches might need to be modified and individualized in a prescriptive manner. For example, early communication intervention for children with Down syndrome might focus in part on improving intelligibility because of the frequently reported speech problems associated with Down syndrome (Stoel-Gammon, 1998). We will discuss the degree to which intervention research has supported prescriptive interventions based on a child's diagnosis.

Participants in research on communication interventions for children with developmental disabilities differ not only in their diagnoses, but also in the severity of impairments. That is, within a given diagnosis, such as autism or Down syndrome, children of the same age often vary greatly in terms of their cognitive, social and communicative development. Thus, our second question is: *How should a child's cognitive and/or social development impact the intervention approach that is applied?* The relationship between communication interventions and a child's development in cognitive and social domains has been studied extensively (Cole, Coggins, & Vanderstoep, 1999; Cole, Mills, & Kelley, 1994; Curcio, 1978; Kelly & Dale, 1989; Smolak & Levine, 1984). Much of this research has focused on whether a child's cognitive status should determine the availability and/or type of communication intervention provided. We concur with the position offered by Cole et al. (1994) that children should receive communication intervention if they have unmet needs (regardless of discrepancies between language and cognitive test scores). However, the most effective interventions will often vary according to a child's specific developmental level. For example, two children of the same chronological age may each be diagnosed with autism, but one child may be functioning commensurate with age-matched peers in academics and certain aspects of communication, whereas the other child may be severely delayed in academics and all aspects of communication. Obviously, the interventions should be different to address the individual needs of these two very different children.

Our third question concerns the issue of intervention intensity. *How does the intensity of intervention affect child outcomes?* Intensity usually refers to the amount of intervention within a given period of time. However, other factors also reflect intensity, including the ratio of students to teacher, opportunity for student responding, teacher responsiveness to students, and the evocative power of the responses taught in intervention. For example, an intervention may be very effective if it teaches the child social interaction skills that lead to more frequent communication learning opportunities throughout the day and across settings. Such an intervention may be much less intensive than an intervention that attempts to achieve the same outcome through frequent drill and practice sessions. Surprisingly little research has been reported that specifically addresses intensity. Therefore, our discussion will center on how intensity is reflected in the continuum of interventions recently reported in the literature.

The fourth question is: *How does the child's social environment affect communication intervention?* Specifically, how does a child's interactions with others support or inhibit progress in communication intervention? Communication takes place within a broader social context and research has investigated the degree to which certain aspects of these social interactions facilitate or discourage communication growth. For example, the degree to which mothers respond to their children's communication attempts appears to be positively correlated to children's communication developments (Brady & McLean, 1997; Brazelton, Koslowski, & Main, 1974; Masur, 1981). In addition, recent research indicates that children's progress in intervention may be predicted by the history of maternal responsiveness prior to and during intervention (Yoder & Warren, 2001). Our review will focus on the implications of recent research regarding the influence of social interactions on future communication intervention research. We suggest that exemplary research in the future should account not only for the child's diagnosis and development, as suggested in previous paragraphs, but also for the history of social interactions that precede the most recent attempts at communication intervention.

II. INTERVENTIONS FOR CHILDREN WITH MENTAL RETARDATION ASSOCIATED WITH VARIOUS DIAGNOSES

How should intervention be adapted to the child's specific diagnosis? More and more communication intervention studies include participants that have the same specific diagnosis. A comparison of literature references in the *psyc info* database serves to illustrate this trend. We compared search results from two time periods, 1982–1992 and 1992–2001. A search on both "language intervention" and "mental retardation" yielded 32 records from 1982–1992 and only 16 records from 1992–2001—a 50% reduction. A search for articles pertaining to both "language intervention" and "autism,"

TABLE I

Results from Searches of the Psyc Info Database for Language Intervention and Specific Disability Types

Disability type	1982–1992	1992–2001
Mental retardation	32	16
Autism	10	20
Down syndrome	2	9
Fragile X syndrome	0	1
Williams syndrome	0	1
Total	44	47

however, showed a doubling from 10 records between 1982 and 1992 to 20 records from 1992 to 2001. A similar increase was seen for intervention articles about children with Down syndrome. Table I shows our comparison of search results across the two time periods.

These data are consistent with a trend toward describing research participants according to their specific diagnoses (e.g., Down syndrome, autism, fragile X syndrome), rather than according to the degree of mental retardation that accompanies the etiology. There are several reasons why research might increasingly focus on specific etiologies or diagnoses. One reason is that the ability to diagnose different disorders is improving, allowing communication researchers greater accuracy in describing their populations. In addition, families' concerns may have led to increased attention to specific diagnoses. Family support groups (e.g., NDSS, NAAR, FRAXA) have aligned with researchers interested in specific etiologies. Together, these groups have become assertive in lobbying for research pertaining to specific etiologies.

The most compelling reason for the increased emphasis on specific etiologies within intervention research, however, is that individuals with different diagnoses may have different language and communication characteristics. Intervention researchers now have more information about behavioral phenotypes associated with certain disorders. These phenotypes often include characteristic profiles of strengths and weaknesses in the area of communication. Differentiating children's interventions according to their etiologies should facilitate the interpretation and extension of results to clinical practice. Presumably there is greater likelihood that the same intervention will be effective with children with the same diagnosis, assuming they are at the same developmental level. Research is needed to verify this assumption, however.

In reviewing research on children with specific etiologies, we examined the degree to which the studies focused the intervention on identified communication characteristics (both strengths and deficits) of the target population. Although there is growing evidence of specific communication characteristics associated with diagnoses such as fragile X syndrome (Abbeduto & Hagerman, 1997) and Williams syndrome (Mervis, Morris, Bertrand, & Robinson, 1999), intervention research has focused primarily on two diagnoses: Down syndrome and autism. This is probably due to the relatively high frequency of these disorders in the general population.

A. Down Syndrome

The speech and language characteristics of children with Down syndrome have been described extensively elsewhere (Miller & Leddy, 1998), including in this volume (Chapman). Children with Down syndrome tend to develop intelligible speech much later than typically developing children. Because of this, two approaches have been used to facilitate communication development during this period of unintelligibility: teaching the child an alternative form of communication (Bondy & Frost, 1994; Kay-Raining Bird, Gaskell, Dallaire Babineau, & Macdonald, 2000) and teaching early pre-speech communication skills, such as natural gestures and communicative vocalizations (Warren & Yoder, 1998).

Alternative means of communication, such as sign language or graphic communication systems, may be easier than speech for young children with Down syndrome to learn. Producing signs requires gross movements that are easier to prompt through imitation or physical guidance than precise articulatory gestures. Sign language is often a temporary form of communication for children with Down syndrome because its use typically drops off as children's speech improves (Kay-Raining Bird et al., 2000; Layton & Savino, 1990). Augmentative and alternative communication is discussed more thoroughly by Romski & Sevcik (this volume).

Another way to improve communication skills in nonspeaking children with Down syndrome is to focus on early pre-speech communication behaviors expressed through conventional gestures, joint attention and pre-speech vocalizations. Children with Down syndrome frequently communicate through natural gestures, such as giving objects and pointing to objects (Franco & Wishart, 1995; Mundy, Kasari, Sigman, & Ruskin, 1995). Compared to early speech production, gesture use appears to be a relative strength of prelinguistic children with Down syndrome. Coordinated joint attention (alternating attention between person and referent) also appears to be a relative strength. In particular, Kasari, Freeman, Mundy, and Sigman (1995) found no differences in coordinated joint attention between children with Down syndrome and typically developing children matched for language levels. Participants with Down syndrome ranged in age from 13 to 42 months and in mental age from 9 to 27 months.

The co-occurrence of gesture, coordinated joint attention, and vocalizations precedes spoken language development in typically developing children (Bates, Camaioni, & Volterra, 1975; Tomasello & Farrar, 1986) and predicts language outcomes in children with disabilities (Calandrella & Wilcox, 2000; Harris, Kasari, & Sigman, 1996; McCathren, Warren, & Yoder, 1996). Linking gestures and joint attention to speech-like vocalizations may improve communication abilities for children with Down syndrome. For example, in our ongoing work aimed at increasing children's prelinguistic communication, we have observed that parents are more likely to respond to their children's communication attempts if they include a vocalization. Thus, we frequently teach children with Down syndrome to produce vocalizations, particularly canonical (i.e., speech-like) vocalizations, during communication attempts.

Children with Down syndrome typically begin to produce canonical vocalizations later than typically developing children (Oller, Steffens, Levine, Basinger, & Umbel, 1995). In addition to the obvious benefit to eventual speech, canonical vocalizations are related to social communication developments. Oller et al. (1995) found that infants who began producing speech-like vocalizations earlier had higher social communication scores at 27 months of age. These data are only correlational, however, and additional research is needed to demonstrate a causal link. That is, one would need to determine whether interventions that increase canonical vocalizations result in improved social communication development.

Another reason to focus on speech-like sound production skills in early intervention is that speech intelligibility continues to be a primary issue as children with Down syndrome begin talking. The speech of children with Down syndrome is often difficult to understand, possibly due to increased tongue size (relative to the oral cavity) and hypotonia in the oral musculature (Kumin & Bahr, 1999). Miller and Leddy (1998) speculate that many of the language problems observed in children with Down syndrome are secondary to poor speech intelligibility. Children with Down syndrome's sentences tend to be short and of poor syntactic structure. These children may attempt shorter and simpler sentences or phrases in an effort to increase the likelihood that they will be understood.

The research on speech and language characteristics of children with Down syndrome indicates that interventions aimed at improving their communication should address both speech and language concerns. For example, Kumin, Goodman, and Councill (1996) described a comprehensive treatment program for school-aged children with Down syndrome. In their program, intervention targeted receptive and expressive communication and speech skills. Studies on the effectiveness of communication interventions with children with Down syndrome often focus more narrowly on language production, however (e.g., Girolametto, Weitzman, & Clements-Baartman, 1998; Yoder & Warren, 2001).

B. Autism Spectrum Disorders

Our search for language intervention studies yielded more studies involving children with autism than any other diagnostic category. The relatively high number of interventions aimed at improving communication in children with autism reflects the pervasiveness and severity of their communication disorders. Impairments of communication are among the defining characteristics of autism (American Psychiatric Association, 1987). Communication impairments associated with autism include delayed or absent speech development (particularly spontaneous speech), echolalia, unusual prosody, use of challenging behaviors in lieu of more acceptable communicative behaviors, and poor joint attention (Wetherby, Prizant, & Schuler, 2000). The term joint attention has been used to refer to coordinated attention between objects and people, such as when a mother and child are both attending to the same referent (as indicated by talking about the same object or looking at the same object) (Akhtar, Dunham, & Dunham, 1991). In isolation or combination, these impairments manifest most strongly in the social aspects of communication (Dissanayake & Sigman, 2001; Kasari, Sigman, Mundy, & Yirmiya, 1990; Loveland, Landry, Hughes, Hall, & McEvoy, 1988; Mundy & Crowson, 1997; Prizant, Wetherby, & Rydell, 2000).

Several of these communication impairments are characteristic of children with autism; that is, they occur proportionally more often in children with autism than in other children. Poor joint attention, for example, has been added to the list of behaviors used to identify children with autism at a young age (Baron-Cohen, Allen, & Gillberg, 1992). Poor joint attention skills manifest themselves in infrequent communications for the purpose of sharing information with others. Young children with autism frequently do not point at objects to share interest with adults and may not even follow the points of others (Baron-Cohen, 1989; McArthur & Adamson, 1996). This disturbance in pointing may be an early manifestation of the impairment in social communication that continues to be present in one form or another throughout life for most individuals with autism.

Mundy and Crowson (1997) have suggested that early intervention for children with autism would be most beneficial if the intervention focused specifically on impairments in nonverbal social communication, including joint attention. They suggested that improved joint attention might prevent future secondary disturbances in social communication. Nevertheless, only a few studies have directly targeted joint attention. Lewy and Dawson (1992) compared the effectiveness of two different types of play behaviors on joint attention in children with autism. Participants included 20 preschool-aged children with autism whose mean receptive language age was 20.4 months. Children showed more joint attention during toy play when the experimenter matched the children's activities than when the experimenter did not match the activities of the child. Results of an ongoing investigation by Kasari and colleagues also indicate that joint attention improves after direct intervention specifically targeting this behavior (Kasari, Freeman, & Paparella, 2001). In addition to targeting joint attention in intervention, Mundy and Crowson (1997) suggest that joint attention should be used as an outcome variable in analyzing the effectiveness of any communication intervention for young children with autism.

One of the difficulties associated with teaching joint attention and other aspects of social communication is that effective intervention requires that the child be motivated by the social consequences provided by their partner. Interventions described by Prizant and colleagues as *developmental social interaction* approaches have attempted to increase the value of social interactions for children with autism by having interventionists initially following the child's lead and be responsive to all communication attempts, even if the form of the attempt is atypical (Prizant et al., 2000). A variety of people are used as agents of such intervention, including peers and family members.

Parents, peers and teachers have also been included in other approaches to teaching social communication to children with autism. In a study by Kaiser, Hancock, and Nietfeld (2000), parents implemented an intervention described as enhanced milieu therapy, which focused on arranging the environment, increasing the responsiveness of the parent to the child's communication attempts, and providing opportunities for communication in naturally occurring contexts. Six mother–child dyads participated. Children were aged 32–54 months and had language abilities at the 20- to 28-month level. Consistent with the suggestions of Prizant et al. (2000), Kaiser and colleagues speculated that the responsiveness component is particularly important for children with autism because they often resist direct social approaches and direct instructions.

Peers were included in an intervention aimed at improving the social communication of two children with autism in a study by Pierce and Schreibman (1995). The children with autism were both 10-year-olds and functioned at around a 3 to 4-year developmental level. Peers learned to give choices, model appropriate social and verbal behaviors, verbally reinforce any attempt at social interaction, extend conversation and take turns. They were also instructed to withhold desired play objects until the child with autism verbalized about the object. Both of the children with autism increased their initiations of social interactions and their word use after participating in this intervention, and they maintained these gains over an additional 10 sessions. Teachers also rated the children's school behavior as improved.

Several studies have also shown that social, conversational speech can be improved using the traditional behavioral methods of prompting target phrases and then gradually reducing the teaching prompts (Buffington, Krantz, McClannahan, & Poulson, 1998; Matson, Sevin, Box, & Francis, 1993; Stevenson, Krantz, & McClannahan, 2000). These studies illustrate how, even within highly structured behavioral approaches, researchers are now targeting the deficits in social communication that are characteristic of autism.

Stevenson et al. (2000) taught four boys with autism (10–15 years) to imitate conversational phrases emitted from a pre-recorded tape loop. The children were taught specific responses by following a recorded script. The use of the script was gradually reduced. The children eventually produced some social phrases in other unscripted interactions. Buffington et al. (1998) taught four children with autism to comment about an object while gesturing and looking toward the object. Children were between 4 and 6 years of age and had language age equivalents between 2;2 and 3;4. Teachers presented an object and an instruction such as, "Let's talk about (name of object)." Participants learned several different combinations of gestures and verbal comments and generalized these comments to other highly similar situations. A study by Matson et al. (1993) was specifically aimed at improving spontaneous (self-initiated) communication in three boys with autism (4–5 years). Children were taught to respond to a visual prompt (e.g., a printed word) paired with a stimulus (e.g., a particular person) that should naturally control the response. Teachers gradually delayed the presentation of the visual prompts over successive opportunities until participants were responding to the "natural" stimuli. The participants increased their self-initiated verbalizations with a number of partners as a result of this method. In each of these studies, children produced the targeted social responses not only in the teaching context, but also in other contexts and with other individuals. In most cases however, the generalization contexts were highly similar to teaching contexts. Therefore, further research is necessary to demonstrate generalization to "real world" situations, as well as maintenance over time.

In summary, the research pertaining to the specific diagnostic categories of Down syndrome and autism reflects increased understanding of the specific communication deficits associated with each of these diagnoses. Research on children with Down syndrome has focused on improving intelligibility through both speech and alternative means of communication. In contrast, research on children with autism has increasingly attended to the social communicative deficits characteristic of autism. As we learn more about the specific communication profiles of children with various etiologies, such as fragile X syndrome (Abbeduto & Hagerman, 1997; Roberts, Mirrett, & Burchinal, 2001), we may see intervention studies aimed at addressing these impairments. Nevertheless, as discussed in the following section, individual children's developmental levels may be more important than their diagnostic category in determining the most appropriate course for communication intervention.

III. THE ROLE OF CHILDREN'S LEVEL OF DEVELOPMENT IN IMPLEMENTING COMMUNICATION INTERVENTIONS

How does a child's level of cognitive and social development impact communication intervention? Up to this point, we have described communication intervention research according to strengths and weaknesses associated with different diagnostic categories. Within groups of children with the same diagnoses and similar ages, however, very different levels of developmental progress across language, cognitive and social domains often exist. For example, one 5-year-old child with autism may be nonspeaking and have severely limited social skills, whereas another 5-year-old child with autism may speak and interact reasonably well with others. Further, the communication needs of the 5-year-old child who is nonspeaking may be more similar to the needs of another nonspeaking child who is not diagnosed as having autism. Thus, in addition to the child's diagnosis, intervention research must account for differences in developmental levels of participants.

Appropriate interventions and expected outcomes vary according to a child's developments in multiple areas. A child's developmental level is an important factor in determining what goals to target via intervention. As stated earlier, research supports providing communication interventions to children whose current communication is insufficient to meet their needs, regardless of a child's measured cognitive level (Cole & Fey, 1996). However, goal selection and expectations for treatment outcomes differ according to developmental level. Different outcomes for children at varying levels of cognitive development have been reported. For example, Santarcangelo and Dyer (1988) found that children functioning below a developmental age of 3 years produced more frequent eye gaze in response to a specific pattern of their mother's speech (i.e., child directed speech, or "motherese"), whereas children functioning above 3 years of age did not show this effect.

Similarly, Yoder and colleagues (1998) found differential effects for two therapy approaches according to participants' level of communication development at the outset of intervention. Preschool children with a mean length of utterance (MLU) above 2.5 morphemes responded better to an approach that used primarily expansions and growth recasts as teaching techniques (termed "responsive interaction") than they did to an approach that primarily used elicited production prompts (termed "milieu intervention"). The opposite effect was found for children with MLUs less than 2.0: these children responded better to the milieu intervention. These correlations between outcome and starting MLU were found through retrospective analyses. Nevertheless, they are sensible from a developmental perspective. The use of elicited imitation prompts in milieu teaching takes advantage of constraints in children's attention and memory resources at this stage of development (Nelson, 1989). As the child develops cognitively, responsive interaction approaches become better suited for facilitating the acquisition of higher level morphological and syntactic skills (above MLU 2.5) because growth recasts can make the relatively minor differences between the child's preceding statement and a more complex adult recast of it highly salient to the child. (A growth recast is a specific expansion or modification of the child's immediately preceding utterance in which new syntactic, semantic, or phonological information is added.) However, to be effective, a growth recast requires that the child has reached a developmental level at which she can compare her utterance with the adult's recast (Nelson, 1989).

Based on such findings, Warren and Yoder (1997) have proposed that a major goal for intervention research should be identifying "a continuum of optimally effective, developmentally appropriate communication and language intervention procedures" (p. 360). Comparative research with many children at varying levels of cognitive, linguistic and social development is necessary however, to fully delineate all the pertinent developmental variables. Based on research to date, it seems likely that such continua will apply to children across diagnostic categories. Thus, the task of determining an appropriate course of intervention requires careful consideration of the needs that derive from a child's developmental level as well as from his or her diagnosis.

IV. INTENSITY OF INTERVENTIONS

How does intensity of intervention affect outcomes? The communication needs in children with mental retardation have been addressed via different methods reflecting different treatment philosophies. One of the parameters that differentiates approaches is the prescribed intensity of the intervention. A rarely challenged premise is that more intense interventions will yield greater changes in the targeted behaviors than will less intense interventions. Yet, little empirical evidence is available to support or refute this premise. An alternative possibility is that intensity may interact with other variables, such as teaching context (e.g., incidental conversations vs massed trial), the child's learning history (e.g., lengthy exposure to highly responsive vs low responsive adults), the responsiveness of adults in the child's day-to-day environment (e.g., highly responsive vs low responsive and directive), and the goals selected. For example, attaining some goals may lead to increased opportunities to participate in reinforcing interactions in the future. Thus, targeting these goals in socially responsive contexts may be highly effective, even at relatively low levels of intensity.

"Intensive" has been defined as "exceptionally great concentration, power or force" (Soukhanov & Ellis, 1984). When used to describe interventions, intensive usually refers to the *concentration* part of this definition. Concentration may refer to the amount of time spent in intervention in a given day or week. That is, an intervention provided to a child for 40 h a week is more concentrated than a similar intervention provided 10 h per week. Some intervention programs for children with autism, for example, are quite intensive and include 40 h per week of direct 1 : 1 intervention in a variety of educational domains, including communication (Green, 1996). A more precise measure of concentration would include the average number of teaching episodes or trials for a given unit of time (i.e., per minute, per hour) multiplied by the number of instructional hours (or other time unit) per week, month, etc.

Irrespective of how it is measured, many authors have argued that highly concentrated interventions should be the treatment of choice, particularly for children with autism and other severe developmental disabilities (Green, 1996; Smith, Eikeseth, Klevstrand, & Lovaas, 1997). According to these authors, intensive interventions, particularly when they are provided to young children, may enable the children to eventually participate more fully in their community (Hawkins, 1995). One of the primary targets for such concentrated interventions is improved communication and language.

The number of teaching episodes that can be reasonably delivered at any given point in time will depend at least in part on the interventionist-to-student ratio. More students per teacher usually equates with fewer opportunities for children to respond and receive feedback for their responses. Green (1996) described intensive intervention as 1 : 1 instruction for 30–40 hours per week for at least 2 years. In a study comparing different intensities of intervention, Graff, Green, and Libby (1998) found that the young child with severe disabilities whom they studied showed more treatment gains in imitation when participating in 1 : 1 intervention than when participating in 1 : 2 intervention (one teacher : two students). The child also showed more disruptive behaviors in the 1 : 2 condition. However, the child's productions of spontaneous communicative responses were slightly higher in the 1 : 2 condition. The presence of a peer may have been disruptive for learning imitation but conducive to spontaneous communication. More research is needed to determine the effects of different levels of intensity on social communication goals.

In addition to the concentration of the intervention, intensity also refers to the notion of "power." Some interventions may be powerful, not because they encompass many hours per week, but because they empower the child to acquire many other skills or opportunities to use skills in their natural environment. Such skills have been described by some researchers as "pivotal responses."

An approach described as "pivotal response intervention" (Koegel, Koegel, Harrower, & Carter, 1999) selects target behaviors intended to lead to important collateral changes in the child's behaviors. Pivotal skills "facilitate generalization of an infinite number of behaviors across an infinite number of environments and people" (Koegel & Koegel, 1995, p. 70). For example, Koegel, Koegel, Shoshan, and McNerny (1999) described *initiating social communication* as a pivotal skill for children with autism. Children who learned this skill set had more favorable outcomes in other treatment areas as well as in social communication. Pierce and Schreibman (1995) taught peers to "extend conversation" between themselves and children with autism by asking questions or encouraging conversations centered on objects in the room. Extending conversation was considered a pivotal skill because it increased the opportunities for social interactions in various environments and with different conversation partners.

Although the targeting of pivotal responses seems promising for future communication research, the bases for identifying pivotal skills are unclear. There are not theoretically driven or empirical processes for determining which communication skills should be pivotal for an individual. Instead, most treatment goals are selected because, on their face, they appear to have the potential to lead to important collateral changes. Mundy and Crowson (1997) speculated that nonverbal social communication skills, such as joint attention are pivotal skills for children with autism because "engaging in joint attention with others may contribute to the development of symbolic abilities in children, the development of language abilities in children and the development of general social cognitive processes in children" (p. 667). It may be that "initiating joint attention" is a pivotal skill that leverages large, nonlinear gains in communication development. More research, however, is needed to verify this contention.

Increased joint attention is one of the goals targeted by another approach that facilitates social interactions by targeting a small set of pivotal skills, namely, prelinguistic milieu therapy (PMT) (Warren & Yoder, 1998; Yoder & Warren, 1998). The effectiveness of PMT comes from the power of the targeted skills in eliciting natural opportunities to interact with responsive caregivers that in turn support further growth in child communication and language (Yoder & Warren, 2001, 2002). For example, when children begin producing clear, frequent prelinguistic forms of requests and comments as a result of PMT, parents and care providers become more likely to respond to these communication acts with natural teaching techniques, such as linguistic mapping (Yoder & Warren, 1998, 2001).

Linguistic mapping provides valuable input that will likely impact later language development (Hart & Risley, 1995). In fact, research has indicated that both typically developing children (Tomasello & Farrar, 1986) and atypically developing children (Yoder, Kaiser, Alpert, & Fischer, 1993) acquire vocabulary, particularly object labels, more readily as a result of linguistic mapping. Thus, an intervention that only takes place for 20 min 3–4 times per week (e.g., Yoder & Warren, 1998) can be powerful because of the transactional effects it has on the communication interactions the child experiences throughout the day.

As children develop more language skills, other approaches, such as milieu language intervention have targeted vocabulary that will generate future opportunities for social interaction (Warren, 1992). Although the intervention goals may vary at different points in development, an underlying premise is that communication interventions can be powerful if they focus on child behaviors that are likely to recruit a substantial number of developmentally progressive teaching opportunities throughout the child's day.

In this section, we have contrasted two aspects of intensity of interventions: concentration and power. Different studies have emphasized one or the other of these two aspects of interventions. Both the concentrated (e.g., 40 h per week, 1 : 1 teaching model) and the less concentrated (e.g., pivotal skill, PMT) approaches are designed to provide intense learning experiences. The 1 : 1 concentrated model provides many opportunities for children to practice basic communication responses such as identifying and labeling objects, along with structured opportunities to practice these responses in more natural situations. The less concentrated model derives its power from selecting key target behaviors that will elicit further growth-enhancing input from the environment.

V. THE ROLE OF A CHILD'S CONVERSATION PARTNER IN COMMUNICATION INTERVENTION

How does the child's social environment affect communication intervention? One of the most important outcomes of a successful communication intervention is the improvement of social interactions between the child with mental retardation and others. Communication is an interactive process and the communication style of the people who interact with children may enhance or inhibit progress in intervention. Communication partners may be asked to change their behavior in order to facilitate and support the child's development. Thus, the characteristics of people who interact with children with mental retardation on a regular basis are critical aspects of the environment to consider when planning and evaluating interventions.

The most important people for infants and young children are parents or other primary caregivers. The responsiveness of parents and caregivers to young children's communication attempts has been shown to be an important variable in their progress in intervention. In a randomized control study comparing two interventions for 58 preschool children with developmental disabilities, Yoder and Warren (1998, 2001) found that the degree of responsiveness by parents before early intervention began determined which of two interventions was most beneficial to children's communication development. Responsiveness was defined as the proportion of child communication acts to which the mother responded. Children whose parents were highly responsive to them at the beginning of the study and who participated in Prelinguistic Milieu Teaching (PMT) showed more treatment gains than did children with highly responsive parents who participated in a contrasting therapy, responsive small group (RSG). In RSG, one interventionist worked with three children. Interventionists responded to children's communicative attempts but did not make any demands. Children of parents who were much less responsive at the outset of intervention showed more gains in the RSG intervention than in the PMT intervention. The authors speculated that children of more responsive parents might come to expect that their communication will be responded to and hence will persist in communication exchanges in which the adult prompts for more elaborate responses (as in PMT). In contrast, children of less responsive parents may not have such expectations due to their history of not being responded to and, therefore, they fail to respond to the prompts used in PMT.

Many studies have focused on teaching parents to be more responsive and to make other changes in their interaction styles. Girolametto and colleagues studied the effects of parent participation in a 12-week parent education program (the Hanen Early Language Parent Program) aimed at teaching parents facilitative strategies, such as following the child's lead and imitating children's communication (Girolametto et al., 1998; Tannock, Girolametto, & Siegel, 1992; Tomasello & Farrar, 1986). Although there were large individual differences in mothers' responses to the intervention, the results of these studies were largely positive in achieving a change in maternal behaviors. As a group, mothers increased their child-focused behaviors and were successful in increasing the frequency and duration of interactive engagement with their children (Girolametto, Verbey, & Tannock, 1994). Mothers also learned to label objects within episodes of joint engagement (Girolametto et al., 1998). The generality of these effects may be limited, however, as the participants in these studies were well-educated middle-class families.

Several changes in children's language were also found. Participants in these studies were preschool-age children with delayed language. Some of the children also had Down syndrome. Tannock et al. (1992) reported increases in the children's vocal turns and Girolametto et al. (1998) found increased expressive vocabulary in children who participated (with their mothers) in the intervention group. It should be noted that earlier reports had not found significant differences in children's vocabulary growth (Tannock & Girolametto, 1992; Tannock et al., 1992), hence the intervention used with children with Down syndrome in the Girolametto et al. (1998) study was modified to provide focused stimulation of vocabulary.

Parents have also successfully learned to apply components of enhanced milieu therapy (Alpert & Kaiser, 1992; Kaiser, 1996). The educational levels of parents in these studies were more diverse than in the studies that used the Hanen program, although still biased toward upper SES. With varying degrees of success, parents learned to use environmental arrangement and incidental teaching within a responsive conversational style. The parents' use of milieu therapy strategies was associated with gains in target language skills, including semantic combinations, intentional communication and number of words used. As in the studies of the Hanen program, however, children's responses to parent implemented milieu intervention were not always positive. Children were, for the most part, preschool-age children with varying degrees of developmental disability. Some children showed little improvements in targeted communication goals. It would be valuable to thoroughly compare the successful vs the unsuccessful dyads in order to determine variables correlating with success. Characteristics of parents and children may interact with style variables reflected in the targeted interaction to affect the outcome of parent-implemented communication interventions.

Lee and Kahn (2000) reported results of an intervention program aimed at improving parenting skills in parents of children who were either already diagnosed as having developmental delays or were at risk for developmental delay. Thirty-three parent–infant dyads participated in a 15-month program and their interactions were observed every 5 months. The authors used the Parent–Infant Interaction Scale (Clark & Seifer, 1986) to measure parent–child interactions during a free play observation. Using survival analysis, the authors found that successful interactions were most likely to occur during the period from the 6th to the 10th month after intervention began. These results suggest that parent behavior should be an ongoing focus of intervention and that interventionists should expect to invest a large amount of time to achieve optimum gains. Studies such as this are important because they not only indicate that an intervention was effective but also suggest the length of time required for meaningful changes in development.

Researchers have also reported positive changes in children's language after teaching peers to be more responsive (Goldstein, English, Shafer, & Kaczmarek, 1997; Pierce & Schreibman, 1995). Goldstein and colleagues found that preschool children without disabilities increased their interactions with eight peers with disabilities after they were specifically taught to do so. The range of expressive language ages for the children with disabilities was 20–39 months. Peers participated in "buddy training" during which they learned to stay in proximity of their buddy, to play with their buddy and talk about ongoing play activities and to respond to their buddy's communicative attempts. Peers demonstrated mastery of all three of these strategies without prompting. After the trained peers began using these strategies with target children, children communicated with each other more often. In addition, a group of social validation observers judged the social interactions after intervention as significantly higher than before intervention.

Pierce and Schreibman (1995) taught peers to implement components of pivotal response training (described in the Intensity section (IV) of this chapter). Peers were given a manual describing strategies, such as encouraging conversation, taking turns, and providing choices to the children with autism ($n = 2$). Peer training included therapist modeling of the strategies and peer role-playing with other peers. Peer training lasted approximately one month. The results indicated increases in child engagement with objects and others after peer PRT.

Although children can be effectively taught to facilitate communication use by their peers with disabilities, these procedures have not been used extensively in practice. Sustaining the behavior changes by peers after the contingencies of intervention are removed may be difficult. However, an alternative explanation for the infrequent use of peers in communication intervention is that education settings undervalue peer interactions and the social communication that occurs within such interactions. In addition, traditional classroom settings may discourage the type of peer interactions necessary to implement peer interventions. Educational models that incorporate cooperative group learning strategies in inclusive environments should be more conducive to peer interventions.

The studies described above demonstrate that teaching caregivers and friends to alter their interaction styles can enhance children's communication development and use. However, the variables affecting differential outcomes and the long-term sustainability of these altered interaction patterns need to be more thoroughly investigated.

VI. CONCLUSION

In this chapter, we have discussed recent research on communication interventions for children with mental retardation that addressed four questions: (1) What is the relationship between participants' diagnoses and intervention? (2) How does a child's cognitive and social development impact communication intervention? (3) How does intervention intensity affect child outcomes? (4) How do the interaction styles of a child's communication partners affect communication intervention?

For each question, we can provide only a partial answer replete with numerous constraining qualifiers. A careful review of the research base relevant to these questions makes it clear that steady progress has been made in response to each question. However, the amount of research on these questions has remained modest over the past two decades, and thus progress is modest as well. For example, beyond Down syndrome and autism, we know surprisingly little about the relation of etiology to effective intervention. Perhaps most disconcerting is how little we know about the relationship between intensity and effectiveness. This is a difficult issue to study for a variety of methodological reasons. Nevertheless, the overwhelming importance of the issue should support a much more active research agenda.

Relative to the effects of specific etiology and intensity of intervention, we know much more about the relationship of different intervention approaches to developmental level and the relationship of communication style to intervention effectiveness. For example, it's clear that degree of parental responsiveness can be an important variable in optimizing the effects of communication and language intervention. Furthermore, it's clear that different intervention approaches are not equally effective across development. Certain approaches (e.g., milieu teaching) seem to be relatively more effective early in development, whereas others (e.g., direct instruction, focused stimulation) appear more effective later.

This is not to say that these other questions have been fully addressed. In fact, a great deal more research is needed regarding all four questions. Communication research should continue to reflect different theoretical perspectives but there should be a unified effort toward achieving high standards in terms of describing participants, intervention, procedures, fidelity of implementation and measures of intensity. The modest level of research on language and communication in children with mental retardation has been noted for some time now (Goldstein, 1990) and limits the abilities of clinicians and teachers to provide optimal treatments. More and better communication intervention research is needed, not only to inform clinical practice, but also to inform researchers investigating the causes of various etiologies associated with mental retardation. Greater understanding of phenotypic communication behaviors, including the effects of intervention and other environmental variables on these behaviors is key to understanding the nature and causes of mental retardation.

Although we have dealt with each question in turn, interventionists and intervention researchers must consider all four questions when selecting an intervention or when designing a study to investigate an intervention. For example, researchers often opt to study the effects of an intervention on a group of children with the same diagnosis and similar cognitive and linguistic developmental levels. Doing so facilitates interpretation of results by the field. For example, a teacher or speech language pathologist may decide to implement an intervention if it was successful with children similar to the child or children whom she or he teaches.

Practitioners must also decide whether to replicate the intensity of the intervention studied, and this decision may require evaluation of the available resources. Creative approaches to increasing resources include the use of college students and parents as primary interventionists for highly concentrated interventions (Smith, Buch, & Gamby, 2000). An alternative way to increase intensity without huge investments of resources is to teach pivotal skills that will facilitate development beyond the intervention context.

Resources also come into play when considering the role of the communication partners in intervention. Interventionists may feel they lack adequate resources and training to evaluate and facilitate the interaction style of a child's communication partner(s). Yet, this aspect of intervention appears to be of great importance for affecting lasting changes in children's communication. Future research should be designed to develop better models for interventions aimed at improving both child and partner communication skills. There appear to be "pivotal" partner interaction skills, such as responsiveness to the child's communication attempts, that can enable parents to facilitate multiple aspects of communication in a number of contexts.

Future studies should further our understanding of answers to each of the four questions posed in this chapter. In particular, biological advances will no doubt continue to propel research on children whose mental retardation is associated with identified etiologies. As more etiologies are diagnosed at earlier ages, comparative research across participants with different etiologies will be possible. Comparative research may help clarify whether particular interventions are well suited to children with specific diagnoses. For example, it may be that an intervention that relies on providing imitative models is more helpful to children with a specific diagnosis and less helpful to children with other diagnoses.

We have discussed the etiologic question in terms of whether research with participants who share a diagnosis leads to better communication interventions for children with the specified diagnosis. However, another purpose of such research is to learn more about the underlying etiology shared by the participants. The ability of children to overcome known deficits in communication associated with a particular etiology can yield vital information about the etiology itself. Studies that seek to demonstrate changes in children's brain activity following specific interventions may lead to greater understanding of the relationship of neurodevelopmental functioning and communication and language development in children with mental retardation.

REFERENCES

Abbeduto, L., & Hagerman, R. J. (1997). Language and communication in fragile X syndrome. *Mental Retardation and Developmental Disabilities Research Reviews*, *3*(4), 313–322.

Akhtar, N., Dunham, F., & Dunham, P. J. (1991). Directive interactions and early vocabulary development: the role of joint attentional focus. *Journal of Child Language*, *18*, 41–49.

Alpert, C., & Kaiser, A. (1992). Training parents as milieu language teachers. *Journal of Early Intervention*, *16*, 31–52.

American Psychiatric Association (1987). *Diagnostic and statistical manual of mental disorders* (4th ed.). Washington, DC: Author.

Baron-Cohen, S. (1989). Perceptual role taking and protodeclarative pointing in autism. *British Journal of Developmental Psychology*, *7*, 113–127.

Baron-Cohen, S., Allen, J., & Gillberg, C. (1992). Can autism be detected at 18 months? The needle, the haystack, and the CHAT. *British Journal of Psychiatry*, *161*, 839–843.

Bates, E., Camaioni, L., & Volterra, V. (1975). The acquisition of performatives prior to speech. *Merrill-Palmer Quarterly*, *21*, 205–226.

Bondy, A. S., & Frost, L. A. (1994). The picture exchange communication system. *Focus on Autistic Behavior, 9*, 1–19.

Brady, N., & McLean, L. (1997). *Parent–child interaction patterns and communication development in children with severe mental retardation.* Paper presented at the 30th Annual Gatlinburg conference on Research and Theory in Mental Retardation and Developmental Disabilities, Riverside, California.

Brazelton, T. B., Koslowski, B., & Main, M. (1974). The origins of reciprocity: the early mother–infant interaction. In L. Rosenblum (Ed.), *The effect of the infant or its caregiver* (pp. 49–76). New York: Wiley.

Buffington, D. M., Krantz, P., McClannahan, L. E., & Poulson, C. L. (1998). Procedures for teaching appropriate gestural communication skills to children with autism. *Journal of Autism and Developmental Disorders, 28*(6), 535–545.

Calandrella, A. M., & Wilcox, M. J. (2000). Predicting language outcomes for young prelinguistic children with developmental delay. *Journal of Speech, Language, and Hearing Research, 43*, 1061–1071.

Clark, G. N., & Seifer, R. (1986). *Parent–infant interaction scale: A manual for analysis of videotapes of unstructured play.* East Providence, RI: E.P. Bradley Hospital.

Cole, K., Coggins, T., & Vanderstoep, C. (1999). The influence of language/cognitive profile on discourse intervention outcome. *Language, Speech and Hearing Services in Schools, 30*, 61–67.

Cole, K., & Fey, M. (1996). Cognitive referencing in language assessment. In K. Cole, P. Dale, & D. Thal (Eds.), *Assessment of communication and language* (pp. 143–161). Baltimore: Paul H. Brookes.

Cole, K., Mills, P., & Kelley, D. (1994). Agreement of assessment profiles used in cognitive referencing. *Language, Speech, and Hearing Services in Schools, 25*, 25–31.

Curcio, F. (1978). Sensorimotor functioning and communication in mute autistic children. *Journal of Autism and Childhood Schizophrenia, 8*, 281–292.

Dissanayake, C., & Sigman, M. (2001). Attachment and emotional responsiveness in children with autism. In L. M. Glidden (Ed.), *International review of research in mental retardation: Autism* (pp. 239–266). San Diego: Academic Press.

Franco, F., & Wishart, J. G. (1995). Use of pointing and other gestures by young children with Down syndrome. *American Journal on Mental Retardation, 100*, 160–182.

Girolametto, L., Verbey, M., & Tannock, R. (1994). Improving joint engagement in parent–child interaction: an intervention study. *Journal of Early Intervention, 18*(2), 155–167.

Girolametto, L., Weitzman, E., & Clements-Baartman, J. (1998). Vocabulary intervention for children with Down syndrome: parent training using focused stimulation. *Infant-Toddler Intervention, 8*(2), 109–125.

Goldstein, H. (1990). The future of language science: a plea for language intervention research. *American Speech and Hearing Association Reports, 20*, 41–50.

Goldstein, H., English, K., Shafer, K., & Kaczmarek, L. (1997). Interaction among preschoolers with and without disabilities: effects of across-the-day peer intervention. *Journal of Speech, Language, and Hearing Research, 40*(1), 33–48.

Goldstein, H., & Hockenberger, E. H. (1991). Significant progress in child language intervention: an 11-year retrospective. *Research in Developmental Disabilities, 12*, 401–424.

Graff, R., Green, G., & Libby, M. (1998). Effects of two levels of treatment intensity on a young child with severe disabilities. *Behavioral Interventions, 13*, 21–41.

Green, G. (1996). Early behavioral intervention for young children with autism: what does research tell us? In C. Maurice, G. Green, & S. C. Luce (Eds.), *Behavioral intervention for young children with autism: A manual for parents and professionals* (pp. 29–44). Austin: Pro Ed.

Harris, S., Kasari, C., & Sigman, M. D. (1996). Joint attention and language gains in children with Down syndrome. *American Journal on Mental Retardation, 100*(6), 608–619.

Hart, B., & Risley, T. (1995). *Meaningful differences in the everyday experience of young American children*. Baltimore: P.H. Brookes.

Hawkins, D. (1995). Spontaneous language use. In R. Koegel & L. K. Koegel (Eds.), *Teaching children with autism: Strategies for initiating positive interactions and improving learning opportunities* (pp. 43–53). Baltimore: Paul H. Brookes.

Kaiser, A. (1996). Parent-implemented language intervention: an environmental system perspective. In A. Kaiser, & D. Gray (Eds.), *Enhancing Children's Communication: Research Foundations for Intervention* (pp. 63–85). Baltimore: Brookes Publishing Co.

Kaiser, T., Hancock, T., & Nietfeld, J. (2000). The effects of parent-implemented enhanced milieu teaching on the social communication of children who have autism. *Early Education and Development, 11*(4), 423–446.

Kasari, C., Freeman, F., & Paparella, T. (2001). *Early Communication Development in Young Children with Developmental Delays*. Paper presented at the 34th Annual Gatlinburg Conference on Research and Theory in Intellectual and Developmental Disabilities, Charleston, South Carolina.

Kasari, C., Freeman, S., Mundy, P., & Sigman, M. D. (1995). Attention regulation by children with Down syndrome: coordinated joint attention and social referencing looks. *American Journal on Mental Retardation, 100*, 128–136.

Kasari, C., Sigman, M., Mundy, P., & Yirmiya, N. (1990). Affective sharing in the context of joint attention. *Journal of Autism and Developmental Disorders, 20*, 87–100.

Kay-Raining Bird, E., Gaskell, A., Dallaire Babineau, M., & Macdonald, S. (2000). Novel word acquisition in children with Down syndrome: does modality make a difference? *Journal of Communication Disorders, 33*, 241–266.

Kelly, C. A., & Dale, P. S. (1989). Cognitive skills associated with the onset of multiword utterances. *Journal of Speech and Hearing Research, 32*, 645–656.

Koegel, R., & Koegel, L. (1995). Motivating communication in children with autism. In E. Schopler, & G. Mesibov (Eds.), *Learning and Cognition in Autism* (pp. 73–87). New York: Plenum.

Koegel, L., Koegel, R., Harrower, J., & Carter, C. (1999). Pivotal response intervention: Overview of approach. *Journal of the Association for Persons with Severe Handicaps, 24*(3), 174–185.

Koegel, L., Koegel, R., Shoshan, Y., & McNerney, E. (1999). Pivotal response intervention II: Preliminary long-term outcome data. *Journal of the Association for Persons with Severe Handicaps, 24*(3), 186–198.

Kumin, L., & Bahr, D. (1999). Patterns of feeding, eating and drinking in young children with Down syndrome with oral motor concerns. *Down Syndrome Quarterly, 4*(2), 1–8.

Kumin, L., Goodman, M., & Councill, C. (1996). Comprehensive speech and language intervention for school-aged children with Down syndrome. *Down Syndrome Quarterly, 1*(1), 1–8.

Layton, T. L., & Savino, M. A. (1990). Acquiring a communication system by sign and speech in a child with Down syndrome: a longitudinal investigation. *Child Language Teaching and Therapy, 6*, 59–76.

Lee, S., & Kahn, J. (2000). A survival analysis of parent–child interaction in early intervention. *Infant-Toddler Intervention, 10*(3), 137–156.

Lewy, A., & Dawson, G. (1992). Social stimulation and joint attention in young autistic children. *Journal of Abnormal Child Psychology, 20*(6), 555–566.

Loveland, K. A., Landry, S. H., Hughes, S. O., Hall, S. K., & McEvoy, R. E. (1988). Speech acts and the pragmatic deficits of autism. *Journal of Speech and Hearing Research, 31*, 593–604.

Masur, E. F. (1981). Mothers' responses to infants' object-related gestures: influences on lexical development. *Journal of Child Language*, *9*, 23–30.

Matson, J., Sevin, J., Box, M., & Francis, K. (1993). An evaluation of two methods for increasing self-initiated verbalizations in autistic children. *Journal of Applied Behavior Analysis*, *26*, 389–398.

McArthur, D., & Adamson, L. (1996). Joint attention in preverbal children: autism and developmental language disorder. *Journal of Autism and Developmental Disorders*, *26*(5), 481–496.

McCathren, R., Warren, S. F., & Yoder, P. J. (1996). Prelinguistic predictors of later language development. In K. N. Cole, P. S. Dale, & D. J. Thal (Eds.), *Assessment of communication and language* (pp. 57–76). Baltimore, MD: Paul H. Brookes Publishing Co.

Mervis, C., Morris, C., Bertrand, J., & Robinson, B. (1999). Williams syndrome: Findings from an integrated program of research. In H. Tager-Flusberg (Ed.), *Neurodevelopmental disorders* (pp. 65–110). Cambridge, MA: MIT Press.

Miller, J. F., & Leddy, M. (1998). Down syndrome: the impact of speech production on language development. In R. Paul (Ed.), *Exploring the speech–language connection* (Vol. 8, pp. 163–177). Baltimore: Brookes Publishing.

Mundy, P., & Crowson, M. (1997). Joint attention and early social communication: implications for research on intervention with autism. *Journal of Autism and Developmental Disorders*, *27*(6), 653–676.

Mundy, P., Kasari, C., Sigman, M., & Ruskin, E. (1995). Nonverbal communication and early language acquisition in children with Down syndrome and in normally developing children. *Journal of Speech and Hearing Research*, *38*, 157–167.

Nelson, K. E. (1989). Strategies for first language teaching. In M. L. Rice, & R. L. Schiefelbusch (Eds.), *The teachability of language* (pp. 263–310). Baltimore: Paul H. Brookes.

Oller, D. K., Steffens, M. L., Levine, S. L., Basinger, D. L., & Umbel, V. (1995). Onset of speech-like vocalizations in infants with Down syndrome. *American Journal on Mental Retardation*, *100*(1), 68–86.

Pierce, K., & Schreibman, L. (1995). Increasing complex social behaviors in children with autism: Effects of peer-implemented pivotal response training. *Journal of Applied Behavior Analysis*, *28*(3), 285–295.

Prizant, B., Wetherby, A., & Rydell, P. (2000). Communication intervention issues for children with autism spectrum disorders. In A. Wetherby, & B. Prizant (Eds.), *Autism spectrum disorders: A transactional developmental perspective* (Vol. 9, pp. 193–225). Baltimore: Paul H. Brookes.

Roberts, J. E., Mirrett, P., & Burchinal, M. (2001). Receptive and expressive communication development of young males with fragile X syndrome. *American Journal on Mental Retardation*, *106*(3), 216–231.

Santarcangelo, S., & Dyer, K. (1988). Prosodic aspects of motherese: Effects on gaze and responsiveness in developmentally disabled children. *Journal of Experimental Child Psychology*, *46*, 406–418.

Smith, T., Buch, G., & Gamby, T. (2000). Parent-directed, intensive early intervention for children with pervasive developmental disorder. *Research in Developmental Disabilities*, *21*, 297–309.

Smith, T., Eikeseth, S., Klevstrand, M., & Lovaas, O. I. (1997). Intensive behavioral treatment for preschoolers with severe mental retardation and pervasive developmental disorder. *American Journal on Mental Retardation*, *102*(3), 238–249.

Smolak, L., & Levine, M. P. (1984). The effects of differential criteria on the assessment of cognitive–linguistic relationships. *Child Development*, *55*, 973–980.

Soukhanov, A., & Ellis, K. (1984). *Webster's II new Riverside University dictionary*. Boston: Riverside Publishing Company.

Stevenson, C., Krantz, P., & McClannahan, L. (2000). Social interaction skills for children with autism: a script-fading procedure for nonreaders. *Behavioral Interventions*, *15*, 1–20.

Stoel-Gammon, C. (1998). Sounds and words in early language acquisition: the relationship between lexical and phonological development. In R. Paul (Ed.), *Exploring the speech–language connection* (pp. 25–53). Baltimore: Paul H. Brookes.

Tannock, R., & Girolametto, L. (1992). Reassessing parent-focused language intervention programs. In S. Warren, & J. Reichle (Eds.), *Causes and effects in communication and language intervention* (Vol. 1, pp. 49 81). Baltimore: Paul H. Brookes.

Tannock, R., Girolametto, L., & Siegel, L. S. (1992). Language intervention with children who have developmental delays: effects of an interactive approach. *American Journal on Mental Retardation*, *97*, 145–160.

Tomasello, M., & Farrar, M. J. (1986). Joint attention and early language. *Child Development*, *57*, 1454–1463.

Warren, S. F. (1992). Facilitating basic vocabulary acquisition with milieu teaching procedures. *Journal of Early Intervention*, *16*(3), 235–251.

Warren, S. F., & Yoder, P. J. (1997). Communication, language, and mental retardation. In W. MacLean (Ed.), *Mental retardation* (pp. 379–403). Mahwah: Lawrence Erlbaum Associates.

Warren, S. F., & Yoder, P. J. (1998). Facilitating the transition from preintentional to intentional communication. In A. Wetherby, S. Warren, & J. Reichle (Eds.), *Transitions in Prelinguistic Communication* (Vol. 7, pp. 365–385). Baltimore: Brookes.

Wetherby, A., Prizant, B., & Schuler, A. (2000). Understanding the nature of communication and language impairments. In A. Wetherby, & B. Prizant (Eds.), *Autism spectrum disorders: A transactional developmental perspective* (pp. 109–143). Baltimore: Paul H. Brookes Publishing Co.

Yoder, P., Kaiser, A., Alpert, C., & Fischer, R. (1993). Following the child's lead when teaching nouns to preschoolers with mental retardation. *Journal-of-Speech-and-Hearing-Research*, *36*(1), 158–167.

Yoder, P. J., & Warren, S. F. (1998). Maternal responsivity predicts the prelinguistic communication intervention that facilitates generalized intentional communication. *Journal of Speech, Language and Hearing Research*, *41*, 1207–1219.

Yoder, P., & Warren, S. (2001). Relative treatment effects of two prelinguistic communication interventions on language development in toddlers with developmental delays vary by maternal characteristics. *Journal of Speech, Language, and Hearing Research*, *44*, 224–237.

Yoder, P., & Warren, S. (2002). Effects of prelinguistic milieu teaching and parent responsivity education on dyads involving children with intellectual disabilities. *Journal of Speech, Language and Hearing Research*, *45*(6), 1158–1175.

Augmentative and Alternative Communication for Persons with Mental Retardation

MARYANN ROMSKI, ROSE A. SEVCIK, and AMY HYATT FONSECA

DEPARTMENT OF COMMUNICATION, GEORGIA STATE UNIVERSITY
ATLANTA, GEORGIA

I. INTRODUCTION

The ability to communicate permits an individual to express basic wants and needs, thoughts, and feelings as well as to interact independently with others. Communication provides a window into our inner selves and often is the basis by which others perceive us. The importance of communication to development and self-determination is no more striking than in children and adults with mental retardation who exhibit great difficulty learning to communicate via speech. When an individual encounters substantial difficulty communicating, it often results in an inability to express one's self, maintain social contact with family, develop friendships, and function successfully in school. As the individual develops and moves into adulthood, an inability to communicate continues to compromise his or her ability to participate in society, limiting access to more advanced education and employment and closing off many leisure activities and personal relationships. Skills that appear effortless for most typically developing children and achievable with the aid of spoken language intervention for the majority of children and adults with mental retardation are never attained by a relatively low incidence sub group of individuals with mental retardation. Typically, these are individuals who have received some speech and language intervention and still have not made significant advances communicating through speech.

Augmentative and alternative communication, or AAC as it is more commonly known, is an intervention approach that provides an avenue by which to replace or augment existing spoken communication skills. In this article, we provide an overview of AAC and summarize key advances on the

0074-7750/2003 $35.00

use of AAC with persons with mental retardation. We also look ahead to the opportunities and challenges that face us in future research efforts. It should be noted that AAC research spans a broad range of disability groups. For the purposes of this review, we will only examine AAC research that focuses on children and adults with mental retardation. And, because AAC is a relatively young field, we will place the research findings in a historical perspective. One other comment is necessary regarding terminology: AAC is an inclusive term that replaces the previously used terms "non-speech" and "nonverbal."

II. THE NATURE OF AUGMENTATIVE AND ALTERNATIVE COMMUNICATION

AAC encompasses many forms of communication from simple gestures, manual signs and picture communication boards to American Sign Language and sophisticated computer-based devices that can speak in phrases and sentences on behalf of their users. The American Speech-Language-Hearing Association (ASHA, 1991) defines AAC as an area of research, clinical, and educational practice that attempts to compensate, either permanently or temporarily, for the impairment and disability patterns of individuals with severe expressive and receptive communication disorders that affects spoken, gestural, and/or written modes of communication. It is comprised of a system of four integrated components: symbols, aids, techniques, and strategies. Visual, auditory, and/or tactile symbols are used to represent vocabulary and are referred to as aided or unaided. An aided AAC symbol involves the use of an external medium (e.g., photographs, pictures, line drawings, objects, Braille, written words), whereas an unaided AAC symbol involves use of the individual AAC user's body (e.g., sign language, eye pointing, vocalizations). An aid is an object used to transmit or receive messages and includes, for example, communication boards, speech-generating devices, and computers. A technique is an approach or method for selecting messages as well as the types of displays used to view messages. Messages are selected via direct selection or scanning. Direct selection permits an individual to communicate messages from a large set of options using, for example, manual signing or pointing with a finger or headstick to a symbol. Scanning is used when message choices are presented to the child in a sequence and the child makes his or her selection by linear scanning, row-column scanning, or encoding. Displays are either fixed (i.e., the symbol remains the same before and after activation) or dynamic (i.e., the symbol visually changes on selection). Strategies are the specific intervention approaches in which AAC symbols, aids, and techniques are used to facilitate or develop language and communication skills via AAC (see ASHA, 1991, for a complete definition).

A. Individuals with Mental Retardation Who Use AAC

The use of AAC by individuals with mental retardation is not specific to an etiology category. Instead, the use of AAC focuses on the individual's presenting behavior; specifically, a lack of expressive language skills that are understandable by familiar and unfamiliar communication partners. Depending on the individual's chronological age and disability severity, communication profiles may range from unintelligible speech to a very limited number of words (e.g., less than 10) or no speech at all. Thus, individuals with mental retardation who can benefit from AAC are a heterogeneous group who span medical etiologies, physical abilities, and are usually identified based on communication profiles. Medical etiologies can include, but are not limited to, Down syndrome, autism, pervasive developmental disorder, dual sensory impairments, cerebral palsy, seizure disorder, and often times, an etiology that is unknown. Individuals who experience such a considerable level of difficulty communicating are, for the most part, those with the most significant degrees of mental retardation. For them, AAC provides a means by which to develop receptive and expressive language skills. Occasionally, there are some individuals with mild or moderate degrees of mental retardation who have developed speech but exhibit substantially reduced speech intelligibility and may benefit from the use of an AAC intervention. They range in age from very young children just beginning their communication development to adults with a broad range of life-span experiences, including a history of institutionalization.

B. Roles for AAC in Language Intervention

The original rationale for employing AAC with individuals with mental retardation was a modest one; namely, to provide individuals with an alternative output mode so that they would be able to communicate (Fristoe & Lloyd, 1979). This approach presumed that the individual's difficulty acquiring spoken language was specifically related to deficits in motor speech-output. Even after such experience, however, many individuals with mental retardation continued to evidence difficulty learning to speak. Deficits affecting the acquisition of spoken language may include: processing dimensions of the auditory input signal, coordinating fine-motor movements, and more generalized receptive and expressive language acquisition impairments (Romski & Sevcik, 1997).

Current perspectives suggest that the functions AAC can play in language and communication development are broader than the original rationale for AAC use. These functions vary depending on the individual's chronological age, degree of disability, and specific environmental needs. In addition to providing a means by which individuals can convey information, AAC can augment existing speech and vocalizations, provide an input mode as well as an output mode for communication for individuals with limited speech comprehension skills, and serve as a language teaching tool (Beukelman & Mirenda, 1998). AAC can also replace or mitigate an individual's socially unacceptable behaviors, such as screaming or hitting, with conventional means of communication (Donnellan, Mirenda, Mesaros, & Fassbender, 1984; Doss & Reichle, 1991; Mirenda, 1997).

III. RESEARCH ON AAC AND PERSONS WITH MENTAL RETARDATION

Early investigations, employing manual signs and visual-graphic symbols, focused on demonstrating the feasibility of employing AAC with children and adults with mental retardation (e.g., Berger, 1972; Carrier, 1974; Deich & Hodges, 1977; Rumbaugh, 1977). In general, these investigations, many involving outgrowths of methods developed to teach language skills to great apes, found that when children and adults were provided with manual signs or visual-graphic symbols, they learned to communicate expressively using the skills they had been taught. The publication of the edited volume *Nonspeech language and communication: Analysis and intervention* (Schiefelbusch, 1980) marked the first synthesis of a newly emerging area of investigation focused on the development of language and communication through alternative means for children and adults with mental retardation. Since that time, AAC has matured into an integral component of language and communication intervention programs for children and adults with mental retardation who encounter significant difficulty learning to speak (e.g., Beukelman & Mirenda, 1998; Mirenda, Iacono, & Williams, 1990; Reichle, York, & Sigafoos, 1991; Romski & Sevcik, 1997). In this section, we examine a number of areas of research that have advanced the field, first focusing on issues related to choice and then moving to discuss a broad range of factors that impact intervention outcomes or are outcomes themselves.

A. Selection Criteria for AAC

For some time, it was presumed that an individual was required to meet specific criteria in order to begin to use AAC (Chapman & Miller, 1980).

These criteria included a history of unsuccessful spoken language intervention, at least some receptive language skills, and cognitive development at Piagetian sensorimotor stage V or VI. The literature on typical language development has linked these sensorimotor skills with the beginning stages of language development. Kahn (1996) examined the role of stage V performance on the *Ordinal Scales of Infant Development* (Uzgiris & Hunt, 1975) in predicting how 34 children with severe and profound mental retardation learned manual signs over a 4-year period of time. Of the 21 children who exhibited stage V or VI functioning on the Uzgiris and Hunt scales, 13 of them used at least one sign independently after 4 years. All but one of these 13 children used at least three signs independently, with one child using ten. Five of the 21 children used two-sign combinations and eight used spoken words. Taken at face value, the Kahn findings suggest that sensorimotor stage V performance is necessary but not sufficient for the learning of manual signs. There was, however, very little control over the fidelity of the manual sign interventions provided across the 4-year intervention time period. Kahn acknowledged that the teachers used manual signs predominately only during direct instruction or after they thought that the child had learned the sign. Given the lack of control over the consistency of the interventions' implementation, it is difficult to conclude that this study supports the importance of sensorimotor stage V or VI for AAC use.

Most of the empirical evidence suggests, however, that persons with even very limited cognitive and receptive language skills can use AAC successfully. Reichle and Yoder (1985), for example, taught preschoolers with severe disabilities, who functioned at sensorimotor stage IV, to label objects using visual symbols. In another study, Romski, Sevcik, and Pate (1988) reported that two young adults with severe mental retardation who were nonspeaking and lacked receptive language skills learned to use visual-graphic symbols to request foods and objects. Romski and Sevcik (1996) also reported that four school-aged youths with severe cognitive disabilities developed vocabularies of up to 35 symbols even though they had demonstrated extremely limited receptive language skills at the onset of the study. Together, these intervention studies suggest that neither cognitive development at Stage V or VI nor speech comprehension skills have to be in place for individuals with developmental disabilities to learn initial language skills, such as single word vocabulary items.

B. Communication Modes

Once it is decided that AAC is the intervention approach, there are a number of choices that must be made related to modes of communication from manual signs and communication boards to speech-output communication devices. With the exception of a few early studies (Locke & Mirenda, 1988; Romski et al., 1988; Romski, White, Millen, & Rumbaugh, 1984), manual signs and cardboard communication boards were the AAC systems of choice for persons with mental retardation but without severe physical disabilities. The prevailing belief had been that persons with limited intellectual ability could not benefit "enough" from the use of more sophisticated technologies such as speech-output communication devices to justify the initial fiscal outlay for the purchase of a device (Turner, 1986). Research on manual sign language suggests that although often successful, manual signs may be difficult for communication partners to interpret. A number of more recent studies support the use of speech-output communication devices for language intervention.

Romski and Sevcik (1996) introduced the System for Augmenting Language (SAL) to 13 school-aged youths with moderate or severe mental retardation (mean CA = 12 years, 3 months; mean nonverbal MA = 3 years, 6 months). At the onset of the study, they each demonstrated intentional communication abilities (e.g., gestures, vocalizations), no more than 10 intelligible word approximations and an unsuccessful history of learning to communicate via other means (i.e., speech, manual signs, communication boards). The SAL included five integrated components: (1) a speech-output communication device; (2) an appropriate arbitrary symbol vocabulary; (3) naturalistic communicative experiences during which the youth was encouraged, but not required, to communicate; (4) partners (teachers, parents, and siblings) who were taught how to use the device and how to provide both a symbol model and input via speech + symbols to the youth; and (5) an investigator-provided resource and feedback mechanism to monitor progress across the study. During two years of naturalistic communicative experiences at home and school, the youth had opportunities to employ a range of communicative functions from greeting, requesting, and attention directing, to answering and questioning.

The results indicated that the 13 youths integrated their use of the SAL with their extant vocalizations and gestures, resulting in a rich multi-modal form of communication that they used to effectively communicate with adults (Romski, Sevcik, Robinson, & Bakeman, 1994) and peers (Romski, Sevcik, & Wilkinson, 1994). These youths developed a vocabulary that integrated referential and social-regulative symbols (Adamson, Romski, Deffebach, & Sevcik, 1992). Some of these youths also then developed combinatorial symbol skills (Wilkinson, Romski, & Sevcik, 1994) as well as intelligible spoken words and rudimentary reading skills (Romski & Sevcik, 1996).

Romski and Sevcik argued that the use of a speech-output communication device was a critical component of the successful use of the SAL by their participants. They contended that the speech-output provided a link to the natural auditory world for the participants and was readily understandable by others in the environment. In a follow-up study, Romski, Sevcik, and Adamson (1999) compared the 13 participants' communication performance during structured interactions with and without their speech-output communication devices. With 5 years of SAL experience, the youths were able to convey more conversationally appropriate, clearer (less ambiguous), and more specific information to an unfamiliar adult partner with their devices than without them in this structured communicative interaction. Brady (2000) also examined the effects of a speech-output communication device on the receptive and expressive language skills of two 5-year-old children with developmental delays using multiple baselines across routines. She reported that both children learned to expressively request six different objects using a speech-output communication device. They also increased their comprehension of these six object names. Dicarlo and Banajee (2000) used multiple baselines across participants to evaluate the effects of speech-output communication devices on the communicative initiations of two young children with developmental delays. They reported that both children's use of initiations increased when they employed the device.

These investigations suggest that speech-output communication devices are an appropriate communication mode for individuals with mental retardation and alter the communication interactions for individuals with mental retardation. None of the studies previously described, however, provided a direct comparison of speech-output + symbols with learning symbols alone. In a case study, Iacono and Duncum (1995) directly compared the effects of manual signs alone to manual signs in combination with a speech-output communication device on the language development of a 32-month-old girl with Down syndrome using an alternating treatments design. They reported that the combined use of manual signs and the speech-output communication device was more effective in eliciting single-word production. Schlosser, Belfiore, Nigam, and Blischak (1995) compared the acquisition of visual-graphic symbols coupled with speech-output to the acquisition of visual-graphic symbols alone by three adults with severe mental retardation. They found that the speech-output + visual-graphic symbols resulted in more efficient learning with fewer errors than the visual-graphic symbols alone. Schepis and Reid (1995) examined the effects of a speech-output communication device on the communicative partners of a 23-year-old young woman with severe disabilities. Results indicated that residential staff members interacted with the young woman more frequently when she had access to her device than when the device was not available for her use.

Taken together, these results lend support to Romski and Sevcik's earlier argument that speech-output devices play a critical role in AAC language learning. Additional investigations that replicate these effects across larger samples and a range of age groups are still needed. It seems likely, however, that the inclusion of a speech-output device may actually play a facilitatory role in communication development for individuals with mental retardation.

C. Vocabulary Representation and Selection

Another issue in the clinical and research literature on AAC has been an ongoing discussion of the extent to which features of the medium by which language is represented may affect its learning and use (Sevcik, Romski & Wilkinson, 1991). AAC symbols have been classified as unaided (e.g., manual signs and gestures) or aided (e.g., visual-graphic symbols that range from objects, pictures, and photographs to highly abstract or arbitrary symbols, such as Blissymbols or English orthography; Lloyd & Fuller, 1986). The level of arbitrariness of different symbols, that is, the degree to which a symbol does or does not physically resemble its referent or meaning, has consistently been judged to be an important factor in the choice of a symbol set for children with developmental disabilities (see, for example, Musselwhite & St. Louis, 1982; Romski et al., 1988, Sevcik et al., 1991, for discussions of terms). This judgment is based on the belief that the more a symbol resembles what it represents, the more likely it is to be learned by children with developmental disabilities. This issue has been a complex and, at times, controversial one.

The majority of research on symbol representation, to date, has focused on how children and adults with typical cognitive skills perceive symbols and/or learn the association between symbols and spoken words. The findings from this work have indicated that symbol learning is affected by the level of symbol arbitrariness (e.g., concrete, abstract) and the physical configuration (e.g., complexity, shape) of symbols (e.g., Ecklund & Reichle, 1987; Mizuko, 1987; Musselwhite & Russello, 1984). Some researchers, however, have questioned whether or not these findings may be extended to children with developmental disabilities who are not speaking (see Sevcik, et al., 1991, for a review). Little symbol research has actually been conducted in which individuals with mental retardation who were not speaking serve as participants. Of the studies that have been conducted, the focus of investigation has been on either the representational abilities of the participants or on the ability of the participants to learn symbol meanings (e.g., Mirenda & Locke, 1989; Sevcik & Romski, 1986). This literature has been reviewed in depth elsewhere (see Romski & Sevcik, 1997). Overall, these findings suggest that a number of factors, including the individual's speech comprehension abilities and the degree of arbitrariness of the symbols used, may influence how symbols are learned by persons with mental retardation. Although there has been relatively little new empirical evidence in this area over the last few years, Sevcik (2002) is currently investigating the interaction of symbol arbitrariness with speech comprehension skills as children with mental retardation learn symbol meanings in a computerized environment.

In addition to choosing the mode and type of symbol to employ, using AAC means that vocabulary must be chosen and placed on the display. Thus, vocabulary selection is a significant issue that must be considered (Wilkinson & McIlvane, 2002). One important decision is between using pre-stored language units (i.e., full sentences that are programmed in a symbol) or individual words. Although there is no empirical literature that has explored this issue, using individual words follows a language development model. When single words are chosen, another issue is the type of word that appears on the display. Adamson et al. (1992) reported that youth with severe mental retardation were able to integrate referential and social-regulative symbols into their vocabularies. This type of vocabulary also permitted some of these youth to then develop combinatorial symbol skills (Wilkinson et al., 1994).

Choosing an appropriate communication mode and vocabulary is just the beginning of the AAC intervention process which then must be focused on the long term development of functional language and communication skills. Research has focused on examining a range of factors that may impact intervention outcomes from the instructional approaches employed to the role of speech comprehension skills.

D. Developing Instructional Approaches

The majority of research in AAC has centered on developing instructional approaches that are designed to provide the sole means of communication or augment the existing receptive and expressive communication skills of individuals with mental retardation (see Mirenda, Iacono, & Williams, 1990; Romski & Sevcik, 1997, for reviews). Studies have typically involved a small number of participants, single-subject research designs, and short-term interventions (e.g. Hamilton & Snell, 1993; Kaiser, Ostrosky, & Alpert, 1993). These investigations includes studies that have focused on assessing approaches for teaching communicative functions, such as requesting, protesting, and commenting (e.g., Reichle & Johnston, 1999; Sigafoos & Roberts-Pennel, 1999), as well as examining the effects of adapting spoken language intervention strategies (such as matrix training and milieu teaching) for AAC use (see Romski, Sevcik, Hyatt, & Cheslock, 2002 for an overview). Although the studies differ in the AAC mode (e.g., manual signs, communication board) and selection technique employed, as well as in the characteristics of the children studied, they consistently reported positive and significant effects for most participants. Such positive findings appear to be the case whether intervention outcomes focused on pragmatic skills (e.g., requesting objects and information) or semantic skills (e.g., vocabulary development, semantic relations). The literature suggests that well established spoken language approaches have had some utility for adaptation to AAC use. Studies, to date, however, have focused on beginning communicators who are functioning at or close to symbolically. Much less evidence is available about the communication development of beginning communicators who are not functioning symbolically.

Although we are accumulating a substantial portfolio of information about short-term instructional approaches that work with a small number of participants, a number of areas of investigation are lacking. We have, to date, few empirical studies that compare interventions across larger samples of participants. Rowland and Schweigert (2000), for example, began to address this issue in the 3-year longitudinal study they conducted, which focused on the use of tangible symbols by 41 children with various disabilities including mental retardation. At the onset of the study, participants demonstrated meaningful and spontaneous use of 10 or fewer abstract symbols for expressive communication. The children's performance was documented and follow-up observations were conducted to investigate the maintenance and long term potential and use of tangible symbols. Three types of performance were identified. Group 1 acquired no symbols at all, Group 2 acquired one or more forms of tangible symbols, and Group 3 acquired tangible symbols and one or more forms of abstract symbols. In summary, Rowland and Schweigert provided evidence about the effects of experience with tangible symbols on the children's communication skills. Romski, Sevcik, Adamson, and Cheslock (2002) are currently studying the relative effects of three language interventions including AAC with toddlers with developmental disabilities. Additional research about the relative effects of instructional approaches is essential to understanding the effects of AAC intervention on the language and communication development of individuals with mental retardation. Further, we know very little about the broader long-term effects of AAC experience on development and learning. We also have not considered the role that the child's development plays in the learning and use of AAC systems.

E. Role of Language Comprehension in AAC Interventions

AAC has typically provided an output mode so that an individual can produce communications and engage as a speaker in conversations with others to express his or her wants, needs, feelings, and ideas. Although this role is essential and permits the individual to have a visible communicative effect upon his or her environment, it does not exist in isolation (Sevcik & Romski, 2002). There is the presumption that the individual who can produce communication can also take on the role of listener, or receiver of messages, in a conversation. To assume the role of message receiver, the individual must be able to understand the information that is being conveyed to him or her by a range of communicative partners. Individuals with mental retardation who are learning AAC may be in the early stages of language development. They may not yet be able to switch between the speaker and listener roles.

As part of their language profile, individuals with mental retardation may evidence speech comprehension skills that range from no or minimal comprehension to comprehension skills equivalent to, in rare cases, their chronological age (Nelson, 1992). Individuals who do comprehend some speech may have knowledge about the relationship between words and their referents in the environment (Romski & Sevcik, 1993). Consequently, their auditory processing skills may be quite distinct from the individual who does not have such a foundation upon which to build AAC skills. Individuals who do not understand spoken words confront a very different task. They must establish conditional relationships between the visual symbols to be learned and their real world referents while relying, almost exclusively, on the visual modality (Romski & Sevcik, 1996). AAC systems then can serve as both input and output modes for such individuals. Not all individuals with mental retardation who employ AAC comprehend speech. A primary focus on production may actually make learning to communicate via AAC systems extremely difficult for some individuals. That is, the individual is asked to produce communications with the assumption that he or she has an adequate foundation of understanding upon which to build these AAC productions.

Sevcik and Romski (1997) described two distinct paths (beginning and advanced) to symbol acquisition for the youth with moderate and severe mental retardation they have studied. The extant spoken language comprehension skills some of the "advanced" youth brought to the language learning task allowed them to rapidly acquire and use symbols for communication. Their performance was in sharp contrast to youth who did not evidence such speech comprehension skill at the onset. Romski and Sevcik suggested that the extant spoken language comprehension skills the advanced achievers brought to the language learning task allowed them to rapidly acquire and use symbols for communication. Their performance was in sharp contrast to the "beginning" achievers, who did not evidence testable speech comprehension skill at the onset of the study. These participants learned to comprehend symbols but did not produce them. If only symbol production performance had been measured, it would have been concluded that the beginning achievers had learned no symbol vocabulary meanings. Additional support for this achievement distinction was provided by Romski et al. (1988) who studied older adolescents and young adults with severe cognitive disabilities. The participants were explicitly taught visual-graphic symbol production skills without speech-output. Distinct symbol acquisition and generalization patterns that were linked to the participants' extant speech comprehension skills were reported.

Another aspect of speech comprehension is the language learning environment to which individuals with mental retardation are exposed. Sevcik, Romski, Watkins, and Deffebach (1995) examined the quantity and quality of the AAC symbol input employed by the partners of the 13 youth in their intervention at three points across one school year (beginning, middle, end). They reported that only a small percentage (mean = 9.6%, $SD = 6.99$) of the partners' overall spoken communicative utterances directed to the youth contained symbol input. The sophistication of the youth's speech comprehension skills, however, differentially affected the amount of AAC symbol input they received from their adult partners. Partners used more AAC symbol input with the beginning SAL achievers who had poor speech comprehension skills (mean = 12.8%) than with the advanced SAL achievers who demonstrated comprehension skills at or greater than 24 months of age (mean = 7.7%). Symbol input in the spoken utterances of the adults were significantly more likely to occur in the final position of an utterance than in either the beginning or middle position of the utterance regardless of the youth's achievement pattern. Not surprisingly, school partners (most often teachers) were more directive in their use of augmented input than home partners (most often parents), whose communications were evenly divided between directive and facilitative. The other important result of this study was that home and school adult partners with relatively modest amounts of instruction in how to provide SAL input were quite skilled in presenting the augmented input in a salient and facilitative manner to the youth.

Comprehension skills can serve as the foundation not only for productive symbol learning but also as a vehicle for language instruction. Peterson, Bondy, Vincent, and Finnegan (1995) assessed the effects of interventions in three communicative input modalities on the task performance and frequency of target behaviors of two boys with autism and challenging behaviors (7 and 9 years of age). The three different communicative inputs were spoken language input alone, pictorial or gestural communicative input, and augmented input (pictorial or gestural input plus spoken input). They reported that spoken input alone did not facilitate performance as well as did the augmented input for either child. In fact, they suggested that spoken input alone may actually have increased challenging behaviors.

More recently, Romski et al. (1999) completed a pilot study to examine the effects of a parent-implemented augmented input intervention focused on teaching a parent to use augmented input in her communications with a 34-month-old toddler with disabilities including partial Trisomy 13, cerebral palsy, and significant developmental delay. This child had speech comprehension skills determined to be at about 15 months on the *Sequenced Inventory of Communication Development* (SICD; Hendrick, Prather, & Tobin, 1984). His expressive communication skills on the SICD were at the 6-month level and he had some undifferentiated vocalizations and a laugh that was not employed communicatively. At the outset, he did not comprehend the meanings of any of the visual-graphic symbols to be taught (e.g., more, all done, book, snack, drink, bubbles, jack-in-the-box).

A 10-week intervention protocol was implemented in a structured environment focused on teaching the parent to provide augmented communication input using visual-graphic symbols and a speech-output communication device to her child. There were two 30-minute sessions per week for a total of 20 sessions. The intervention increased his symbol and speech comprehension skills for the target vocabulary items from 0 to 10 words across the 10-week period. After 6 weeks, there was also a steady increase in his spontaneous use of symbols to communicate messages though there was no comparable change in spoken language production skills over the course of the intervention period (Romski, Sevcik, & Forrest, 2001).

This pilot study provides preliminary evidence that augmented communication input intervention may serve at least three distinct functions. First, it yields increased symbol and sometimes speech comprehension skills. Second, it provides an intervention that is comfortable for parents/partners to implement. And, third it may facilitate productive communicative use of symbols. This was only a pilot study that could not rule out the role of the child's development. Additional studies of augmented input interventions are needed to evaluate the effects of utilizing AAC input as an intervention strategy for AAC communicators.

Romski et al. (2002) are currently assessing the relative effects of this augmented input intervention strategy described above in comparison to two other early communication intervention strategies, one focused on augmented communication output and the other focused on communication interaction with no augmentation. In this ongoing longitudinal study, a total of 60 toddlers (24–36 months) are being recruited and randomly assigned to one of these three interventions. Each child and his or her parent (primary caregiver), participate in a 12-week parent-implemented intervention protocol and then are followed at 3, 6, and 12 months post intervention. The intervention protocol for all three interventions is focused on teaching the parent to implement specific communication strategies at home during daily routines. Each 30-min intervention session includes three 10-min routines around play, book-reading, and snack. Parents first observe the child and an interventionist using the intervention strategies prior to implementing the interaction themselves with coaching from the interventionist. To date, participant recruitment and data collection are underway with approximately 30 participants at some phase of data collection. In this context, we expect to be able to articulate the effects of the augmented input intervention approach for young children with severe communication disabilities with a range of speech comprehension skills at the onset of the intervention.

In summary, there has been, at best, a modest amount of research on the role of speech comprehension in the communication development process. There has been even less research that has focused on the role of augmented input as an intervention approach for individuals who are at a variety of different stages of the language development process.

F. Effects of AAC on Speech Development

The fear of many parents, and some practitioners, is that AAC will become the individual's primary communication mode and take away the motivation to speak. The empirical data to date, though limited, does not support this fear. In fact, it suggests just the opposite. There are a modest number of empirical studies that report improvement in speech skills for some individuals after AAC intervention experience (e.g., Fulwiler & Fouts, 1976; Kouri, 1988; Miller & Miller, 1973; Romski & Sevcik, 1996; Romski et al., 1988; Romski, Sevcik, Robinson, & Wilkinson, 1990; Yoder & Layton, 1988). There are no studies that support the belief that AAC intervention hinders the development of speech.

G. Replacing Socially Unacceptable Behaviors

An area that has seen a substantial focus over the past decade is that of the relationship between the development of AAC use and a decrease in socially unacceptable behaviors (Reichle & Wacker, 1993; Wacker, Berg, & Harding, 2002). This area of research has focused on the development of interventions to replace socially unacceptable behaviors (i.e., agression, self-injury) with socially acceptable communication using AAC. Often the functions of socially unacceptable behaviors are communicative when an individual does not have a conventionally interpretable way to express wants, needs, and desires. Functional communication training (FCT) comes from a behavior analysis tradition and first assesses the function of the problem behavior and then teaches the individual to use a more socially appropriate form of that behavior to serve the same function (Carr & Durand, 1985; Durand, 1990). Mirenda (1997) reviewed the growing body of empirical literature in this area and suggested that there is strong empirical support that this intervention approach is effective across individuals who present with such behaviors. In this tradition, additional studies have been conducted to lend further support to the effectiveness of this intervention at home and with a range of children (e.g., Brown et al., 2000; Derby et al., 1997; Drasgow, Halle, & Ostrocky, 1998).

H. Advances in Development of Technology for Communication

One striking characteristic of the AAC field today is the rapid development of new technologies (Beukelman & Mirenda, 1998). Changes in the types of communication devices that are available occur so frequently that it can be difficult to keep abreast of every device on the market today. Although AAC in general has developed as a field, people with mental retardation have not always been included in the mainstream of that development (Wehmeyer, 1995). In the early 1980s, The Arc created a bioengineering initiative to evaluate available assistive technology (AT) in terms of its applicability to the needs of children and adults with mental retardation and to develop new devices to address the unmet needs of individuals with mental retardation (Mineo, 1985). These developments have led to a number of technological advances in AAC that have opened up new possibilities for individuals with mental retardation. Recent additions to the AAC device market are able to provide a range of capabilities within one device that may enable a child or adult to use one piece of equipment for a more extended period of time. Technological advances such as the speed of computer-based communication, dynamic graphic symbol displays, and speech recognition technology have the potential to further facilitate the inclusion of individuals with significant mental retardation into society. Research that evaluates the effects of these technological advances on learning is only beginning to be conducted. For example, Reichle, Dettling, Drager, and Leiter (2000) examined the efficiency of fixed versus dynamic symbol displays for one AAC user. They found that the AAC user employed the dynamic active displays faster and more accurately than the fixed or passive displays. These differences increased as the size of the vocabulary expanded. Though preliminary in nature, these findings suggest that the effects of these technological advances on learning and use of AAC devices should continue to be explored.

I. Chronological Age at the Onset of AAC Intervention

Clinically, chronological age has been used as an exclusionary criteria for participating in AAC intervention. Individuals have been judged as too young or too old to benefit from communication, including AAC, intervention (NJC, 2002). For individuals with mental retardation, chronological age is often linked to language development level and together these two factors may influence the outcomes of AAC interventions in complex ways. The majority of research about individuals with mental retardation who employ AAC interventions is with individuals who are at least school-aged. There has been little empirical investigation about the use of AAC interventions with very young children. The more significant the developmental delay, the more important it may be to initiate intervention early in childhood to ensure steady developmental progress (Shonkoff, Hauser-Cram, Krauss, & Upshur, 1992). A significant delay in communication development affects all aspects of the child's development. Existing research and practice have focused attention on developing spoken language skills (Fey, 1986) or teaching prelinguistic skills (e.g., Warren, Yoder, Gazdag, Kim, & Jones, 1993; Yoder & Warren, 1993). Developing functional intelligible speech production skills is the ultimate goal for any young child with significant developmental disabilities. Approaches that focus on speech, however, can frustrate the child and his or her family, sometimes resulting in challenging behaviors because they do not provide a way to communicate while the child is slowly, and sometimes unsuccessfully, learning to talk. Teaching prelinguistic skills focuses on establishing a strong intentional communicative foundation on which to build spoken linguistic skills. Even with such a prelinguistic base, often the young child with a severe communication disorder does not smoothly make the transition from intentional communication to spoken language skills. If these young children had a conventional mode by which to first take in linguistic information and then intentionally communicate early in childhood, perhaps their overall communicative interaction skills and adaptive behavior skills might not lag as far behind other children without such experience. Schiefelbusch (1984, 1985) and others have speculated that if young children at significant risk for receptive and expressive language development difficulties received AAC experience early in the course of their development, the young child's communication skills might follow a more "normalized" developmental route. With the aid of an AAC system, symbol comprehension and production skills may emerge earlier than they would through other therapeutic approaches that focus on speech alone.

For toddlers who are not speaking and at significant risk for not developing speech and language skills, early augmented language experiences may facilitate communication development, prevent the emergence of challenging behaviors, and facilitate social interactions with adults and peers. Very little is known about the process of language and communication development in very young children with significant developmental delays who engaged in early augmented language experience.

J. Perceptions of Competence

In general, speech and language impairments negatively affect how others perceive children and adults. Rice, Hadley, and Alexander (1993) reported, for example, that adults showed systematic negative biases towards children with limited oral communication abilities. With respect to individuals who do not speak, Gorenflo and Gorenflo (1991) reported that the use of computer-based communication devices, coupled with additional information about the individual, increased favorable attitudes of observers towards individuals using augmented communication systems. In a followup study, Gorenflo, Gorenflo, and Santer (1994) investigated the effects of four different voice synthesizers on the attitudes of adults towards adult AAC users. More favorable attitudes were noted when the synthetic voice was easier to listen to, though a voice consistent with the user's gender did not produce more favorable attitudes from the listeners. Blockberger, Armstrong, O'Connor, and Freeman (1993) examined the attitudes of fourth-grade children toward a nonspeaking peer using three different types of communication techniques. They found that a positive attitude was influenced by gender, reading ability and experience with children with disabilities. Beck and Dennis (1996) investigated the attitudes of fifth graders toward a similar-aged peer who was nonspeaking. Their findings, consistent with those of Blockberger and her colleagues, were that females and children who had experience with children with disabilities had more positive attitudes toward the child who communicated through augmented means. Beck, Fritz, Keller, and Dennis (2000) presented a reliable and valid tool to measure the attitudes of elementary school-aged children towards peers using AAC. Their recent findings replicate the earlier studies and suggest a developmental trend in attitude. Lilienfeld and Alant (2002) extended these findings to early adolescence (youth ages 11–13). They reported that girls' attitudes were more favorable than boys' attitudes and that overall children's attitudes were more favorable when the same-aged peer employed a speech-output communication device. Williams, Romski, Sevcik, and Adamson (2003) are currently examining the perceptions of naive adults about the communication competence of individuals with mental retardation with and without their speech-output communication devices.

Overall, then, these studies suggest that among the factors that influence perception is the speech-output communication device and the perceiver's individual experiences. It appears that devices can enhance not only ongoing communication with partners but also judgments of competence by familiar as well as unfamiliar observers. AAC has the potential to raise expectations of competency, which, in turn, influence how individuals are viewed as a potential communicative partners. These increased expectations may support more varied and complex communicative patterns and by extension, facilitate inclusion in society as well.

IV. AUGMENTATIVE COMMUNICATION FOR PERSONS WITH MENTAL RETARDATION: SUMMARY, IMPLICATIONS, AND FUTURE RESEARCH

In summary, there has been substantial growth in research on the use of AAC with children and adults with mental retardation. Many assumptions about which individuals can benefit from AAC and how they can be taught have been eliminated. The acquisition of communication skills can be the key to unlocking the world for every child and adult with mental retardation (Mirenda et al., 1990; Romski & Sevcik, 1996). Its use can change the quality of a child's or adult's life by enhancing communication in inclusive settings, in transitions from school to work, in family interactions, and in the perceptions and attitudes of others towards children and adults who do not speak (Romski & Sevcik, 1996). The field's focus has moved away from an assessment of who can use what type of device and a concentration on the technology alone and towards the development of effective interventions and the broader outcomes of their implementation and use. There is still a substantial amount of uncharted territory that must be studied in the future.

A. Implications

The implications are that AAC interventions are a viable intervention approach for a broad range of individuals with mental retardation from very young children to aging adults. The AAC device is a tool, a means to an end—functional language and communication skills—not the end. Incorporating AAC for individuals with mental retardation requires a focus on language and communication development within the context of the AAC mode. AAC is sometimes thought of as a separate area of practice and thus clinicians do not always incorporate the information they know about language and communication development as they consider AAC assessment and intervention. It is imperative that these two areas be linked.

AAC use can be the key to unlocking the world for children with significant developmental disabilities (Mirenda et al., 1990; Romski & Sevcik, 1996). Its use can change the quality of a child's life by facilitating communication in inclusive settings (Heller et al., 1996), transitions from school to work, family interactions and the perceptions and attitudes of others towards children who do not speak (Romski & Sevcik, 1996). Finally, AAC permits individuals with mental retardation to communicate, which must be closely associated with quality of life issues and facilitating self-determination (Wehmeyer, 1996, 1998).

B. Future Research Directions

Because children and youths with more severe developmental disabilities are a low incidence population, they have not been a major focus of study for the field of mental retardation. The majority of language-related mental retardation research has focused on individuals who speak (Rosenberg & Abbeduto, 1993). Future research must tackle important methodological considerations.

Studies typically have used fairly sophisticated verbal tasks to probe an individual's knowledge and thus omitted individuals who did not speak. With the development of AAC intervention approaches, researchers can now include children and adults who do not speak in a traditional sense, but who do communicate through AAC modes in a wide range of behavioral studies such as investigations that examine aspects of word learning, attention, memory, and problem solving. Romski, Sevcik, Robinson, Mervis, and Bertrand (1996), for example, were able to assess the abilities of 12 school-aged youths to "fast map" the meanings of novel nonsense words + symbols through the use of a speech-output communication device and visual-graphic symbols. They found that these youth were able to learn the novel vocabulary on a single exposure and argued that fast mapping may be one explanation for how these youths developed extensive symbol vocabularies.

One particularly important, yet challenging, area of research need is that of language and communication measurement tools (Sevcik, Romski, & Adamson, 1999). Attention must be focused on the development of assessment tools that provide a fine-grained analysis of the child's language and communication skills across modes and that measure a range of intervention outcomes over time. Some outcomes of using AAC go beyond the development of specific comprehension and production vocabulary and even grammatical skills and have been somewhat elusive to quantitative measurement. Access to communication through AAC use can change the quality of an individual's life in inclusive settings from school to work, family interactions, and the perceptions and attitudes of others towards individuals who do not speak (Romski & Sevcik, 1996). Such communication access can also prevent the emergence of secondary disabilities (e.g., challenging behaviors). Tools that permit measurement of these secondary outcomes are important.

The development of language and communication skills, regardless of the mode, also sets the stage for the development of literacy skills. Although literacy is an extremely important area of emphasis, it is only in its infancy for children and adults with mental retardation (Connors, this volume; Koppenhaver, Pierce, & Yoder, 1995). This is an area of investigation that requires a strong plan that is built on what we know about developmental reading disorders and considers the unique aspects of AAC use.

Another area of investigation that is becoming increasingly feasible is detailing the relationships between brain structure and function and language behavior in individuals with mental retardation who use AAC. Molfese, Morris, and Romski (1990) recorded the Auditory Evoked Responses (AERs) of six school-aged children with severe mental retardation as they were shown individually meaningful and nonmeaningful visual-graphic symbols. They found that the AER activity recorded from the left hemisphere frontal and temporal electrode sites successfully discriminated between the meaningful and nonmeaningful symbols. Continued examinations of these relationships, using newly available techniques such as fMRI, will permit a careful assessment of the neural underpinnings to language and communication in these individuals and the effects of interventions on biology as well as behavior.

Much work remains in understanding the communication development of children and adults with mental retardation who use AAC. Researchers must continue to examine the contributions and interactions of a range of factors to communication and language development including age at onset of instruction, speech comprehension, instructional conditions, and the partners with whom they communicate.

V. CONCLUSION

In conclusion, using AAC interventions children and adults with mental retardation and severe spoken communication disabilities have demonstrated communication achievements far beyond those the early clinical expectations afforded them. Essential research and resultant recommended practices continue to expand our views about the communication abilities of children and adults with mental retardation who require supports and accommodations to communicate.

ACKNOWLEDGMENTS

Preparation of this manuscript was supported by National Institutes of Health grants NIDCD-03799 and NIDCD-03766 and a Research Program Enhancement Grant from Georgia State University.

REFERENCES

Adamson, L. B., Romski, M. A., Deffebach, K. P., & Sevcik, R. A. (1992). Symbol vocabulary and the focus of conversations: augmenting language development for youth with mental retardation. *Journal of Speech and Hearing Research*, *35*, 1333–1344.

American Speech-Language-Hearing Association. (1991). Report: Augmentative and alternative communication, *ASHA*, *33* (Suppl. 5): 9–12.

Beck, A. R., & Dennis, M. (1996). Attitudes of children toward a similar-aged child who uses augmentative communication. *Augmentative and Alternative Communication*, *12*, 78–87.

Beck, A. R., Fritz, H., Keller, A., & Dennis, M. (2000). Attitudes of school-aged children toward their peers who use augmentative and alternative communication. *Augmentative and Alternative Communication*, *16*, 13–26.

Berger, S. (1972). A clinical program for developing multimodal language responses with atypical deaf children. In J. McLean, D. Yoder, & R. L. Schiefelbusch (Eds.), *Language intervention with the retarded: Developing strategies* (pp. 212–236). Baltimore: University Park Press.

Beukelman, D. R., & Mirenda, P. (1998). *Augmentative and alternative communication.* Baltimore: Paul H. Brookes Publishing Co.

Blockberger, S., Armstrong, R. W., O'Connor, A., & Freeman, R. (1993). Children's attitudes toward a nonspeaking child using various augmentative and alternative communication techniques. *Augmentative and Alternative Communication*, *9*, 243–258.

Brady, N. C. (2000). Improved comprehension of object names following voice output communication aid use: two case studies. *Augmentative and Alternative Communication*, *16*, 197–205.

Brown, K., Wacker, D., Derby, K., Peck, S., Richman, D., Sasso, G., Knutson, C., & Harding, J. (2000). Evaluating the effects of functional communication training in the presence and absence of establishing operations. *Journal of Applied Behavior Analysis*, *33*, 53–71.

Carr, E. G., & Durand, V. M. (1985). Reducing behavior problems through functional intervention training. *Journal of Applied Behavior Analysis*, *18*, 111–126.

Carrier, J. (1974). Nonspeech noun usage training with severely and profoundly retarded children. *Journal of Speech and Hearing Research*, *17*, 510–517.

Chapman, R., & Miller, H. (1980). Analyzing language and communication in the child. In R. L. Schiefelbusch (Ed.), *Nonspeech language and communication: Analysis and intervention* (pp. 159–196). Baltimore: University Park Press.

Deich, R., & Hodges, P. (1977). *Language without speech.* NY: Brunner/Mazel.

Derby, K., Wacker, D., Berg, W., DeRaad, A., Ulricj, S., Asmus, J., Harding, J., Prouty, A., & Laffery, P. (1997). The long-term effects of functional communication training in a home setting. *Journal of Applied Behavior Analysis*, *30*, 507–531.

Dicarlo, C. F., & Banajee, M. (2000). Using voice output devices to increase initiations of young children with disabilities. *Journal of Early Intervention*, *23*, 191–199.

Donnellan, A., Mirenda, P., Mesaros, R., & Fassbender, L. (1984). Analyzing the communicative functions of aberrant behavior. *Journal of the Association for Persons with Severe Handicaps*, *9*, 141–150.

Doss, S., & Reichle, J. (1991). Replacing excess behavior with an initial communicative repertoire. In J. Reichle, J. York, & J. Sigafoss (Eds.), *Implementing augmentative and alternative communication: Strategies for learners with severe disabilities* (pp. 215–238). Baltimore: Paul Brookes.

Durand, V. M. (1990). *Severe behavior problems: A functional communication training approach.* New York: Guiliford Press.

Drasgow, E., Halle, J. W., & Ostrocky, M. M. (1998). Effects of differential reinforcement delays. *Journal of Applied Behavior Analysis, 31*, 357–374.

Ecklund, S., & Reichle, J. (1987). A comparison of normal children's ability to recall symbols from two logographic systems. *Language, Speech and Hearing Services in Schools, 18*, 34–40.

Fey, M. (1986). *Language intervention with young children.* San Diego, CA: College-Hill Press.

Fristoe, M., & Lloyd, L. (1979). Nonspeech communication. In N. R. Ellis (Ed.), *Handbook of mental deficiency: Psychological theory and research* (pp. 401–430). Hillsdale, NJ: Lawrence Erlbaum Associates.

Fulwiler, R. L., & Fouts, R. S. (1976). Acquisition of American Sign Language by a noncommunicating autistic child. *Journal of Autism and Childhood Schizophrenia, 6*, 43–51.

Gorenflo, C., & Gorenflo, D. (1991). The effects of information and augmentative communication technique on attitudes towards nonspeaking individuals. *Journal of Speech and Hearing Research, 34*, 19–26.

Gorenflo, C., Gorenflo, D., & Santer, S. (1994). Effects of synthetic voice output on attitudes toward the augmented communicator. *Journal of Speech and Hearing Research, 37*, 64–68.

Hamilton, B. L., & Snell, M. E. (1993). Using the milieu approach to increase spontaneous communication book use across environments by an adolescent with autism. *Augmentative and Alternative Communication, 9*, 259–272.

Heller, K. W., Allgood, M., David, B., Arnold, S., Castelle, M., & Tabor, T. (1996). Promoting nontask-related communication at vocational sites. *Augmentative and Alternative Communication, 12*, 169–178.

Hendrick, D., Prather, E., & Tobin, A. (1984). *Sequenced Inventory of Communication Development.* Los Angeles, CA: Western Psychological Services.

Iacono, T., & Duncum, J. (1995). Comparison of sign alone and in combination with an electronic communication device in early language intervention: a case study. *Augmentative and Alternative Communication, 11*, 249–259.

Kaiser, A. P., Ostrosky, M. M., & Alpert, C. L. (1993). Training teachers to use environmental arrangement and milieu teaching with nonvocal preschool children. *Journal of the Association for the Severely Handicapped, 18*, 188–199.

Kahn, J. V. (1996). Cognitive skills and sign language knowledge of children with severe and profound mental retardation. *Education and Training in Mental Retardation and Developmental Disabilities, X*, 162–168.

Koppenhaver, D., Pierce, P., & Yoder, D. (1995). AAC, FC, and the ABCs: Issues and relationships. *American Journal of Speech-Language Pathology, 4*, 5–14.

Kouri, T. A. (1988). Effects of simultaneous communication in a child-directed treatment approach with preschoolers with severe disabilities. *Augmentative and Alternative Communication, 4*, 222–232.

Lilienfeld, M., & Alant, E. (2002). Attitudes of children toward an unfamiliar peer using an AAC device with and without voice output. *Augmentative and Alternative Communication, 18*, 91–101.

Lloyd, L. L., & Fuller, D. (1986). Towards an augmentative an alternative communication system taxonomy: a proposed superordinate classification. *Augmentative and Alternative Communication, 2*, 165–171.

Locke, P., & Mirenda, P. (1988). A computer supported communication approach for a nonspeaking child with severe visual and cognitive impairments. *Augmentative and Alternative Communication, 4*, 15–22.

Miller, A., & Miller, E. E. (1973). Cognitive-developmental training with elevated boards and sign language. *Journal of Autism and Childhood Schizophrenia, 3*, 65–85.

Mineo, B. (1985). Technology for the future: A report from the ARC Bioengineering Program. *Exceptional Parent, 15*, 11–15.

Mirenda, P. (1997). Supporting individuals with challenging behavior through functional communication training and AAC: research review. *Augmentative and Alternative Communication, 13*, 207–225.

Mirenda, P., Iacono, T., & Williams, R. (1990). Communication options for persons with severe and profound disabilities: State of the art and future directions. *Journal of the Association for Persons with Severe Handicaps, 15*, 3–21.

Mirenda, P., & Locke, M. (1989). A comparison of symbol transparency in nonspeaking persons with intellectual disabilities. *Journal of Speech and Hearing Disorders, 54*, 131–140.

Mizuko, M. (1987). Transparency and ease of learning of symbols represented by Blissymbols, PCS, and Picsyms. *Augmentative and Alternative Communication, 3*, 129–136.

Molfese, D., Morris, R. D., & Romski, M. A. (1990). Semantic discrimination in nonspeaking youngsters with moderate or severe retardation: electrophysiological correlates. *Brain and Language, 38*, 61–74.

Musselwhite, C., & St. Louis, K. (1982). *Communication programming for the severely handicapped.* San Diego: College-Hill Press.

Musselwhite, C. R., & Russello, D. M. (1984). Transparency of three communication symbol systems. *Journal of Speech and Hearing Research, 27*, 436–443.

National Joint Committee on the Communication Needs of Individuals with Severe Disabilities (2002). Position Statement and Report on Access to Communication Services and Supports: Concerns Regarding the Application of Restrictive "Eligibility" Policies. Unpublished manuscript.

Nelson, N. (1992). Performance is the prize: language competence and performance among AAC users. *Augmentative and Alternative Communication, 8*, 3–18.

Peterson, S., Bondy, A., Vincent, Y., & Finnegan, C. (1995). Effects of altering communicative input for students with autism and no speech: two case studies. *Augmentative and Alternative Communication, 11*, 93–100.

Reichle, J., Dettling, E. E., Drager, K, & Leiter, A. (2000). Comparison of correct responses and response latency for fixed and dynamic displays: Performance of a learner with severe developmental disabilities. *Augmentative and Alternative Communication, 16*, 154–163.

Reichle, J., & Johnston, S. S. (1999). Teaching the conditional use of communicative requests to two school-age children with severe developmental disabilities. *Language, Speech and Hearing Services in Schools, 30*, 324–334.

Reichle, J., & Wacker, D. (1993). *Communication alternatives to challenging behavior: Integrating functional assessment and intervention strategies.* Baltimore, MD: Paul H. Brookes Publishing.

Reichle, J., & Yoder, D. (1985). Communication board use in severely handicapped learners. *Language, Speech, Hearing Services in Schools, 16*, 146–157.

Reichle, J., York, J., & Sigafoos, J. (1991). *Implementing augmentative and alternative communication: Strategies for learners with severe disabilities.* Baltimore: Paul H. Brookes Publishing Co.

Rice, M., Hadley, P., & Alexander, A. (1993). Social biases toward children with speech and language impairments: a correlative causal model of language limitations. *Applied Psycholinguistics, 14*, 445–471.

Romski, M. A., & Sevcik, R. A. (1993). Language comprehension: considerations for augmentative and alternative communication. *Augmentative and Alternative Communication*, *9*, 281–285.

Romski, M. A., & Sevcik, R. A. (1996). *Breaking the speech barrier: Language development through augmented means*. Baltimore: Paul H. Brookes Publishing Co.

Romski, M. A., & Sevcik, R. A. (1997). Augmentative and alternative communication for children with developmental disabilities. *Mental Retardation and Developmental Disabilities Research Reviews*, *3*, 363–368.

Romski, M. A., Sevcik, R. A., & Adamson, L. B. (1999). Communication patterns of youth with mental retardation with and without their speech-output communication devices. *American Journal on Mental Retardation*, *104*, 249–259.

Romski, M. A., Sevcik, R. A., Adamson, L. B., Browning, J., Williams, S., & Colbert, N. (1999). *Augmented communication input intervention for toddlers: A pilot study*. Poster presented at the Annual Meeting of the American Speech-Language-Hearing Association, San Francisco, CA.

Romski, M. A., Sevcik, R. A., Adamson, L. B., & Cheslock, M. (2002, August), *Exploring communication development in toddlers who are not speaking*. Paper presented at the biennial meeting of the International Society for Augmentative and Alternative Communication, Odense, Denmark.

Romski, M. A., Sevcik, R. A., & Forrest, S. (2001). Assistive technology and augmentative communication in inclusive early childhood programs. In M. Guralnick (Ed.), *Early childhood inclusion: Focus on change* (pp. 465–479). Baltimore, MD: Paul H. Brookes.

Romski, M. A., Sevcik, R. A., Hyatt, A., & Cheslock, M. B. (2002). Enhancing communication competence in beginning communicators: identifying a continuum of AAC language intervention strategies. In J. Reichle, D. Beukelman, & J. Light (Eds.), *Implementing an augmentative communication system: Exemplary strategies for beginning communicators* (pp. 1–23). Baltimore, MD: Paul H. Brookes.

Romski, M. A., Sevcik, R. A., & Pate, J. L. (1988). The establishment of symbolic communication in persons with mental retardation. *Journal of Speech and Hearing Disorders*, *53*, 94–107.

Romski, M. A., Sevcik, R. A., Robinson, B. F., & Bakeman, R. (1994). Adult-directed communications of youth with mental retardation using the System for Augmenting Language. *Journal of Speech and Hearing Research*, *37*, 617–628.

Romski, M. A., Sevcik, R. A., Robinson, B. F., Mervis, C. B., & Bertrand, J. (1996). Mapping the meanings of novel visual symbols by youth with moderate or severe mental retardation. *American Journal of Mental Retardation*, *100*, 391–402.

Romski, M. A., Sevcik, R. A., Robinson, B. F., & Wilkinson, K. M. (1990, November), *Intelligibility and form changes in the vocalizations of augmented language learners*. Paper presented at the annual meeting of the American Speech-Language-Hearing Association, Seattle, WA.

Romski, M. A., Sevcik, R. A., & Wilkinson, K. M. (1994). Peer-directed communicative interactions of augmented language learners with mental retardation. *American Journal on Mental Retardation*, *98*, 527–538.

Romski, M. A., White, R., Millen, C. E., & Rumbaugh, D. M. (1984). Effects of computer-keyboard teaching on the symbolic communication of severely retarded persons: five case studies. *The Psychological Record*, *34*, 39–54.

Rosenberg, S., & Abbeduto, L. (1993). *Language and communication in mental retardation: Development, processes, and intervention*. Hillsdale, NJ: Lawrence Erlbaum Associates.

Rowland, C., & Schweigert, P. (2000). Tangible symbols, tangible outcomes. *Augmentative and Alternative Communication*, *16*, 61–76.

Rumbaugh, D. (1977). *Lana.* New York: Academic Press.

Schepis, M., & Reid, D. (1995). Effects of a voice output communication aid on interactions between support personnel and an individual with multiple disabilities. *Journal of Applied Behavior Analysis, 28*, 73–77.

Schiefelbusch, R. L. (1980). *Nonspeech language and communication: Analysis and intervention.* Baltimore: University Park Press.

Schiefelbusch, R. L. (1984). Speech, language and communication disorders of the multiply handicapped. *Folia Phoniatrica, 36*, 8–23.

Schiefelbusch, R. L. (1985). *Risk conditions for the development of speech and language.* Unpublished manuscript, University of Kansas, Lawrence, KS.

Schlosser, R., Belfiore, Nigam, R., & Blischak, D. (1995). The effects of speech output technology in the learning of graphic symbols. *Journal of Applied Behavior Analysis, 28*, 537–549.

Sevcik, R. A. (2002). *Factors in visual-graphic symbol acquisition and use.* Unpublished manuscript, Georgia State University, Atlanta, GA.

Sevcik, R. A., & Romski, M. A. (1986). Representational matching skills of persons with severe retardation. *Augmentative and Alternative Communication, 2*, 160–164.

Sevcik, R. A., & Romski, M. A. (1997). Comprehension and language acquisition: evidence from youth with severe cognitive disabilities. In L. B. Adamson, & M. A. Romski (Eds.), *Communication and Language Acquisition: Discoveries from Atypical Language Development* (pp. 184–201). Baltimore: Paul H. Brookes Publishing.

Sevcik, R. A., & Romski, M. A. (2002). The role of language comprehension in establishing early augmented conversations. In J. Reichle, D. Beukelman, & J. Light (Eds.), *Implementing an augmentative communication system: Exemplary strategies for beginning communicators* (pp. 453–474). Baltimore, MD: Paul H. Brookes.

Sevcik, R. A., Romski, M. A., & Adamson, L. B. (1999). Measuring AAC interventions for individuals with severe developmental disabilities. *Augmentative and Alternative Communication, 15*, 38–44.

Sevcik, R. A., Romski, M. A., Watkins, R., & Deffebach, K. P. (1995). Adult partner-augmented communication input to youth with mental retardation using the System for Augmenting Language (SAL). *Journal of Speech and Hearing Research, 38*, 902–912.

Sevcik, R. A., Romski, M. A., & Wilkinson, K. (1991). Roles of graphic symbols in the language acquisition process for persons with severe cognitive disabilities. *Augmentative and Alternative Communication, 7*, 161–170.

Shonkoff, J., Hauser-Cram, P., Krauss, M., & Upshur, C. (1992). Development of infants with disabilities and their families: Implications for theory and service delivery. *Monographs of the Society for Research in Child Development, 57* (6, Serial No. 230). Chicago: University of Chicago Press.

Sigafoos, J., & Roberts-Pennel, D. (1999). Wrong-item format: A promising intervention for teaching socially appropriate forms of rejecting to children with developmental disabilities. *Augmentative and Alternative Communication, 15*, 135–140.

Turner, G. (1986). Funding VOCAs for the lower cognitive functioning. *Closing the Gap, 5*, 26.

Uzgiris, I., & Hunt, J. McV. (1975). *Assessment in Infancy: Ordinal Scales of Psychological Development.* Urbana: University of Illinois Press.

Wacker, D., Berg, W., & Harding, J. (2002). Replacing socially unacceptable behavior with acceptable communication responses. In J. Reichle, D. Beukelman, & J. Light (Eds.), *Implementing an augmentative communication system: Exemplary strategies for beginning communicators* (pp. 97–121). Baltimore, MD: Paul H. Brookes.

Warren, S., Yoder, P., Gazdag, G., Kim, K., & Jones, H. (1993). Facilitating prelinguistic communication skills in young children with developmental delay. *Journal of Speech and Hearing Research, 36*, 83–97.

Wehmeyer, M. L. (1995). The use of assistive technology by people with mental retardation and barriers to this outcome: A pilot study. *Technology and Disability*, *4*, 195–204.

Wehmeyer, M. L. (1996). Self-determination for youth with significant disabilities: From theory to practice. In L. E. Powers, G. H. Singer, & J. Sowers (Eds.), *On the road to autonomy: Promoting self-competence in children and youth with disabilities* (pp. 115–134). Baltimore: Paul H. Brookes.

Wehmeyer, M. L. (1998). Self-determination and individuals with significant disabilities: Examining meanings and misinterpretations. *JASH*, *23*, 5–16.

Wilkinson, K. M., & McIlvane, W. (2002). Considerations in teaching graphic symbols to beginning communicators. In J. Reichle, D. Beukelman, & J. Light (Eds.), *Implementing an augmentative communication system: Exemplary strategies for beginning communicators* (pp. 273–321). Baltimore, MD: Paul H. Brookes.

Wilkinson, K. M., Romski, M. A., & Sevcik, R. A. (1994). Emergence of visual-graphic symbol combinations by youth with moderate or severe mental retardation. *Journal of Speech and Hearing Research*, *37*, 883–895.

Williams, S., Romski, M. A., Sevcik, R. A., & Adamson, L. B. (2003). Perceptions of the communicative competence of three groups of communicators with mental retardation by naive observers. Manuscript in preparation.

Yoder, P., & Layton, T. (1988). Speech following sign language training in autistic children with minimal verbal language. *Journal of Autism and Developmental Disorders*, *18*, 217–229.

Yoder, P., & Warren, S. (1993). Can developmentally delayed children's language development be enhanced through prelinguistic intervention? In A. Kaiser, & D. Gray (Eds.), *Enhancing children's communication: Research foundations for intervention* (pp. 35–62). Baltimore: Paul H. Brookes.

Atypical Language Development in Individuals with Mental Retardation: Theoretical Implications

JEAN A. RONDAL

LABORATORY FOR PSYCHOLINGUISTICS
UNIVERSITY OF LIEGE, LIEGE, BELGIUM

I. INTRODUCTION

Near-normal language acquisition seems to be possible despite serious intellectual impairment. The bulk of the argument comes from the study of a small number of cases of exceptional language development in mental retardation (MR) in the recent literature. These cases are summarized in Section II. The findings are powerful arguments against the claim that the acquisition of grammar is determined by prior nonlinguistic cognitive achievements, as discussed in Section III. Section IV is devoted to the difficult question of explaining the existence of atypical cases of language development in MR.

II. ATYPICAL LANGUAGE DEVELOPMENT IN INDIVIDUALS WITH MENTAL RETARDATION

Table I lists a number of cases of exceptionally favorable language development in individuals with MR (for a full review, including the specification of the numerous language and nonlanguage tests and tasks used by the researchers to operationalize the participants' performance, see Rondal, 1995, and Rondal & Edwards, 1997). It is seldom the case, however, that a comprehensive assessment of nonlinguistic cognitive abilities is undertaken (with the exception of my case study of Françoise; Rondal, 1995). At the same time, the sheer number of these cases across time makes them

INTERNATIONAL REVIEW OF RESEARCH IN MENTAL RETARDATION, Vol. 27

0074-7750/2003 $35.00

TABLE I

ATYPICAL CASES OF LANGUAGE DEVELOPMENT AND FUNCTIONING IN INDIVIDUALS WITH MR

Study	Subjects	Etiology	CA [a]	IQ [b]	MA [c]	MLU [d]	Cognitive level
1. Curtiss (1989); Yamada (1990)	Antony	Unknown	6	50	2.9 years		Preoperatory [e]
	Rick	Unknown	15				Preoperatory
	Laura	Unknown	16	32			Preoperatory
2. Cromer (1991, 1993)	DH	Unknown	Adolescent	<35			Severely retarded
3. O'Connor and Hermelin (1991); Smith and Tsimpli (1995)	Christopher	Unknown	29	42–67 [f]			Severe problems in spatial cognition; failure on tasks of conservation of number
4. Seagoe (1965)	Paul	DS [g]	13	60			
5. Vallar and Papagno (1993); Papagno and Vallar (2001)	FF	DS	23 30 [h]	63			Grossly defective in executive functions, reasoning, and visuospatial abilities
6. Rondal (1995)	Françoise	DS	32	60	5.8 years	12.24	Late preoperatory to early operatory
7. Rondal et al. (1998)	Claudine	DS	27	57	5.4 years	15.39	Preoperatory

[a]CA: chronological age (in years) at beginning of the study.
[b]IQ: nonverbal intellectual quotient according to standard intellectual scales.
[c]Mental age (in years and months).
[d]Mean length of utterance (computed in a number of words plus inflectional morphemes).
[e]According to Piagetian criteria and with reference to Piaget's cognitive developmental theory.
[f]Christopher was given the WAIS (Wechsler, 1958) several times with the resulting IQ varying between 42 and 67. The median note was 52.
[g]Down syndrome (all cases of standard trisomy 21).
[h]CA of FF at the time of the study by Papagno and Vallar (2001).
Unnumbered. Empty boxes in table correspond to pieces of information not supplied by the authors in the original sources.

compelling despite the limitations that may be found with the study of any individual such case.

The three participants with mental retardation studied by Curtiss (1989) and Yamada (1990) exhibited extreme dissociations between cognitive and language levels. Antony's speech was well-formed phonologically and morphosyntactically appropriate with fully elaborated inflectional and derivational bound morphology and free grammatical morphemes. It included syntactic structures involving movement, embedding, and complementation. In contrast, his language was semantically deficient. Antony often used words incorrectly and failed to grasp the full meaning of his own and other's utterances. He had poorly developed topic maintenance skills, was only moderately sensitive to the interests of his interlocutors, and apparently little concerned with the need to be relevant or informative in conversation.

Rick's language paralleled that of Antony. Rick had well-developed phonological, morphological, and syntactic abilities, alongside poorly developed lexical and semantic abilities. He had difficulties in understanding the meaning of the utterances addressed to him and made numerous errors in his lexical and propositional realizations.

Laura's linguistic profile is similar to those of Rick and Antony, with the proviso that her lexicon was richer, particularly in its inclusion of more quantifiers and adverbs. Laura's age-equivalent score on the PPVT was 6 years and 1 month. Despite her larger vocabulary, she presented semantic, pragmatic, and discursive deficiencies akin to those of Rick and Antony. However, Laura's expressive language was phonologically correct, fully elaborated morphologically, and contained complex and well-formed syntactic structures. She produced full passives, sentences with coordinated and subordinated clauses, including WH-relatives, multiple embeddings, infinitival complements, and complement-containing participial forms. Receptively, however, the picture was very different. Laura demonstrated genuine grammatical difficulties in comprehension. On the Curtiss–Yamada Comprehensive Language Evaluation (CYCLE, 1992), her receptive performance was poor in the domain of syntax. She performed at or below the 2-year-old level on most subtests, including the object manipulation version of various tasks (e.g., active and passive voice word order, WH-questioning of grammatical subject and object in relativization tests). In her spontaneous speech, Laura produced many of the structures that she failed to understand on the comprehension tests. On the Token Test (De Renzi & Vignolo, 1962), which evaluates the ability to understand sentences of varying syntactic complexity, Laura scored below the mean score of typically developing (TD) children aged 3 years, 6 months. Her comprehension of grammatical morphemes likewise was reduced. On the CYCLE battery of morphology, she demonstrated mastery over only two grammatical morphemes (i.e., the tense/aspect marker -ing and comparative -er). It is remarkable that she spontaneously and correctly produced some of same forms that she could not understand in controlled receptive tasks.

Cromer (1991, 1993) has reported the case of DH, an adolescent girl with spina bifida and arrested hydrocephalus. DH was unable to learn to read and write, and she had severe MR. In contrast, her speech was fluent and correctly articulated. DH's language was meaningful and contained elaborated noun and verb phrases, conditional, subordinate, and embedded clauses. Her grammatical morphology was judged to be normal.

Christopher, a young adult with MR, was first studied by O'Connor and Hermelin (1991). The case was further analyzed by Smith and Tsimpli (1995). Christopher was diagnosed as brain-damaged at the age of 6 weeks. No etiology was determined. Christopher was described by his family as having an almost obsessive interest with languages from an age of about 6 years. His articulatory skills were normal except for a minor speech defect. His receptive and expressive command of English was within normal range. This claim is based on Christopher's performance on a variety of structures including declaratives, passives, negatives, interrogatives, relatives, and structures involving variations in agreement and word order. Christopher could also make complex metalinguistic judgments. He was able to translate and to converse to some extent in 13 different languages (Danish, Dutch, Finnish, French, German, Greek, Hindi, Norwegian, Polish, Portuguese, Russian, Spanish, and Welsh) with varying degrees of ability depending on the language. His "lexical IQs" on the German, French, and Spanish adaptations of the PPVT, were 114, 110, and 89, respectively (population mean score 100). However, his mastery of the syntax of languages other than English was approximate. On tests of production and judgment, he tended to generalize structural principles from English to other languages. His multilingual ability appears to be based on a capacity to acquire lexical entries in a number of languages together with their morphological characteristics.

Paul's case is different from those considered thus far in that the report by Seagoe (1965) is almost exclusively concerned with written language. Seagoe only mentions that Paul's oral language level was similar to that of TD 5-year-old children, admittedly an above-average achievement for a person with Down syndrome (DS). Paul kept a diary from age 11 to 43 years. Seagoe's report contains excerpts of this diary. I have analyzed one randomly selected excerpt (cf. Rondal, 1995). The mean length of utterance (MLU; computed in a number of words plus inflectional morphemes) is 16.75, which by all standards is remarkable, even admitting that written language tends to be longer than oral language. Several sentences are composed of coordinated or subordinated clauses. Very few syntactic errors are committed. From this excerpt, and others supplied by Seagoe (1965), it is clear that Paul's linguistic ability was well developed.

FF, the young woman with DS studied by Vallar and Papagno (1993), demonstrated correct articulation with occasional stuttering. She had developed a good mastery over Italian, her native language. FF had also acquired some knowledge of French and English that she could use in everyday conversation. She had been exposed to these languages when she was living with her parents until the age of 6 years in a NATO military base in Belgium. FF's Italian expressive morphosyntax has been described as close to normal. Receptively, she scored 31 out of a maximum score of 36 on a shortened version of the Token Test (De Renzi & Faglioni, 1978). In a second and more recent study, Papagno and Vallar (2001) have retested FF's (aged 30 years) phonological, syntactic, and visuospatial abilities confirming the previous report, but adding new data on a tendency to erroneously treat the first noun as the agent in nonreversible passives (Batteria per l'Analisi dei Deficit Afasici; Miceli, Laudanna, & Burani, 1990) and on the severity of her visuospatial impairment. Additionally, they investigated FF's capacity to understand metaphors and idioms, only to find out that despite her good literal language she was severely restricted as to her nonliteral language comprehension.

Another interesting case is that of Françoise (Rondal, 1995). Her speech was fluent with correct sound articulation and normal intonation. Tonic and stress accents were correctly distributed. The sentences produced were complete (except for regular ellipses) and conventional French word order followed. Declarative, interrogative (WH- and Yes-No subtypes), imperative, emphatic, and exclamative sentences were used either affirmatively or negatively. Reflexive constructions were frequent and correctly formed. Full syntactic and lexical passives were used. Coordinated as well as subordinated clauses were produced, including nominal subordinates (subject and object completives), relatives and circumstantial subordinates (temporal, comparative, causal, consequential, and conditional ones). Simple and, at times, multiple embeddings were noted. Tense agreement between main and subordinate clauses was properly marked. The various phrases (nominal, verbal, prepositional, adjectival, and adverbial) were correctly formed. Some of her utterances were quite complex, with the use of coordination, determiners, modifiers, and embedded or chained relative clauses. Large portions of Françoise's free conversational speech were analyzed using Halliday's functional grammar (1985) adapted for the French language. Halliday's specifications regarding clause level, below the clause (groups and phrases), and above the clause (clause and complex sentences) were found to apply perfectly to Françoise's language productions, which may be considered a bona fide demonstration of the basic normality of this aspect of her language.

Additional analyses showed that Françoise's speech correctly incorporated the grammatically free and bound morphemes obligatory in French. Articles were properly marked for number, gender, and for the contrast between specific and nonspecific reference. Personal pronouns were correctly marked for number, gender, person, and case. They were regularly positioned with respect to the verbs. Pronominal coreference was clear. Possessive pronouns and adjectives were correctly marked for person, gender, and number. Epithets were correctly marked for number and gender, where applicable. Demonstrative pronouns and adjectives were correctly used with respect to number, gender, and the proximal–distal contrast. This, together with the proper use of personal and possessive pronouns, attests to Françoise's mastery of the deixis function of language. Relative and interrogative pronouns and adjectives were correctly marked for number, gender, and case (where applicable). Verbs were correctly inflected for mood, tense, aspect, number, and person, including the French polite plurals. Auxiliaries and modals were properly used.

Françoise's advanced morphosyntactic capacity was confirmed on a number of receptive tasks. Reversible as well as nonreversible relative clauses were correctly understood, whether embedded or derived on the right side of the main clause. Causal subordinates were correctly understood, whether the subordinate clause embodying the causal argument preceded or followed the main clause. Temporal subordinates were correctly understood, whether or not the clause order matched the order in which the events referred to were happening or would be happening. The mechanism of coreference in the case of anaphoric personal pronouns also proved to be mastered. Françoise was able to make systematic use of the number and gender correspondence between pronouns and nouns to establish anaphoric coreference in paragraphs.

Françoise correctly interpreted 95% of the active and passive sentences presented to her. She could correctly identify the underlying grammatical subject or the underlying grammatical object in irrealis sentences with low-transitivity verbs (Hopper & Thompson, 1980) (e.g., The book is imagined by the box), with no pragmatic and semantic support. She could even handle irrealis sentences that would turn realis were they reversed (e.g., The man is imagined by the book), thereby going against a possible pragmatic interpretative tendency.

Françoise's lexical usage was globally appropriate. She made occasional mistakes, such as, incomplete locutions, incorrect word forms and adverbial derivations. Françoise was given the Test de Vocabulaire

Actif et Passif (TVAP) (a test of expressive and receptive lexical ability; Deltour & Hupkens, 1980), the Test des Relations Topologiques (TRT) (a test assessing expressive and receptive knowledge of lexicalized topological spatial relations; Deltour, 1982), and Boehm's Test of Basic Concepts (Boehm, 1971). The picture labeling and pointing scores indicated delayed lexical development, particularly concerning the locative expressions. On a word definition task (WAIS, Vocabulary subtest), Françoise scored one standard deviation below the population mean, suppling incorrect definitions for a number of terms. Another limitation in her language ability regarded the discourse level. She followed the usual given–new information structure throughout her clauses (Halliday, 1985). However, although her discourse at the level of the speech turn and the paragraph was coherent, the cohesion was often reduced. Textual cohesion was distinct from the grammatical, the thematic or the information level of the clause and depended on making explicit external relationships between clauses or groups of clauses. Normally, textual cohesion is achieved by relying on the following processes: reference (an element introduced at one place in text can be taken as a reference point for something that follows), ellipsis, conjunction, and lexical cohesion (choice of words, repetition of the same words, or use of related words to insure semantic continuity). The conjunctive process was limited in Françoise's discourse. She made use of conjunctive forms, often located at the beginning of the utterances, but not really making clear relationships between clauses or utterances.

Regarding metalinguistic abilities, Françoise could detect and correct word order errors appearing in grammatically incorrect but semantically appropriate sentences. She proved capable of detecting and repairing grammatically correct but semantically abnormal sentences. She was not sensitive to inflectional morphological errors, however, which is curious, as grammatical morphology was not a problem in her spontaneous speech.

Regarding nonlinguistic cognitive abilities, Françoise's computational capacity proved limited. She could correctly read and write the first 1000 numbers and beyond. She knew the first 10 multiplication tables and could correctly perform multiplication and division operations on numbers contained in the tables, albeit slowly and often counting on her fingers. Beyond table 10, any mental operation of multiplication or division was very slow and often yielded an incorrect result.

Françoise's visual perception was judged to be normal based on her performance on Poppelreuter's Test of the "Figures enchevêtrées" (1985) and on left–right discrimination. Her visuographic abilities were assessed using several tests. On the Complex Figure of Rey (1966), Françoise exhibited serious difficulties in interpreting the macrostructure of the drawing to be reproduced, and she proved unable to draw according to perspective. On the Bender-Gestalt Test revised (Santucci & Galifret-Granjon, 1960), she scored at the median level for 6-year-old children.

On a task of concentrated attention (The Barrage Subtest of the KLT scale) (Kettler, Laurent, & Thireau, 1964), on which eight types of small drawings alternating along rows have to be discriminated, Françoise scored within the lower quartile of the TD population. However, confronted with a more demanding attention task, involving two visually closed letters (*p* and *b*) accompanied by quotation marks and apostrophes in varying spatial combinations (Test D2 of Hogrefe, 1962/1966), Françoise scored within the bottom 2nd percentile of the reference population.

Regarding episodic memory, Françoise exhibited little ability on a classical task of learning paired-associate French words presented auditorily. She could correctly associate only two words with their respective stimulus word in a series of eight pairs after four presentations of the series. She was also administered a modified version (Gilon, 1988) of the cued recall and selective reminding task of Buschke (1973, 1984). Comparison data were obtained from TD adults and "typical" DS adult individuals (Gilon, 1988). Françoise, like the TD adults, made frequent spontaneous use of spatial cues in free recall, a retrieval strategy completely lacking in most DS adults. Nevertheless, Françoise's episodic memory learning fell short of the corresponding performance of TD adults.

Lastly, Françoise's visuo-spatial short-term memory (VS-STM) was assessed using the Block-Tapping Test (Smirni, Villardita, & Zappalia, 1983), in which blocks displayed in front of the participant are hit in a sequence that is to be reproduced following demonstration. Françoise demonstrated a span of four, which is surpassed by 92% of the TD population according to reference data supplied by Smirni et al. (1983). Françoise was also administered the visual reproduction task from the Scale of Wechsler (1974). In this paper-and-pencil task, the participant is requested to reproduce three relatively simple abstract drawings from immediate memory after a 10-second exposure to each drawing. Françoise's global score placed her in the very low end of the TD adult distribution on this test.

Quite clearly, Françoise's level of computational ability, attention–concentration, episodic memory, and visuo-spatial cognition, although often better than those of most DS individuals, falls markedly short of what is usually observed in TD adults. She, therefore, may be described as exhibiting a profound dissociation between formal language and nonverbal abilities.

Another case of favorable language development in a person with DS, that of Claudine (also French speaking), has been documented by Rondal, Comblain, and Deboever (1998). Claudine's receptive lexical ability, measured on the Vocabulary scale of the Epreuves Differentielles d'Efficience Intellectuelle (Perron-Borelli & Misès, 1974), fell within the range typical of adults with DS. Her productive language was well developed with relatively long and grammatical sentences. She was able to produce well-formed temporal, causal, and relative subordinates, even though her speech on the whole tended to be more parataxic than that of Françoise.

The four individuals with DS listed in Table I are of the standard trisomy 21 type (genotype 47, XX, + free 21). Considerable intellectual variation has been reported in mosaic trisomy 21 (Clarke, Edwards, & Smallpiece, 1961; Fishler & Koch, 1991; Kohn, Tayse, Atkins, & Mellman, 1970; Rosencrans, 1968); including a case of mosaic trisomy 21 (3% rate of trisomic cells) with a global IQ of 99, reported by de Moreira, San Juan, Pereira, and de Souza (2000). Languagewise, however, mosaic trisomy 21 are not different from other individuals with DS except for a slight superiority in receptive lexical ability (Fishler & Koch, 1991).

III. ISSUES IN THE COGNITION–LANGUAGE RELATIONSHIP

What is the bearing of the above data on the cognition–language issue in the ontogenesis of language? Traditional conceptions have stressed the dependence of language development upon cognitive development (e.g., Bever, 1970; Slobin, 1973; the Piagetian lineage: e.g., Sinclair, 1971, 1987; see Maratsos & Matheny, 1994, and Tomasello, 1995, for affiliative restatements). Bever (1970) endeavored to demonstrate that there was less innate structure to language than believed at the time. He proposed a number of universal strategies (perceptual, semantic, and syntactic) rooted in cognitive structures, which by interacting with the psychological projection of linguistic universals would be responsible for language development. Slobin (1973) specified a series of cognitive principles purportedly used by children to reconstruct the meanings and the forms of their language. Piaget (1963; Furth, 1969) denied that children are endowed with innately specified linguistic structures. He posited that language's basic structures are a generalization from sensorimotor schemata and cognitive structures. Particular cognitive acquisitions are preconditions for the emergence of grammar. Conceptual links and semantic relations are the prime movers of language acquisition, with syntax being derivative from these.

It is dubious, however, that individuals with MR, some with severe retardation, could reach advanced levels of grammatical development if the cognitive achievements advocated above were stringent prerequisites to such development. It is not clear how people with MR, unable to decentrate cognitively, with little logico-mathematical ability and poor spatial cognition, could develop mastery over complex morphosyntactic structures if grammar were as cognitively rooted as claimed by Piagetians.

An approach distinct from "the strong cognition hypothesis" in language acquisition has been proposed by Bates and MacWhinney (1987) and MacWhinney (1987) under the name of "competition model." It deserves a complementary analysis. These authors assume that distributional regularities available in children's input play a major role in language learning. The model has two distinguishing factors: (1) lexicality, referring to the assumption that grammatical knowledge is represented by connections in the lexicon; and (2) competitiveness, i.e., the view that lexical items in some way compete with each other during language comprehension and expression (e.g., competition of nouns for grammatical roles). Learning is considered to take place through the shaping of connections between lexical items on the basis of positive instances from language input.

From a language pathology point of view, the insertion of grammatical knowledge in the lexicon of the language regardless of its validity and/or sufficiency as a theoretical proposal—which I will not discuss—in no way renders the task of learning language easier for individuals with MR nor does it help explain the remarkable grammatical levels reached by the exceptional individuals with MR described in the previous section. As indicated previously, lexical development, on the whole, is not particularily outstanding in these individuals, with the apparent exception of Christopher. It is often in closer connection with the conceptual level than with morphosyntactic abilities. It is hard to see, therefore, how lexicality could "resist" the data on language-exceptional individuals with MR better than does a Piagetian type of approach to grammatical development.

The competition model also uses a set of general cognitive principles (i.e., not specific to language processing) assumed to provide the learner with the tools necessary to achieve input-sensitive language learning. Even a sketchy presentation of the above type (see Rondal, 1995, for a more detailed analysis), is sufficient to realize the ubiquity of the cognitive participation in grammar acquisition according to the competition model. It is easy to understand why individuals with moderate or severe MR would fail to develop grammatical regulations properly according to this model, given that they have major difficulties in performing cognitive tasks of the type demanded by such a model (i.e., short-term memory (STM) limitations, attentional problems, poor organization of semantic memory, retrieval difficulties, etc.). However, the language-atypical individuals with MR mentioned above all have serious cognitive shortcomings, and about to the same extent as typical individuals with MR. The implication is that the competition model, inasmuch as it relies heavily on cognitive principles for its complementation, can account for the exceptional cases of language development documented in individuals with MR no more than can any other "cognition drives grammar" model.

It could, perhaps, be contended, that atypical individuals with MR are "simply" demonstrating language abilities corresponding to their cognitive levels (E. Moerk, personal communication, October 15, 1994). E. Bates (personal communication, May 19, 1997) maintains that basic grammatical development in TD children is complete by 4–5 years of age. Hence, one should expect MR individuals with MAs of 4 or 5 years to exhibit well-developed conceptual and formal language abilities. If general cognition at a 4–5 year level were a sufficient condition for explaining advanced formal language abilities, typical MR individuals with corresponding MAs (and there are many of them) should exhibit well-developed morphosyntactic skills. Unfortunately for them and for the above claim, most such individuals display severely impoverished grammatical development despite often receiving systematic language intervention (Rosenberg & Abbeduto, 1993; Rondal & Edwards, 1997; Rondal & Comblain, 2002). Alternatively, if one refuses the idea that grammatical development is complete by 4–5 years of age in TD children, but insists that it goes on until 9–10 years for a number of complex syntactic structures, then the levels reached by the atypical MR individuals cannot be explained by relying on general cognitive variables. These individuals exhibit grammatical levels well beyond what may be considered typical for an MA of 4–5 years (see Smith & Tsimpli, 1995). In short, the cognition hypothesis is falsified either by the data on typical individuals with MR or those on atypical individuals with MR, depending on how one wants to set the timing for completion of grammatical development in TD children and given the obvious fact that one cannot have it both ways.

Bates also argues that in order to prove that cognitive abilities are unnecessary for grammatical development (which is not my position, see below), one would have to find a case in which grammar is acquired in the absence of the particular cognitive abilities that 2-year olds have at their disposal. It is true that this demonstration has not been provided (although some participants listed in Table I are not far from such a cognitive situation). The reverse is observed, however. Typical individuals with moderate and severe MR reach and go beyond 2 years MA but fall far short of developing full grammar.

Reviews of the abundant literature on language development in people with MR (Barrett & Diniz, 1989; Cromer, 1991; Dodd, 1976; Fowler, 1988, 1990, 1998; Fowler, Gelman, & Gleitman, 1994; Leifer & Lewis, 1984; Rosenberg & Abbeduto, 1993; Rondal, 1975, 1984, 1995; Rondal &

Edwards, 1997; Tager-Flusberg & Sullivan, 1998) show that in most of these individuals, basic lexical, semantic-structural, and pragmatic developments follow with increasing chronological age (CA) and MA (which should not be taken to mean that these developments are fully similar to those of TD children nor that general cognitive level is a sufficient condition for lexical production, for instance—cf. Fayasse, Comblain, & Rondal, 1992). However, most typical individuals with MR (i.e., those without exceptionally favorable language abilities) present important delays and deficiencies, both productive and receptive, in the phonological, grammatical-morphological, and syntactic organization of language going beyond what can be predicted on the basis of MA (also Vicari, Caselli, & Tonucci, 2000), particularly with respect to sophisticated aspects of grammatical development (e.g., comprehension and production of function words, gender and number agreement, double object construction, reversible passives, comprehension and production of temporal clauses and temporal relationships between clauses). These discrepancies between components of the language system, and between general cognitive level and the phonological and grammatical subsystems of language in typical individuals with MR, reveal the same dissociative trends as those exemplified in atypical cases. The difference between the two sets of observations is that the dissociations go in opposite directions for the typical and the atypical persons with MR. The former have lower phonological and grammatical levels from what can be expected based on MA; the converse is true for the latter.

The preceding sections beg the question of what is meant exactly by atypical (and hence typical) individuals with MR from a language perspective. By "language-atypical individuals with MR," witness the cases reviewed above, I mean individuals with language abilities (either globally or for some language component and/or modality) close to or at the level of age-matched TD individuals. When this is not the case, I suggest the label "language-typical," no matter whether the language aspect(s) considered is (are) below, at the level, or ahead of MA.

A double dissociation between formal aspects of language and cognitive functioning also holds between children with specific language impairment (SLI) and language-atypical individuals with MR. SLI children display typical nonverbal intellectual capacities. They exhibit important phonological and grammatical problems (Clahsen, 1989; Leonard, 1992). Language-atypical individuals with MR have serious intellectual impairments but develop sophisticated phonological and grammatical abilities. Double dissociations are suggestive of domain specificity.

There also are indications that the dissociation between cognition and language in individuals with MR intervenes at a point in development after important early cognitive acquisitions. Those language-atypical individuals for whom we have sufficiently early developmental histories—Curtiss' Rick, Yamada's Laura, Seagoe's Paul, Christopher studied by O'Connor and Hermelin, and by Smith and Tsimpli, Vallar and Papagno's FF, as well as Françoise and Claudine, and my participants with DS—were markedly delayed in language onset. Françoise was only producing one word (/to/ for couteau, knife) at CA 4 years, worse than many typical children with DS at the same age. She developed her formal language abilities between approximately 5 and 10 years. These observations are consistent with the view that a cognitive-semantic basis amounting to what is known by TD children around 20–24 months and children with moderate and severe MR around CA 4–5 years (and MA around 24 months) is needed for the grammatical component to start working.

Such a theoretical view, defining a limited cognitive-semantic basis for grammatical learning, is different from the "cognition-drives-grammar" position described above and some of its more extreme formulations (e.g., Beilin, Lust, & Sack, 1975; Ferreiro, 1971; Ferreiro, Othenin Girard, Chipman, & Sinclair, 1976; Sinclair & Ferreiro, 1970; Sinclair, Sinclair, & de Marcellus, 1971) according to which a number of grammatical forms require the prior attainment of particular logical notions and operations. Acknowledging that thematic roles stem from cognitive notions is not equivalent to accepting that children move directly from these notions onto morphosyntactic regulations.

The preceding discussion should not be taken to mean that particular mechanisms of a cognitive nature could not have a role in language development. A candidate in point for such a status is STM (Baddeley, 1990). Given its possible importance and the fact that the STM variable has been advocated, at least by one researcher (see below), to explain language atypicality in DS, this topic deserves particular attention.

Gathercole and Baddeley (1993) have suggested that auditory-vocal short-term memory (AV-STM)—one of the basic components, together with VS-STM, and a central executive and attentional system, in Baddeley's (1990) working memory model—is directly involved in several aspects of language acquisition. Correlational evidence for a link between nonword repetition ability (hypothesized to depend on the proper functioning of the phonological loop, a subcomponent of AV-STM) and size of receptive vocabulary in children and teenagers, has been reported (e.g., Gathercole, Willis, Emslie, & Baddeley, 1992; Laws, 1998; see Bowey, 1996, 1997, however, for a criticism).

A mechanism possibly accounting for this relationship is that the longer the new word is held in short-term storage, the greater its chance of being learned. This might help explain the difficulty of language-disordered children in learning new words despite normal conceptual development

(Gathercole & Baddeley, 1990). These children could have poor short-term phonological storage capacities, which would render learning new words more difficult. The same reasoning may be applied to most individuals with MR (Jarrold, Baddeley, & Phillips, 1999). Typical children, adolescents, and adults with moderate and severe MR have important limitations in AV-STM (Mackenzie & Hulme, 1987; Rondal, 1995; Rondal & Comblain, 1999), which could be responsible in part for their difficulties in vocabulary learning. A noisier functioning of the phonological loop (Numminen, Service, Ahonen, & Ruappila, 2001), less efficient rehearsal strategies (whether purely articulatory, auditory, or both; cf. Gupta & MacWhinney, 1995), and slower speech rhythm (Rondal, 1995), could render unstable the organization of phonological representations of new words in STM, which could hinder the construction of long-term memory representations. These difficulties would add to the conceptual deficits to make vocabulary development problematic.

However, Jarrold, Baddeley, and Hewes (2000) have expressed doubts regarding the sufficiency of the limitations cited in order to account for poor verbal memory. They suggest an additional explanation, i.e., encoding difficulties. If the information entering the phonological store is of a lower quality, recall would necessarily be poorer even if the phonological loop and the AV-STM processes were intact. Jarrold et al. correctly acknowledge that an encoding deficit of this sort places the locus of impairment partially or totally outside of the STM system. I have long suspected that articulatory difficulties and early lexical limitations negatively interact with AV-STM development in individuals with DS. One should not exclude quicker trace fading, modality notwithstanding, given that VS-STM in individuals with DS is similarly reduced or only slightly better than AV-STM (Jarrold & Baddeley, 1997; Marcell & Armstrong, 1982; Marcell & Weeks, 1988; Rondal, 1995, 1998; Rondal & Comblain, 1999). Extrapolating to TD children, one could hypothesize that speech encoding and even language development as a whole play as important a role in the development of working memory as the components charted in Baddeley's standard model.

Considering language-atypical individuals with MR, it is unlikely that the same phonological memory limitations as for typical participants with MR could be advocated to explain their lexical limitations. Curtiss' Antony and Rick have AV-STMs at the 6–7 years old level. Yet they demonstrate marked productive and receptive lexical difficulties. Françoise's AV-STM span is four items (digits, words, nonwords). She has near-normal AV-STM processes (attested by phonological similarity, word-length, and Brown-Peterson effects, when recalling verbal material—cf. Baddeley, 1990) and she uses rehearsal strategies relying on semi-private speech. It follows that the relative underdevelopment of her lexicon cannot be explained in terms of phonological memory limitations. Nor can it be suggested (following Jarrold et al., 2000) that the lexical limitations of Françoise and those of other atypical-language individuals with MR stem (even partially) from speech encoding or language difficulties. My interpretation is that the lexical deficits exhibited by Curtiss' participants, as well as the milder lexical limitations of Françoise, must be traced primarily to conceptual shortcomings. Mutatis mutandis for typical individuals with MR/DS, this suggests that the impact of the conceptual limitations on vocabulary development are underestimated in Jarrold et al.'s (2000) analysis.

Regarding the difference between Françoise's expressive and receptive lexical abilities and those of typical individuals with DS, it is conceivable that her better functioning with respect to the phonological loop of the AV-STM system—itself a reflection of better speech and faster speech rate—may have at least partial explanatory value. However, neither Françoise's AV-STM span nor her levels of receptive and productive vocabulary are comparable to those of typically developing individuals. Claudine's case is similar to that of Françoise. She has an AV-STM span of four items with normal-like working memory processes. Her speech rate is lower than that of typically developing adults but higher than that of typical adults with DS. Claudine's levels of productive and receptive vocabulary are close to those of language-typical individuals with DS. Vallar and Papagno (1993) claimed that their participant FF's better AV-STM span (5.75) and articulatory rehearsal explain her good acquisition of the Italian vocabulary. This is not convincing in the absence of systematic vocabulary assessment. A positive contribution of AV-STM to vocabulary development, due to a better functioning of the phonological loop, cannot be ruled out in some language-atypical individuals with MR. Given all the data, however, such a contribution must be conceived of as quite limited.

Working memory has also been claimed to play a role in language comprehension (Baddeley, 1990). The phonological store might have a buffering role in retaining strings of incoming words for a period of time pending the construction of more durable representations of the sentence. This could prove particularly important with longer sentences. Baddeley and Wilson (1988) have reported the case of a brain-damaged patient with a sentence span of three words, who showed no difficulty in comprehending short sentences, but had increasing problems as sentence length increased. However, other brain-damaged patients with limited STM spans, studied by Butterworth, Campbell, and Howard (1986) and by Butterworth, Shallice, and Watson (1990), exhibited no comprehension difficulties with long and complex sentences. Butterworth et al. (1990) argue that since a span of, say, three words is sufficient for regular sentence comprehension, it may be assumed that the AV-STM contribution to this task is only three words or so. Working spaces containing the information for dealing with semantic and syntactic information must be assumed to play the major role, and comprehension difficulties, when present, have to be primarily attributed to a deficit with these latter systems (also Caplan & Hildebrandt, 1988).

The data regarding Françoise are congruent with Butterworth et al.'s suggestion. As indicated, her AV-span is 4 units. Françoise's sentence span is 14 words, however. At times, she can repeat correctly sentences containing up to 20 words. This is near-normal functioning (Craik & Massani, 1969). Butterworth et al. (1986) presented university students with sentences 15–21 words long for immediate recall. The students recalled 60% of these sentences perfectly. Most of the errors were omissions and word substitutions. Very few word order errors were recorded. Such was also the case with Françoise for most of the sentences containing more than 14 words. In contrast, typical adults with DS, used as controls, could not repeat correctly sentences containing more than 5–8 words. In controlled tasks, Françoise had no problem correctly interpreting (center-) embedded subject and object relatives when the relative pronouns and their coreferring nouns were separated by several incoming words. Nor did she have difficulties in establishing pronominal coreference across sentences in nonambiguous paragraph interpretation or with personal pronouns and coreferring nouns separated by incoming words. The contribution of Françoise's immediate phonological memory to sentence comprehension may be considered minimal. Her capacity to deal with complex sentence material mainly depends on implicit linguistic knowledge and operations stored in longer-term stores.

In conclusion, any hypothesis postulating too important a cognitive basis for grammar is bound to fail when confronted with exceptionally favorable development in individuals with MR. Of course, particular cognitive mechanisms, such as auditory-vocal short-term memory, could have a role in grammatical development. But the evidence to date for the language-atypical individuals with MR is not overwhelming.

IV. EXPLAINING INTRASYNDROMIC VARIATION: A NEURO-GENETIC PERSPECTIVE

Language atypicality in individuals with MR demands an explanation. This risky exercise hopefully may bring us closer to important variables in language ontogenesis. There is no clear indication that particular remedial procedures or family contexts were directly responsible for the formal language abilities of the atypical individuals with MR.

However, it is correct to point out that we do not know much about the educational or family context of the atypical cases. Seagoe (1965) mentions that Paul's familial environment was particularly stimulating. He was fully accepted as a functioning part of all the activities of his family, including frequent travels. A tutor was available to him on a 24-hour basis. The familial environment of Françoise also was favorable. At $4\frac{1}{2}$ years, she started language intervention twice a week at the Speech Clinic of the University of Liège. Compared to today when early intervention (prior to 4 years) is available to numerous DS children in the developed countries, this would not seem particularly remarkable. Additionally, educational intervention has not proven effective to the point of fully compensating for language difficulties in MR children, especially regarding the phonological and morphosyntactic aspects. Parent–child verbal interactions with MR children have been shown to be basically normal when by normal it is meant the type and quantity of linguistic input and feedback received by TD children at corresponding levels of language development (Buckhalt, Rutherford, & Goldberg, 1978; Gutmann & Rondal, 1979; Rondal, 1977, 1978; O'Kelly-Collard, 1978; see Marfo, Dedrick, & Barbour, 1998; Rondal, 1985; Rondal & Edwards, 1997; for reviews). If adaptations of this sort were key factors in determining language atypicality in individuals with MR, one should record many more similar cases. It remains, however, that an interaction between a spared language capacity and a favorable environment cannot be ruled out.

Yamada (1990) has suggested that the language atypicality of her participant Laura could be related to Laura's left cerebral hemisphere dominance for processing speech stimuli. This suggestion demands further discussion and a brief reminder of the nature of brain specialization in typical MR individuals. Dichotic-listening studies indicate a left ear/right hemisphere (RH) advantage for speech reception in individuals with DS (not found in control groups of TD and people with MR of other etiologies) (Elliott, Weeks, & Elliott, 1987). People with DS exhibit the expected right ear/left hemisphere (LH) superiority in speech production (e.g., dual-task studies, Elliott, Edwards, Weeks, Lindley, & Carnahan, 1987; Kinsbourne & Hiscock, 1983). Elliott et al. (1987) have suggested that the language problems of persons with DS may be related to a dissociation between cerebral areas responsible for speech perception and production causing difficulties of communication between organic systems that normally overlap.

The language-atypical individuals with MR for whom relevant data are available (i.e., Yamada's Laura and Françoise) are LH dominant for the speech functions (receptive as well as expressive). Yamada (1990) has suggested that this could explain Laura's particular language abilities.

Things, however, may be more complex. I have reported (Rondal, 1995) data for 24 DS adults with typical language abilities for DS (15 males and 9 females, aged 21–36 years) in a dichotic-listening task and 19 of the same adults in a dual-task study. A large number of these participants showed interference between verbalization and right-hand movements in the dual task, compatible with the hypothesis of a LH dominance for speech production. In the dichotic-listening task, three females exhibited a right-ear advantage (from 30 to 70%), suggesting LH dominance for speech reception. Six males exhibited also a right-ear advantage (from 10 to 63%). Retaining those individuals for whom the right-ear advantage was equal to or in excess of 50%, one had two female and one male individuals. All three participants demonstrated a positive relative amount of interference in the dual task, suggesting LH dominance for speech production. They could be considered homogeneous as to cerebral hemispheric dominance for the speech functions. This was also the case of Françoise. However, the language abilities of the above three adults with DS were typical for DS persons. LH dominance may be a necessary condition for advanced language development. LH dominance, however, cannot be a sufficient condition for atypical language development in people with MR.

The left cerebral hemisphere, as a sequential analyzer, is dominant in around 95% of typically developing right-handed individuals (Bresson, 1991), particularly (perhaps exclusively) for the formal aspects of language. It is admitted, however, that the right hemisphere, more of a parallel distributed processor, participates in semantic, pragmatic, and discourse processing (Eisele, 1991; Koenig, Wetzel, & Caramazza, 1992). Having reviewed the clinical literature on semantic impairments as well as a series of PET and fMRI (functional magnetic resonance imaging) studies of normal brain activity, Saffran and Sholl (1999) suggested that semantic information is distributed over a number of brain areas bilaterally, some of these regions (e.g., inferotemporal cortex) lying outside of the area usually considered to be committed to language function (see below).

Language, therefore, can be understood as a function involving both hemispheric specialization and bi-hemispheric coordination. Hence one should pay attention to possible callosal problems in language-impaired cohorts. Typical individuals with DS exhibit callosal anomalies and a reduction in frontal projections from the corpus callosum, in addition to a number of other brain anomalies (see below) and myelination problems affecting intracortical fibers between frontal, parietal, and temporal lobes, and long association and intercortical fibers (Horwitz, Shapiro, Grady, & Rapoport, 1990; Nadel, 1996; Shapiro, Haxby, & Grady, 1992; Wang, Doherty, Hesselink, & Bellugi, 1992; Wisniewsky, Kida, & Brown, 1996). Callosal anomalies and atypical myelinization are likely to reduce the degree of interaction between the two cerebral hemispheres and jeopardize complex information processing (Banisch & Brown, 2000; Hagelthorn, Brown, Amano, & Asarnow, 2000).

I have suggested (Rondal, 1998) that the major determinants of morphosyntactic and phonological differences between atypical and typical individuals with MR operate at the brain level.

The brain areas responsible for the expressive and receptive processing of the formal aspects of language in typically developed adults involve the posterior perisylvian sector of the left-cerebral hemisphere with respect to the processing of speech sounds, phoneme assembly into words, and selection of word forms; and the anterior perisylvian sector of the left hemisphere with respect to receptive and expressive morphosyntax (Damasio & Damasio, 1989). Reviews of functional brain electrophysiological, PET scan, fMRI, and hemodynamic (regional cerebral blood flow) studies by Stowe et al. (1994) and Hagoort, Brown, and Osterhout (1999) point to the involvement of the left-cerebral hemisphere extrastriate cortex and superior temporal cortex in lexical access; Brodmann's areas 41, 42, and mid-Brodmann's 22 in phonological processing; the left-superior temporal cortex in conceptual action with other left-perisylvian areas in the various aspects of syntactic processing; and the inferior frontal gyrus, the mid and inferior temporal gyri, Brodmann's area 8, and the temporal lobes in discourse analysis. Neocerebellar structures (e.g., vermis and cerebellar hemispheres) may also be involved in speech and language regulations; for example, coordination of complex articulatory sequences, as suggested by Leiner, Leiner, and Dow (1986, 1991, 1993). They may function in interaction with the frontal lobe system and the anterior perisylvian language zone (Ackerman & Hertrich, 2000). PET scan studies show that the right-cerebellar hemisphere, directly connected to the left-cerebral hemisphere, is activated during word production tasks (Marien, Engelborghs, Pickut, & De Keyn, 2000). Other subcortical structures, such as the basal ganglia and the thalamus of the left hemisphere, participate in neural circuits controlling word selection and phonemic production (Crosson, 1992, 1999; Fabbro, 1999).

Brain studies in persons with DS have revealed major anomalies, including slowing down of maturation of neurons and synapses some time around birth, reduced brain weight and neuronal densities, decreased synaptic density and presynaptic length, hypoplasia of frontal lobes, narrowed superior temporal gyri, and, as already indicated, delayed myelination of associative intra- and inter-cortical fibers between frontal, parietal, and temporal lobes, hypothalamic and hipocampal abnormalities, and diminished size of brain stem and neocerebellum (Bellugi et al., 1990; Nadel, 1996; Wang, 1992; Wisniewsky et al., 1996). Horwitz et al.'s (1990)

PET scan studies of cerebral metabolism in young adult participants with DS indicate smaller correlations for region-pairs within and between frontal and parietal lobes. One brain region particularly affected is the inferior frontal gyrus including Broca's area. The thalamus shows smaller correlations with the temporal regions in the DS groups compared to controls. Shapiro et al. (1992), also using PET scan, report a corresponding disruption of neuronal interactions between frontal and parietal lobes.

The macroscopic brain structures devoted to the treatment of the formal aspects of language (as opposed to the more conceptual aspects) may be spared to a large extent in those MR individuals with atypical language abilities, whereas the same brain structures remain underdeveloped in typical people with MR. I further suggest that atypical MR individuals with genetic syndromes escape the latter fate for reasons related to favorable phenotypic effects of genetic variation. Geneticists agree that there is substantial variation at the genetic level between people within DS, Williams syndrome (WS), and other genetic causes of MR (Dykens, 1995). Most genetic influences on phenotypes are not discrete. The inheritance patterns may be a blend between single gene and polygenic influences (Smith, Pennington, & DeFries, 1996). Complex traits show a quantitative variation in their presentation. Major sources of variation are: (a) major genes involved in a phenotype showing variable penetrance (i.e., the proportion of indiviuals affected with a given susceptibility); (b) variable expression of a single major gene or of a number of genes involved in a phenotype, due to the modifying influence of other genes or environmental factors; (c) a major gene can have several possible mutations (alleles) that may differentially affect the corresponding phenotype; and (d) imprinting effects, i.e., variability of gene expression associated with parental origin (father vs mother) of the genetic material.

Genetic research is yielding more precise gene identification and mapping of a number of chromosomes. Korenberg et al. (1994) have suggested that DS, etiologically linked to chromosome 21, is a contiguous gene syndrome. This augurs against any single chromosomal region being responsible for the DS features. DS and its phenotypes are the result of the overexpression and subsequent interactions of a subset of the genes located on chromosome 21. Korenberg et al. (1994) assign a region of 2–20 megabases between region p11.2 and 22.3 on the distal part of the long arm of chromosome 21, as containing the genes responsible for 25 features considered typical of DS. This conception is consistent with the rich variety of phenotypes and the variability in both penetrance and expression of the DS features.

It is conceivable that there could be significant within-syndrome variability at the brain level in the language area of DS, WS, and other genetic syndromes, consequent upon genetic variation. The brain–gene perspective defined here has the advantage of proposing a single explanation for the variability observed in the language of typical MR people and the extremes of such variability in atypical cases. Of importance, is the observation that language-exceptional persons with MR are atypical only with respect to the phonological and morphosyntactic aspects of language. Their lexical abilities are less impressive (with the possible exception of Christopher). Formal language deficiencies may not be inherent in MR qua MR. The conceptual and the formal language difficulties of people with MR have different roots. The former originate in their cognitive limitations and are unavoidable as such. The latter do not stem from limitations in general cognition, as proved a contrario by the atypical cases. They arise from a basic impairment in devoted brain structures.

What is the nature and the origin of the linguistic knowledge exhibited by the language-atypical individuals with MR? Assuming representational nativism (e.g., Pinker, 1995, 1996) to be empirically valid (which is not my position, see below), one would expect to be spared in the exceptional cases the linguistic notions ascribable to innate properties of the human mind (e.g., phrase structure rules, movement rules, close-class elements operating with respect to tense, aspect, modality, case, and negation, and grammatical categories, such as noun, verb, article, and preposition; or, more succinctly, in the minimalist program (Chomsky, 1995), word semantics and morpho-phonology, word features, and operations fixing together or merging words and word complexes). This is the bulk of Smith and Tsimpli's interpretation of Christopher's talents. I made a similar suggestion in my 1995 book: "A reasonable explanation is that this procedural knowledge [the one displayed by Françoise] is the product of a specific predisposition of the type postulated by Chomsky and others under the name of universal principles of core grammar interacting with minimal epigenetic learning.... It could be argued that [in language-regular MR participants] true linguistic capacities are strictly limited (...) because of a probable lack of adequate expression of the genetically coded phonological and grammatical information" (Rondal, 1995, p. 268).

I now believe such a hypothesis to be of a low degree of plausibility (also Tomasello, 1995). Representational nativism can be challenged on logical, mathematical, and neurobiological grounds (see Elman et al., 1996 for a detailed exposition). It is becoming clear that linguistic representations are constructed on the basis of people's experience with language. Most likely, language-atypical individuals with MR enjoy preserved brain macrostructures devoted to the formal treatment of language. This indication may be related to Elman et al.'s (1996) notion of architectural constraints at brain level (e.g., cytoarchitecture, transmitter types, number of layers of neurones, packing density, basic cortical circuitry, connections between brain regions). It refers to the innate structuring of the brain information processing system devoted to the acquisition and use of linguistic representations.

The difference between a conception of the above type and representational nativism is not in the belief that humans are biologically prepared for language. It is in the idea that linguistic knowledge is constructed by particular brain structures following regular epigenetic sequences. Phonology and morphosyntax have domain-specific properties. They necessitate devoted learning devices. From the vantage point of the language-atypical MR cases, it is necessary to posit that these devices not only are devoted but largely specific with some fair degree of informational encapsulation with respect to general cognitive mechanisms. This is at variance with a central tenet of connectionism that priviledges distributed over localized and specialized processing. Despite Elman et al.'s (1996) efforts, we are still far from a comprehensive connectionist theory applicable to language acquisition. More traditional connectionist approaches to language learning fail on a number of important aspects of language acquisition (e.g., they cannot explain morphological and phonological regulations) although they may represent interesting implementations of the associative memory component of language, helping people, for instance, to store information about word forms (particularly the irregular ones). It would seem, however, that whatever help language learning might receive from associative networks, it could be as problematic for typical individuals with MR as the proper functioning of their rule-governed processing systems. Regarding the language-atypical cases, no datum is available that would depend on associative networks for its plausible interpretation.

As a concluding statement, for those who might be tempted to discard the exceptional cases as mere curiosities with little bearing on theory, let me enlist Richard Feynman's epistemological reminder: when a scientific law fails to apply if only to a single observation where it should, it is simply false (or, at best, incomplete—my addition) (Feynman, 1963).

REFERENCES

Ackerman, H., & Hertrich, I. (2000). The contribution of the cerebellum to speech processing. *Journal of Neurolinguistics*, *13*, 95–116.

Baddeley, A. (1990). *Human memory*. Hillsdale, NJ: Erlbaum.

Baddeley, A., & Wilson, B. (1988). Comprehension and working memory: a single case neuropsychological study. *Journal of Memory and Language*, *27*, 479–498.

Banisch, M., & Brown, W. (2000). A life-span perspective on interaction between the cerebral hemispheres. *Developmental Neuropsychology*, *18*, 1–10.

Barrett, M., & Diniz, F. (1989). Lexical development in mentally handicapped children. In M. Beveridge, G. Conti-Ramsden, & I. Leudar (Eds.), *Language and communication in mentally handicapped people* (pp. 3–32). London: Chapman and Hall.

Bates, E., & MacWhinney, B. (1987). Competition, variation, and language learning. In B. MacWhinney (Ed.), *Mechanisms of language acquisition* (pp. 157–193). Hillsdale, NJ: Erlbaum.

Beilin, H., Lust, B., & Sack, H. (1975). *Studies in the cognitive basis of language development.* New York: Academic.

Bellugi, U., Bihrle, A., Jernigan, T., Trauner, D., & Doherty, S. (1990). Neuropsychological, neurological and neuroanatomical profile of Williams syndrome. *American Journal of Medical Genetics*, Supplement 6, 115–125.

Bever, T. (1970). The cognitive basis for linguistic structures. In J. Hayes (Ed.), *Cognition and the development of language* (pp. 279–362). New York: Wiley.

Boehm, A. (1971). *The Boehm test of basic concepts.* New York: Psychological Corporation.

Bowey, J. (1996). On the association between phonological memory and receptive vocabulary in five-year-olds. *Journal of Experimental Psychology, 66*, 44–78.

Bowey, J. (1997). What does nonword repetition measure? A reply to Gathercole and Baddeley. *Journal of Experimental Child Psychology, 67*, 295–301.

Bresson, F. (1991). Phylogeny and ontogeny of languages. In G. Piérault le Bonniec, & M. Dolitsky (Eds.), *Language bases and discourse bases* (pp. 11–29). Amsterdam: Benjamins.

Buckhalt, J., Rutherford, B., & Goldberg, K. (1978). Verbal and nonverbal interaction of mothers with their Down syndrome and nonretarded infants. *American Journal of Mental Deficiency, 79*, 52–58.

Buschke, H. (1973). Selective reminding for the analysis of memory and learning. *Journal of Verbal Learning and Verbal Behavior, 12*, 543–556.

Buschke, H. (1984). Cued recall in amnesia. *Journal of Clinical Neuropsychology, 16*, 433–440.

Butterworth, B., Campbell, R., & Howard, D. (1986). The use of short-term memory: a study. *Quarterly Journal of Experimental Psychology, 38A*, 705–738.

Butterworth, B., Shallice, T., & Watson, F. (1990). Short-term retention without short-term memory. In G. Vallar, & J. Shallice (Eds.), *Neuropsychological impairment of short-term memory* (pp. 187–213). Cambridge, UK: Cambridge University Press.

Caplan, D., & Hildebrandt, N. (1988). *Disorders of syntactic comprehension.* Cambridge, MA: M.I.T. Press.

Chomsky, N. (1995). *The minimalist program.* Cambridge, MA: MIT Press.

Clahsen, H. (1989). The grammatical characterization of developmental dysphasia. *Linguistics, 27*, 897–920.

Clarke, C., Edwards, J., & Smallpiece, V. (1961). Trisomy 21 normal mosaicism in an intelligent child with some mongoloid characters. *Lancet*, 1028–1030.

Craik, F., & Massani, P. (1969). Age and intelligence differences in coding and retrieval of word lists. *Bristish Journal of Psychology, 63*, 315–319.

Cromer, R. (1991). *Language and thought in normal and handicapped children.* London: Blackwell.

Cromer, R. (1993). A case study of dissociations between language and cognition. In H. Tager-Flusberg (Ed.), *Constraints on language acquisition: Studies of atypical children* (pp. 141–153). Hillsdale, NJ: Erlbaum.

Crosson, B. (1992). *Subcortical function in language and memory.* New York: Guilford Press.

Crosson, B. (1999). Subcortical mechanisms in language: lexical-semantic mechanisms and thalamus. *Brain & Cognition, 40*, 414–438.

Curtiss, S. (1989). Abnormal language acquisition and the modularity of language. In F. Newmeyer (Ed.), *Linguistics: The Cambridge survey* (Vol. 2, pp. 96–116). Cambridge, UK: Cambridge University Press.

Curtiss, S., & Yamada, J. (1992). *The Curtiss–Yamada Comprehensive Language Evaluation* (CYCLE). Unpublished manuscript, University of California at Los Angeles, Department of Linguistics.

Damasio, H., & Damasio, A. (1989). *Lession analysis in neuropsychology*. Oxford, UK: Oxford University Press.

Deltour, J. J. (1982). *Test des Relations Topologiques*. Issy-les-Moulineaux, France: Editions Psychologiques.

Deltour, J. J., & Hupkens, D. (1980). *Test de Vocabulaire Actif et Passif*. Issy-les-Moulineaux, France: Editions Psychologiques.

de Moreira, L., San Juan, A., Pereira, P., & de Souza, C. (2000). A case of mosaic trisomy 21 with Down's syndrome signs and normal intellectual development. *Journal of Intellectual Disability Research*, *44*, 91–96.

De Renzi, E., & Faglioni, P. (1978). Normative data and screening power of a shortened version of the token test. *Cortex*, *14*, 41–49.

De Renzi, E., & Vignolo, L. (1962). The token test. A sensitive test to detect receptive disturbances in aphasics. *Brain*, *85*, 665–678.

Dodd, B. (1976). A comparison of the phonological systems of mental-age-matched severely subnormal and Down's syndrome children. *British Journal of Disorders of Communication*, *11*, 27–42.

Dykens, E. (1995). Measuring behavioral phenotypes: provocations from the "new genetics." *American Journal on Mental Retardation*, *99*, 522–532.

Eisele, J. (1991). Selective deficits in language comprehension following early left and right hemisphere damage. In I. Pavao Martins, A. Castro-Caldas, H. Van Dongen, & A. Van Hout (Eds.), *Acquired aphasia in children* (pp. 225–238). Boston, MA: Kluwer.

Elliott, D., Edwards, J., Weeks, D., Lindley, S., & Carnahan, H. (1987). Cerebral specialization in young adults with Down syndrome. *American Journal on Mental Retardation*, *91*, 480–485.

Elliott, D., Weeks, D., & Elliott, C. (1987). Cerebral specialization in individuals with Down syndrome. *American Journal on Mental Retardation*, *92*, 263–271.

Elman, J., Bates, E., Johnson, M., Karmiloff-Smith, A., Parisi, D., & Plunkett, K. (1996). *Rethinking innateness: A connectionist perspective on development*. Cambridge, MA: MIT Press.

Fabbro, F. (1999). *The neurolinguistics of bilingualism*. Hove, UK: Psychology Press.

Fayasse, M., Comblain, A., & Rondal, J. A. (1992). Compréhension et production des prépositions spatiales topologiques et projectives chez les sujets handicapés mentaux modérés. *Revue Francophone de la Déficience Intellectuelle*, *3*(2), 91–116.

Ferreiro, E. (1971). *Les relations temporelles dans le langage de l'enfant*. Genève: Droz.

Ferreiro, E., Othenin Girard, C., Chipman, H., & Sinclair, H. (1976). How do the children handle relative clause? A study in comparative developmental psycholinguistics. *Archives de Psychologie*, *44*, 229–266.

Feynman, R. (1963). *Six easy and six not-so-easy pieces: Essentials of physics*. Boston, MA: Addison-Wesley.

Fishler, K., & Koch, R. (1991). Mental development in Down's syndrome mosaicism. *American Journal on Mental Retardation*, *96*, 345–351.

Fowler, A. (1988). Determinants of rate of language growth in children with Down syndrome. In L. Nadel (Ed.), *The psychobiology of Down syndrome* (pp. 217–245). Cambridge, MA: MIT Press.

Fowler, A. (1990). Language & abilities in children with Down syndrome: evidence for a specific syntactic delay. In D. Cicchetti, & M. Beeghly (Eds.), *Children with Down syndrome: A development perspective I* (pp. 302–328). New York: Cambridge University Press.

Fowler, A. (1998). Language in mental retardation: associations with and dissociations from general cognition. In J. Burack, R. Hodapp, & E. Zigler (Eds.), *Handbook of mental retardation and development* (pp. 290–333). New York: Cambridge University Press.

Fowler, A., Gelman, R., & Gleitman, L. (1994). The course of language learning in children with Down syndrome: longitudinal and language level comparisons with young normally developing children. In H. Tager-Flusberg (Ed.), *Constraints on language acquisition* (pp. 91–140). Hillsdale, NJ: Erlbaum.

Furth, H. (1969). *Piaget and knowledge*. Englewood Cliffs, NJ: Prentice-Hall.

Gathercole, S., & Baddeley, A. (1990). Monological memory deficits in language disordered children: Is there a causal connection? *Journal of Memory Language*, *29*, 336–360.

Gathercole, S., & Baddeley, A. (1993). *Working memory and language*. Hillsdale, NJ: Erlbaum.

Gathercole, S., Willis, C., Emslie, H., & Baddeley, A. (1992). Phonological memory and vocabulary development during the early school years. A longitudinal study. *Development Psychology*, *28*, 887–898.

Gilon, S. (1988). *Mémoire et trisomie 21*. Mémoire de licence (unpublished), University of Liège Laboratory for Psycholinguistics.

Gupta, P., & MacWhinney, B. (1995). Is the articulatory loop articulation or auditory? Reexamining the effects of concurrent articulation on immediate serial recall. *Journal of Memory and Language*, *34*, 63–88.

Gutmann, A., & Rondal, J. A. (1979). Verbal operants in mothers' speech to nonretarded and Down's syndrome children matched for linguistic level. *American Journal of Mental Deficiency*, *83*, 446–452.

Hagelthorn, K., Brown, W., Amano, S., & Asarnow, R. (2000). Normal development of bilateral field advantage and evoked potential interhemispheric transmission time. *Developmental Neuropsychology*, *18*, 11–31.

Hagoort, P., Brown, C., & Osterhout, L. (1999). The neurocognition of syntactic processing. In C. Brown, & P. Hagoort (Eds.), *The neurocognition of language* (pp. 273–316). Oxford, UK: Oxford University Press.

Halliday, M. (1985). *An introduction to functional grammar*. London: Arnold.

Hogrefe, C. (1962). *Test D2. Göttingen: Verlag für Psychologie* (French adaptation, R. Brückenchamp, Bruxelles, Editest, 1966).

Hopper, P., & Thompson, S. (1980). Transitivity in grammar and discourse. *Language*, *56*, 251–299.

Horwitz, B., Shapiro, M., Grady, C., & Rapoport, S. (1990). Cerebral subjects: altered intercorrelations between regional rates of glucose utilization. *Journal of Mental Deficiency Research*, *34*, 237–252.

Jarrold, C., & Baddeley, A. (1997). Short-term memory for verbal and visuospatial information in Down's syndrome. *Cognitive Neuropsychiatry*, *2*, 101–122.

Jarrold, C., Baddeley, A., & Hewes, A. (2000). Verbal short-term memory deficits in Down syndrome: a consequence of problems in rehearsal? *Journal of Child Psychology and Psychiatry*, *40*, 233–244.

Jarrold, C., Baddeley, A., & Phillips, C. (1999). Down syndrome and the phonological loop: the evidence for and importance of a specific verbal short-term memory deficit. *Down Syndrome*, *6*, 61–75.

Kettler, A., Laurent, P., & Thireau, B. (1964). *Echelle KLT*. Issy-Les-Moulineaux (France): Editions Scientifiques.

Kinsbourne, M., & Hiscock, M. (1983). Asymmetrics of dual task performance. In J. Hellige (Ed.), *Cerebral hemisphere asymmetry: Method, theory, and application* (pp. 114–129). Hillsdale, NJ: Erlbaum.

Koenig, O., Wetzel, C., & Caramazza, A. (1992). Evidence for different types of lexical representations in the cerebral hemispheres. *Cognitive Neuropsychology*, *9*, 33–45.

Kohn, G., Tayse, K., Atkins, T., & Mellman, W. (1970). Mosaic mongolism. I. Clinical correlations. *Journal of Pediatrics*, *73*, 855–874.

Korenberg, J., Chen, X., Schipper, R., Sun, Z., Gonsky, R., Gerwehr, S., Carpenter, N., Daumer, C., Dignan, P., Distche, C., Graham, J., Hugdins, L., McGillivray, B., Miyazaki, K., Ogasawara, N., Park, J., Pegon, R., Pueschel, S., Sack, G., Fay, B., Schuffenhauer, S., Soukup, S., & Yamanaka, T. (1994). Down syndrome phenotypes. The consequences of chromosomal imbalance. *Proceedings of the United States National Academy of Sciences*, *91*, 4997–5001.

Laws, G. (1998). The use of nonword repetition as a test of phonological memory in children with Down syndrome. *Journal of Child Psychology and Psychiatry*, *39*, 1119–1130.

Leifer, J., & Lewis, M. (1984). Acquisition of conversational response skills by young Down syndrome and nonretarded young children. *American Journal of Mental Deficiency*, *88*, 610–618.

Leiner, C., Leiner, A., & Dow, R. (1986). Does the cerebellum contribute to mental skills? *Behavioral Neuroscience*, *100*, 443–454.

Leiner, C., Leiner, A., & Dow, R. (1991). The human cerebro-cerebellar system: its computing, cognitive, and language skills. *Behavioral Brain Research*, *44*, 113–128.

Leiner, C., Leiner, A., & Dow, R. (1993). Cognitive and language functions of the human cerebellum. *Trends in Neurosciences*, *16*, 444–447.

Leonard, L. (1992). The use of morphology by children with specific language impairment. Evidence from three languages. In R. Chapman (Ed.), *Processes in language acquisition and disorders* (pp. 40–67). Chicago: Mosby.

Mackenzie, S., & Hulme, C. (1987). Memory span development in Down's syndrome, severely subnormal and normal subjects. *Cognitive Neurospychology*, *4*, 303–319.

MacWhinney, B. (1987). The competition model. In B. MacWhinney (Ed.), *Mechanisms of language acquisition* (pp. 249–308). Hillsdale, NJ: Erlbaum.

Maratsos, M., & Matheny, L. (1994). Language specificity and elasticity: brain and clinical syndrome studies. In L. Porter, & M. Rosenzweig (Eds.), *Annual review of psychology* (Vol. 45, pp. 487–516). Palo Alto, CA: Annual Reviews Inc.

Marcell, M., & Armstrong, V. (1982). Auditory and visual sequential memory of Down syndrome and nonretarded children. *American Journal of Mental Deficiency*, *87*, 86–95.

Marcell, M., & Weeks, S. (1988). Short-term memory difficulties and Down's syndrome. *Journal of Mental Deficiency Research*, *32*, 153–162.

Marfo, K., Dedrick, C., & Barbour, N. (1998). Mother–child interactions and the development of children with mental retardation. In J. Burnack, R. Hodapp, & E. Zigler (Eds.), *Handbook of mental retardation and development* (pp. 637–668). New York: Cambridge University Press.

Marien, P., Engelborghs, S., Pickut, B., & De Keyn, P. (2000). Aphasia following cerebellar damage: fact or fallacy? *Journal of Neurolinguistics*, *13*, 145–171.

Miceli, G., Laudanna, A., & Burani, C. (1990). *Batteria per l'Analisi dei Deficit Afasici*. Milano: Associazione per le Richerche Neuropsicologiche.

Nadel, L. (1996). Learning, memory and neural function in Down's syndrome. In J. A. Rondal, J. Perera, L. Nadel, & A. Comblain (Eds.), *Down's syndrome: Psychological, psychobiological and socio-educational perspectives* (pp. 21–42). London: Whurr.

Numminen, H., Service, E., Ahonen, T., & Ruappila, I. (2001). Working memory and everyday cognition in adults with Down's syndrome. *Journal of Intellectual Disability Research*, *45*, 157–168.

O'Connor, N., & Hermelin, B. (1991). A specific linguistic ability. *American Journal on Mental Retardation*, *95*, 673–680.

O'Kelly-Collard, M. (1978). Maternal linguistic environment of Down's syndrome children. *Australian Journal of Mental Retardation*, *5*, 121–125.

Papagno, C., & Vallar, G. (2001). Understanding metaphors and idioms: a single-case neuropsychological study in a person with Down syndrome. *Journal of the International Neuropsychological Society*, *7*, 516–528.

Perron-Borelli, M., & Misès, R. (1974). *Epreuves Différentielles d'Efficience Intellectuelle*. Issy-Les-Moulineaux, France: Editions Psychologiques.

Piaget, J. (1963). *Le language et les opérations intellectuelles*. In *Problèmes de psycholinguistiques* (pp. 51–61). Actes du Symposium de l'Association de Psychologie Scientifique de Langue Française. Paris: Presses Universitaires de France.

Pinker, S. (1995). Facts about human language relevant to its evolution. In J. P. Changeux, & J. Chavaillon (Eds.), *Origins of human brain* (pp. 262–283). Oxford, UK: Oxford University Press.

Pinker, S. (1996). *The language instinct*. New York: Norton.

Poppelreuter, S. (1985). *Test des Figures Enchevêtrées*. Bruxelles: Editest.

Rey, A. (1966). *Connaissance de l'individu par les tests*. Bruxelles: Dessart.

Rondal, J. A. (1975). Développement du language et retard mental: Une revue critique de la littérature en language Anglaise. *L'Année Psychologique*, *75*, 513–547.

Rondal, J. A. (1977). Maternal speech in normal and Down syndrome children. In P. Mittler (Ed.), *Research to practice in mental retardation. Vol. II. Education and Training* (pp. 239–243). Baltimore, MA: University Park Press.

Rondal, J. A. (1978). Maternal speech to normal and Down's syndrome children matched for mean length of utterance. In C. Meyers (Ed.), *Quality of life in the severely and profoundly retarded people: Research foundations for improvement* (pp. 193–265). Washington, DC: American Association on Mental Deficiency.

Rondal, J. A. (1984). Linguistic development in mental retardation. In J. Dobbing, A. D. B. Clarke, J. Corbett, J. Hog, & R. Robinson (Eds.), *Scientific studies in mental retardation* (pp. 323–345). London: The Royal Society of Medicine and Macmillan.

Rondal, J. A. (1985). *Adult child interaction and the process of language acquisition*. New York: Praeger.

Rondal, J. A. (1995). *Exceptional language in Down syndrome. Implications for the cognition–language relationship*. New York: Cambridge University Press.

Rondal, J. A. (1998). Cases of exceptional language in mental retardation and Down syndrome: explanatory perspectives. *Down syndrome*, *5*, 1–15.

Rondal, J. A., & Comblain, A. (1999). Current perspectives on developmental dysphasias. *Journal of Neurolinguistics*, *12*, 181–212.

Rondal, J. A., & Comblain, A. (2002). Language in ageing persons with Down syndrome. *Down Syndrome*, *8*(1), 1–19.

Rondal, J. A., Comblain, A., & Deboever, D. (1998). *Evaluation langagière et cognitive de Claudine*. Unpublished raw data, University of Liège, Laboratory for Psycholinguistics.

Rondal, J. A., & Edwards, S. (1997). *Language in mental retardation*. London: Whurr.

Rosenberg, S., & Abbeduto, L. (1993). *Language and communication in mental retardation. Development, processes, and intervention*. Hillsdale, NJ: Erlbaum.

Rosencrans, C. (1968). The relationship of normal 21 trisomy mosaicism and intellectual development. *American Journal of Mental Deficiency*, *72*, 562–566.

Saffran, E., & Sholl, A. (1999). Clues to the functional and neural architecture of word meaning. In C. Brown, & P. Hagoort (Eds.), *The neurocognition of language* (pp. 241–272). Oxford, UK: Oxford University Press.

Santucci, H., & Galifret-Granjon, N. (1960). *Test Bender-Gestalt*. Bruxelles: Editest.

Seagoe, M. (1965). Verbal development in mongolism. *Exceptional Children*, *6*, 229–275.

Shapiro, M., Haxby, J., & Grady, C. (1992). Nature of mental retardation and dementia in Down syndrome: study with PET, CT, and neuropsychology. *Neurobiology of Aging*, *13*, 723–724.

Sinclair, A., Sinclair, H., & de Marcellus, D. (1971). Young children's comprehension and production of passive sentences. *Archives de Psychologie*, *39*, 1–22.

Sinclair, H. (1971). Sensorimotor action patterns as a condition for the acquisition of syntax. In R. Huxley, & E. Ingram (Eds.), *Language acquisition: Models and methods* (pp. 121–135). New York: Academic.

Sinclair, H. (1987). Language. A gift of nature or a homemade tool? In S. Modgil, & C. Modgil (Eds.), *Noam Chomsky: Consensus and controversy* (pp. 112–129). New York: Falmer.

Sinclair, H., & Ferreiro, E. (1970). Etude génétique de la compréhension, production et répétition des phrases au mode passif. *Archives de Psychologie*, *40*, 1–42.

Slobin, D. (1973). Cognitive prerequisites for the development of grammar. In C. Ferguson, & D. Slobin (Eds.), *Studies of child language development* (pp. 607–619). New York: Halt, Rinehart, & Winston.

Smirni, P., Villardita, C., & Zappalia, G. (1983). Influence of different paths on spatial memory performance in block-tapping test. *Journal of Clinical Neuropsychology*, *5*, 355–379.

Smith, N., & Tsimpli, I. (1995). *The mind of a savant. Language learning and modularity*. Oxford, UK: Blackwell.

Smith, S., Pennington, B., & DeFries, J. (1996). Linkage analysis with complex behavioral traits. In M. Rice (Ed.), *Toward a genetics of language* (pp. 29–44). Mahwah, NJ: Erlbaum.

Stowe, L., Wijers, A., Willemsen, A., Reuland, E., Paans, A., & Vaalburg, W. (1994). PET studies of language: an assessment of the reliability of the technique. *Journal of Psycholinguistic Research*, *23*, 499–527.

Tager-Flusberg, H., & Sullivan, K. (1998). Early language development in children with mental retardtion. In J. Burack, R. Hodapp, & E. Zigler (Eds.), *Handbook of mental retardation and development* (pp. 208–239). New York: Cambridge University Press.

Tomasello, M. (1995). Language is not an instinct. *Cognitive Development*, *10*, 131–156.

Vallar, G., & Papagno, C. (1993). Preserved vocabulary acquisition in Down's syndrome: the role of phenological short-term memory. *Cortex*, *29*, 467–483.

Vicari, S., Caselli, M., & Tonucci, F. (2000). Asynchrony of lexical and morphosyntactic development in children with Down syndrome. *Neuropsychologia*, *38*, 634–644.

Wang, P. (1992, June). *Relationship of neuropsychological and neurobiological profiles in Williams and Down's syndromes*. Communication at the Symposium "Two genetic syndromes of contrasting profiles" of the American Psychological Society, San Diego, CA.

Wang, P., Doherty, S., Hesselink, J., & Bellugi, U. (1992). Callosal morphology concurs with neuropathological findings in two neurodevelopmental disorders. *Archives of Neurology*, *49*, 407–411.

Wechsler, D. (1958). *The measurement and appraisal of adult intelligence*. New York: Baillière, Tindall and Cox.

Wechsler, D. (1974). *Manual for the Wechsler Intelligence Scale for children—Revised*. San Antonio, TX: The Psychological Corporation.

Wisniewsky, K., Kida, E., & Brown, T. (1996). Consequences of genetic abnormalities in Down's syndrome on brain structure and function. In J. A. Rondal, J. Perera, L. Nadel, & A. Comblain (Eds.), *Down's syndrome: Psychological, psychobiological and socio-educational perspectives* (pp. 3–19). London: Whurr.

Yamada, J. (1990). *Laura: A case for the modularity of language*. Cambridge, MA: MIT Press.

Index

Contents of Previous Volumes

Volume 3

Volume 4

Volume 5

Volume 6

Volume 7

Volume 8

Volume 9

Volume 10

Volume 11

Volume 12

Volume 13

Volume 14

Volume 15

Volume 16

Volume 17

Volume 18

Volume 19

Volume 20

Volume 21

Volume 22

Volume 23

Volume 24

Volume 25

Volume 26

ISBN: 0-12-366227-3

90038

9 780123 662279